Practical Veterinary Forensics

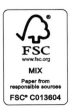

FSC
www.fsc.org
MIX
Paper from
responsible sources
FSC® C013604

For Adam and Jade.

Practical Veterinary Forensics

Edited by

David Bailey

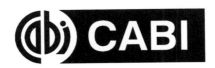

CABI is a trading name of CAB International

CABI
Nosworthy Way
Wallingford
Oxfordshire OX10 8DE
UK

CABI
745 Atlantic Avenue
8th Floor
Boston, MA 02111
USA

Tel: +44 (0)1491 832111
Fax: +44 (0)1491 833508
E-mail: info@cabi.org
Website: www.cabi.org

Tel: +1 (617)682-9015
E-mail: cabi-nao@cabi.org

A catalogue record for this book is available from the British Library, London, UK.

Library of Congress Cataloging-in-Publication Data

Practical veterinary forensics / David Bailey, editor. -- First edition.
   p. ; cm.
  Includes bibliographical references and index.
  ISBN 978-1-78064-294-9 (alk. paper)
  I. Bailey, David (Forensic veterinary surgeon), editor.
  [DNLM: 1. Forensic Medicine--methods. 2. Veterinary Medicine--methods.
3. Animal Welfare--legislation & jurisprudence. SF 769.47]

  SF769.47
  636.0894--dc23

                    2015029404

ISBN-13: 978 1 78064 294 9

Commissioning Editor: Caroline Makepeace
Associate Editor: Alexandra Lainsbury
Production Editor: Lauren Povey

Typeset by SPi, Pondicherry, India.
Printed and bound in the UK by CPI Group (UK) Ltd, Croydon, CR0 4YY.

Contents

Contributors

David Bailey, Department of Forensic and Crime Science, Staffordshire University, Stoke-on-Trent, Staffordshire, UK. E-mail: daysbays@yahoo.co.uk

Rachel Bolton-King, Department of Forensic and Crime Science, Staffordshire University, Stoke-on-Trent, Staffordshire, UK. E-mail: r.bolton-king@staffs.ac.uk

Claire Gwinnett, Department of Forensic and Crime Science, Staffordshire University, Stoke-on-Trent, Staffordshire, UK. E-mail: c.gwinnett@staffs.ac.uk

Jenny Hamilton-Ible, Highcroft Veterinary Group, Bristol, UK. E-mail: jhamiltonible@gmail.com

Karl Harrison, Cranfield Forensic Institute, Cranfield University, Defence Academy UK, Shrivenham, Wiltshire, UK. E-mail: k.harrison@cranfield.ac.uk

Nikolaos Kalantzis, Chartoularios Laboratory of Questioned Document Studies, Piraeus, Greece and Department of Forensic and Crime Science, Staffordshire University, Stoke-on-Trent, Staffordshire, UK. E-mail: nkalantzis@chartoularios.gr

Lucy Leicester, School of Veterinary Medicine and Science, University of Nottingham, Nottinghamshire, UK. E-mail: lucy.leicester@nottingham.ac.uk

Louise MacLeod, Hills Veterinary Surgery, London, UK. E-mail: louiseemacleod@hotmail.co.uk

Lloyd Reeve-Johnson, Institute of Health and BioMedical Innovation, Queensland University of Technology, Brisbane, Australia and Principal Research Fellow, Translational Research Institute, Brisbane, Australia. E-mail: lloyd@goydpark.com

Ernest Rogers, American Board of Forensic Medicine, American College of Forensic Examiners Institute, Springfield, Missouri, USA. E-mail: forensicinvestigations@comcast.net

Deborah Rook, Northumbria Law School, Northumbria University, Newcastle-upon-Tyne, UK. E-mail: debbie.rook@northumbria.ac.uk

Johan Schulze, Veterinary Forensic and Wildlife Services, Germany and Norway. E-mail: schulze@vet-for-wild-serv.eu

Pippa Swan, Clare Veterinary Group, Ballyclare, Co. Antrim, Northern Ireland, UK. E-mail: pippaswan@gmail.com

Adele Wharton, Saphinia Veterinary Forensics, Bottesford, Nottinghamshire, UK. E-mail: adele_wharton@hotmail.co.uk

1 Introduction – What is Veterinary Forensics?

David Bailey*

*Department of Forensic and Crime Science, Staffordshire University,
Stoke-on-Trent, Staffordshire, UK*

*Corresponding author: daysbays@yahoo.co.uk

Live long and prosper.
(Mr Spock, *Star Trek*, Season 2,
Episode 1, 'Amok Time', 1967)

1.1 Introduction

At the time of writing, one is reminded of
the recent passing (27 February 2015) of
Leonard Nimoy, who played the character
of Spock in the *Star Trek* films and television series. The half-human, half-Vulcan
who preferred fact to emotion is a useful re-
minder of the de facto mindset that is required in the world of veterinary forensics.
Being exposed to some of the most challenging crime scenes that involve animals and,
in many cases, the carcasses of animals, the
forensic vet needs a Spock-like skill to filter
out the emotional impact of what they encounter and to be able to articulate, clearly
and without emotion, what has occurred.
This is an important skill to develop if any
longevity is expected in this field.

1.2 Current Projects

The following section is provided as a reference for the reader to appreciate the current
workload of a forensic vet and to provide an
insight into the scale and complexity of the
specialism that is veterinary forensics.

1.2.1 Anti-terrorism

While constructing this introductory chapter
I am preparing for a talk at the Counter Terror
Expo in London, the fourth consecutive year
I have been invited to speak at this event.
The topic for my discussion this year is
'The ability to weaponize biological agents',
and covers the utilization of 'pig bombs' as
a crude but effective device for spreading
biological agents. My audience will be
mainly first responders and UK ambulance
personnel; however, there is a large component of private trainers, ex-military consult-
ants and government operatives. The reason
for my invitation is a linear recognition of my

expertise in antiterrorism and agroterrorism,
the former being a subject module of my
master's degree, and the latter something
that I had applied and developed from my
master's degree training to my veterinary
science degree. Many vets are in the unusual
and unacknowledged position of being able
to discuss the role that animals and animal
products can play in the spread of biological
or chemical hazards.

1.2.2 Forensic analysis of hair

I am currently completing the world's first
data collection of hair samples from Pit Bull
Type (PBT) animals. This research project
aims to identify differences between breeds
of dog by qualitative and quantitative
measurement of microscopic hair features.
It has taken two years and has involved the
sampling and measurement of more than
300 hair samples from 50 dogs in the USA,
UK, Australia and Ireland. Statistical analysis
is currently being conducted on more than
18,000 measurements.

1.2.3 Bitemark analysis

I have been involved in two recent cases involving allegations of dog bites against humans, where I have come up against den-
tists and plastic surgeons who are able to
describe injuries but fail to articulate *how*
the injuries may have occurred.

1.2.4 Teaching and examining

I am preparing to teach and then examine
seven more UK-based veterinarians in a
postgraduate certificate course in veterinary
forensics and law. This is a postgraduate
course that was created in 2010 for vets in
the UK to learn the skills and importantly,
the mindset that accompanies the work of the
veterinary forensic scientist. Many of the
vets on the postgraduate course work for
the Royal Society for the Prevention of
Cruelty to Animals (RSPCA). I am also

involved in the teaching and delivery of the inaugural Veterinary Forensics course in Brazil, where I am going next year to lecture at a veterinary forensics conference.

1.2.5   Contract research

I am currently conducting some contract research in collaboration with Staffordshire University, which is investigating the effect that electronic collars may have on dog skin. The dog skin has been provided from cadavers to assist with claims that have been made by some end users that the use of these devices can cause burn necrosis on their dog's skin. The manufacturers claim that the electronic collars don't cause any type of burning on the dog at all and the preliminary results of this research would support this view. The voltage and amperage involved are too small to cause any detectable damage to the dog skin, even under electron microscope.

Previous contract research has included a review of the chosen methodology used in a large research project involving dog behaviour. Another project assisted in the determination of the provenance of migrating birds through Isotope Ratio Analysis of sampled feathers. A requirement has been identified for rapid determination of the origin of a sick bird in the wake of ongoing worldwide fear about pandemic bird flu.

1.2.6   Expert witness appearance

I have recently completed a particularly onerous court schedule, requiring my presence in a different court (including a Sheriff's court appearance in Scotland) nearly every week for the last three months. These appearances are as an expert witness in cases involving allegations of animal cruelty or claims of injuries received by humans from animals.

1.2.7   Toxicology and chemical analysis

I am in the process of developing a timeline of exposure to hydrocarbons (kerosene) in a group of horses based on examination of their equine tail hair. The hair is helpful in identifying the time of contamination of a number of horses that were exposed to a hydrocarbon leak into their water source from a neighbouring property. It is possible to construct the timeline using the growth rate of equine tail hair, and involves cutting up the hair into small segments (subsampling the hair) and analysing each small segment. Hair at the end of the tail was produced years ago and the level of hydrocarbons in the tip of the hair (if detected) will indicate an exposure at a time in the past, determined by comparing the exact length of the hair with its growth rate. An increase in hydrocarbons from any subsampled region should provide sufficient information to determine that exposure has occurred at that point in time and a timeline can be established, a source–pathway–receptor (SPR) model now exists and culpability should follow.

1.2.8   Veterinary call-out services

I provide investigative, advisory and forensic services for the Police Service of Northern Ireland (PSNI) and the Ulster Society for the Prevention of Cruelty to Animals (USPCA), where I can be called upon to attend to animals that are sick, dead, dying or injured and require veterinary intervention or forensic investigation if an allegation of a crime is being pursued. I am on the board of trustees of the USPCA.

When I'm not working as a forensic vet, I work in clinical practice, where I find emergency medicine particularly satisfying. I also have a fair amount of small and large animal work, including equine, which helps to keep my credentials as an expert witness up to date.

1.2.9   Television and media

I have just completed filming for a one-hour television documentary on the proliferation of puppy farms in Northern Ireland (*The Dog Factory*).

Previously I have been involved in news slots on the subject of animal hoarders in Northern Ireland. I frequently write articles for various veterinary publications around the world on the topic and various subtopics of veterinary forensics.

1.2.10 Report writing

I have written two reports this week on civil claims. One involves a farm labourer who alleges that he was struck by a dairy bull as he was walking through the milking parlour, and the other involves a dispute between a vet and an owner of a dog that had developed heart complications after 'anaesthetic and a dental' – these four words were the sum total of the clinical notes describing the procedure provided by the vet surgery.

1.2.11 Documentary evidence

I have been to premises under police escort and seized documentary evidence that provides a strong probative link between the alleged offender and a crime. Handwriting analysis, document examination and even ink examination can be used to determine whether a crime has been committed in a world dominated by clinical input. A vet can send documentation to a document examiner and then add the document examiner's report to his or her own court report, in a similar way that a clinical pathology or radiology report can be utilized. Many vets need to be reminded that one of the most common causes of a vet being removed from their professional governing body is miscertification, i.e. signing a document that shouldn't have been signed.

1.2.12 Blood pattern analysis

I have been able to determine that a stag transported in a trailer suffered injury in transit. This was through the analysis and correct photography of blood patterns in the seized trailer. Blood pattern analysis is, as will be explained, an analysis of the forces that create the blood pattern and not the blood pattern itself.

1.2.13 Bestiality

I have investigated a claim of sexual contact between a teenage boy and a large Dogue de Bordeaux, where the dog had learned sexual behaviour that was not expected from a dog unless it was being used for stud purposes. Radiographs were able to determine that the dog had genetic anomalies that made him an unsuitable stud animal and when faced with this information the boy confessed to contact with the dog.

1.2.14 Ballistics

I have examined and treated numerous cats that have been shot with an air pellet, and I have examined many dogs and dog carcasses that have been injured or killed by shotgun pellets.

1.2.15 DNA analysis and laboratory competence

I have been involved in a dispute as a defence expert involving the analysis of more than 300 DNA samples. The Department of Agriculture and Rural Development (DARD) in Northern Ireland had charged a farmer with dishonesty over the pedigree claims he had made relating to his cattle. DARD had diligently collected hundreds of blood samples from the cattle and submitted them to an ISO 17025-accredited laboratory for testing. The laboratory and DARD, acting as the prosecution provider, had their substantial accumulation of evidence thrown out of court – an example of poor sample continuity and how forensics can apply in a robust defence of a seemingly open-and-shut case.

1.3   Conceptual Views

1.3.1   Comparison to human forensics

The processing of crime scenes that involve crimes against humans has become very specialized. Different expertise exists in the forensic science school, ranging from crime scene processing to analytical techniques and laboratory compliance. Forensic science is still an emerging specialism in the veterinary world and is heavily dependent on the human discipline as it navigates its way to becoming an established discipline in its own right. The most significant difference between human and veterinary forensics is that in the former the evidence is *physical* but inanimate, and can consist of drugs, glass fragments, fingerprint images and nearly all other forms of physical evidence, while in veterinary forensics, the evidence can be *living*. This small yet significant point is a characteristic of veterinary forensics that can't be replicated, copied or learned from our human colleagues.

As veterinarians, we deal with evidence that gets sick, dies, is already dead or has been killed. Our evidence can become pregnant, improve in body weight or lose body condition. The forensic world, according to the human forensic scientists, is not designed for *living* evidence. Forensic analysis and interpretation is for samples, not pets. Physical handling and manipulation is for forensic data, not restraint and clinical sample extraction from an unyielding and uncooperative animal. Forensic evidence can be bagged, labelled and stored on a shelf for 18 months prior to trial. Not animals. They need to eat and live and go to the toilet. They have a need for companionship *and* they are evidence that cannot be bagged and tagged and placed on a shelf. It is at this point that veterinary forensics cannot rely on the human field for guidance, and it is not surprising that post-seizure is the most probative and evidentially useful period, in terms of how the animal responds to care. It is also the most vulnerable period for the seizing authorities, who can unwittingly commit further offences against the animal by incorrect post-seizure *storage* of *living* evidence.

1.3.2   A definition of veterinary forensics

While some have commented and written on the subject of veterinary forensics, it remains poorly defined. Some have used forensics as a synonym for pathology. Others have used forensics as a tool for prosecution (only) of animal abusers. However, a more accurate definition of veterinary forensics is: *The application of science to the resolution of legal disputes involving animals and animal derivatives.*

1.3.3   Breadth of field

These 'veterinary' disputes usually involve animals or animal keepers, yet they may also include trade in animal products, as well as professional negligence claims against animal health professionals. A forensic vet will tend to deal with cases involving animal cruelty, animal trade, injuries received from animals and the various legal vagaries involved in the application of science to the resolution of these matters. Forensics as a discipline cares not for the likely innocence or guilt of the party concerned, and it is surprising that when asked to define veterinary forensics, many others see it as a tool for the establishment of the prosecution position *only*. The ability to use forensics for both prosecution and defence in legal disputes should force each side to think twice before entering into dispute resolution via an adversarial legal battle.

When dealing with claims of animal cruelty, a vet is inevitably asked to provide comment on any suffering that an animal may or may not have experienced.

It is an anomalous discovery in the UK that there is no currently accepted legal, forensic or veterinary definition of the word *suffering*. This is problematic for a scientific discipline such as forensics that thrives on and utilizes definitions.

A vet who is involved in forensics will often encounter human mental health issues when dealing with cases, and, although we are unqualified mental health experts, we will all too often be a designated de facto social worker, dealing with alcohol abuse, mental health issues (e.g. hoarding), and on the receiving end of verbal and physical abuse. I have attended one court where a defendant had to have their false teeth removed for the duration of proceedings because they chose to bite people who weren't on their 'side'. Another case involved the seizure of 11 dogs from premises of an owner who had developed gangrene in his toes. The dogs had eaten part of his foot without his knowledge and intervention resulted in the seizure of the dogs and the owner having a leg amputated.

The reader may quickly realize that one should add the term 'social work and mental health issues' to any working definition of veterinary forensics, but you will now be running very close to committing the forensic scientist's worst error – straying outside one's area of expertise.

This book isn't the first to attempt to define veterinary forensics. There is already an established a priori expectation that veterinary forensics involves pathology or prosecution (only) of animal abusers, or is a niche term applied to wildlife crime. There is no room in these definitions for the likes of DNA or document analysis, or an understanding of ballistics, and even less interest in defending those accused of animal abuse. To have a prosecution-only definition of any forensic discipline removes 50% of your potential paid work in this field and betrays a 100% understanding of the adversarial nature of the judicial system that we have in the UK, Australia, North America and many Commonwealth countries.

1.3.4 Getting caught

In ancient Sparta, soldiers were encouraged to go out and steal. Stealing was not a crime; however, if you were caught, you were punished, not for stealing, but for *getting caught.*

Veterinary forensics is looking at the people (and their surrounding circumstances) who have been caught in crimes or disputes that involve animals and animal derivatives, and it includes the application of our (clinical and cumulative) knowledge

to the resolution of the dispute that arises out of the evidence.

1.4 Biological Concepts

Charles Darwin has a theory of evolution that still exists in *theoretical format* and has failed to be catapulted into a *law* of biology. Biology then appears to be the only science that has no governing laws. All biological theories start off as *hypothesis* and then, through trial and error and experimentation they become elevated to *theory*, awaiting the one singular event, experience or experiment that prevents them from being cemented into a law. Physics, chemistry and maths have many laws to flaunt at the biological sciences. Veterinary science, as a discipline that is heavily dependent on the biological processes, has only one law, and we don't even exalt it as a law, more of an inconvenience – *All living things will die.*

And here we have biological science competing unfavourably with physics and chemistry and mathematics, which have an abundance of laws and rules to establish precision and, most importantly, predictability.

We can predict and plan events with physics and chemistry, we can build large architectural arrangements and send rockets beyond our solar system with the laws of motion, mathematics and engineering, yet with biology we think we understand evolution but we fail to elevate Darwin's 'theory' into a law that cannot be challenged. Newton and Pascal would laugh at our attempts to describe the biological world as scientific, reliant upon only one theory and no laws.

Biology, it seems, allows us only to look back at all our observations, measurement or data and describe what has already happened. All other forensic science disciplines apart from biology allow you to look forward in time and predict. This is an expected but poorly broadcast observation in a discipline that seeks to apply science to the law, and wants these observations to be beyond reasonable doubt.

Forensic science is all about the utilization of the *physical sciences* with scientific laws to predict outcomes with great accuracy, and *all* of the measuring and analytical tools of forensic science use laws and principles of physics, chemistry or maths – the physical sciences that allow structure and prediction.

'Animals are made up of atoms, anyway' is the infamous quote from a court case where a vet was asked to explain that, despite having never seen a wild Bengal cat, he was able to give expert opinion on the matter as he was a vet and he knew 'all animal breeds and species'.

The reply from the barrister was appropriate for the expert:

'So you claim that veterinary science, then, is applied chemistry?'

'Yes, partly.'

'What part?'

'The chemical part.'

Veterinary science is the study of biological systems, which, at the atomic level of all cells, are obedient to the laws of chemistry and physics, but when these atoms combine together, they coalesce to form cells, organs and bodies – an emergent system of a living thing that is reluctant to yield to any laws, legal or scientific, except one – death.

Problems become apparent when you try to shove a biological sample into one of these analytical devices created by and for the rules of physical science. A square-peg-and-round-hole situation has developed. These devices are created and skilfully crafted to understand physics or chemistry or mathematics and they feel contaminated and dirty with biological samples, and they tend to spit out results that can be measured and compared to a *range of results* that are expected in the biological world. And here we have the first rule of cross-examination when dealing with biological materials. All answers in biology require a range of possible answers except the answer to one question: was it dead?

Everything else requires a spectrum of answers, and the courts dislike this fuzzy approach to truth determination. Courts want the 'beyond reasonable doubt' type of answer and they require certainty, when all we can provide as biologists is reliability. Vets will often attempt to be 100% certain when being almost sure is all that is sanctioned by biological and veterinary sciences, and being unsure is sometimes all that biology provides.

Biologists can produce a very reliable *range* of results that lack the certainty and singular answers of the other physical sciences. A ballistic scientist can tell you that the faster a projectile travels the more energy it will have, and they can provide a formula to assist in this prediction (kinetic energy of an object):

$$E_k = {}_{1/2}M.V^2$$

A vet couldn't tell you what the resultant injury will be in the body of the animal that the projectile hits, yet a ballistic scientist can tell you the *exact* amount of energy the projectile will have on impact if they know the distance the animal is standing from the projectile-delivering device. The physical sciences *predict* events with great accuracy and the forensic scientists embrace this certainty and frontload their analysis, interpretation and mindset with analytical tools that rely on formulae, laws and predictability. The biological and natural sciences *reflect* on what occurred with vague ranges of possible scenarios. The projectile could over-penetrate the animal and cause minimal (or massive) tissue damage; or the energy from the projectile could be dumped and captured completely within the animal, resulting in massive temporary and permanent cavity damage – there is a range of possible results. Courts dislike this. A pathologist can tell you what happened to this animal on this occasion, yet a ballistic scientist can tell you what energy will be imparted from the projectile to every animal, every time. A pathologist, unable to post-mortem every animal, every time, is reduced to giving a range of possible results based on the post-mortem that he or she has performed on other animals of different height, weight, sex and breed, and the problems begin when applying this fuzzy logic and introducing it to the court.

DNA analysis is the one analytical measurement utilized by forensic scientists that uses biological samples and yields accurate results that courts have become comfortable with. This is due to the high utilization of probability and the laws of a mathematical arena that can be applied to biological samples. The courts don't like DNA but they do like the statistics (and the laws of statistics) that compulsorily accompany any reliable DNA result.

Statistics are often used to explain the results, then the forensic scientist has to interpret the result, and the court will determine whether the probability offered is beyond reasonable doubt.

And here a schism develops between biological science and physical sciences, because biology is a science but it is different to all other physical sciences. Darwin is weak when compared to Newton, who has three laws of motions named after him. All Darwin can manage is a *theory* of evolution. Ballistics then is a great descriptor for predicting what will happen when you fire a projectile out of a weapon. There are equations of maths and laws of science that allow you to predict how fast that projectile travels and how much energy it will have when it impacts its intended target. Even blood spatter analysis is less to do with the patterns created by bloodstains and more to do with an understanding of the forces that created those patterns. Forensic science is geared toward the hard sciences, the physical sciences and maths, and not surprisingly the sciences that have laws that are constant and predictable. Biology has no laws, one single theory and does not lend itself easily to interpretation through forensic analysis. We, as forensic scientists, are forced, through discipline and training, to forensically adapt biological samples, including veterinary evidence, into a process that suits physical science evidence. We will see that the judicial and court system is not prepared for this inconvenience: when you consider that a seized animal is, in the view of the court, a piece of evidence, then placing that evidence in a bag and on a shelf where it can remain until the trial is problematic. Our evidence requires food, air and water, it is often alive and the physical chemists, analysts and mathematicians find this life contaminant as difficult to work with as any other sample

adulteration. The evidence, according to the physical scientists and mathematicians, is living. The evidence we provide them with is an intruder into their predictable, formula-driven world.

1.5 Know Yourself

This implement called forensics, then, is the tool and skill necessary to fill that gap between court requirements and veterinary capability, and includes an understanding of veterinary science, sociology, psychology and courtroom procedures, as well as a firm grasp of the separation between biological and physical sciences; along with an increased need to understand legal motives derived from the adversarial system and motives based, in part, on points of fact and points of law. But perhaps the most important tool to have as a forensic vet is a deep sense of self-awareness, as a basis for self-respect. Once in place, these two elements are the chief principles that open the door to self-confidence, which is a prerequisite in most aspects of adversarial life, but particularly in the brutal world of a competitive judicial system, where, regardless of your level of expertise, awareness and knowledge, and the respect you have for yourself and the court, there is always going to be someone who asks you in the most polite, patient, caring and persistently appropriate manner just *how sure* you are. You are perpetually challenged as to your sense of purpose and entitlement to appear in court as an expert. You are challenged by many aspects of adversarial life in the courtroom cross-examination, but the one lingering issue that you are perpetually confronted with is an externally imposed sense of self-doubt. As long as the doubt is not self-imposed then you can feel confident in answering truthfully – the rest *really* is up to the court.

1.6 A Common Thread

The current status of applied veterinary forensics is still heavily reliant upon the human forensic available literature. There is a large amount of available research, knowledge and understanding on ballistics, hair, DNA, blood pattern analysis, documentary evidence, crime scene processing, report writing and courtroom skills that relates to human forensics that can be applied to veterinary forensics but needs to be understood *and applied* as a separate discipline to human forensics.

There are similar themes and consistency of approach that run through each different speciality in forensics and the repetition of each should consolidate learning and understanding of these core elements. A forensic laboratory may be run by a hair analyst who, despite not having any DNA or document analysis experience, can still oversee a laboratory that performs these functions, as there is a common approach to the science of forensic science. Much as a dog and cat vet who has little to do with equines nevertheless understands that a consultation (regardless of species) must start with a thorough knowledge of the individual animal's history.

A deep sense of philosophy is incorporated into the reading of forensic science, with an understanding of history, personal value hierarchies and even sociology, and how these seemingly disparate silos of knowledge combine to provide an emergent property that has an impact upon the understanding and practice of how forensics is incorporated into our work flow and not the other way around. There is an unwritten rule that you must know yourself better than your area of expertise, and this is a natural consequence of having all elements of your work scrutinized in court by a cross-examining barrister who knows little about the subject and cares even less. Barristers have a common approach in an adversarial system – attack the person delivering the evidence, not the subject matter, so a deep understanding of both is necessary.

In modern-day jurisdictions the offence for all crimes is just as the Spartans interpreted them – *getting caught* – and for that you need an understanding of the gathering, presentation and subsequent application of evidence. This is where forensics becomes a speciality. The law provides guidance on what you can and can't do, forensics helps to determine whether you did or did not do it, and the court decides whether you were caught or not and provides appropriate punishment.

1.7　Jones versus Kaney

Jones versus Kaney is a 2011 decision of the Supreme Court of the UK on whether expert witnesses retained by a party in litigation can be sued for professional negligence, or whether they have the benefit of immunity from suit. The case involved a psychologist (Kaney), instructed as an expert witness in a personal injury claim, who was said to have negligently signed a statement of matters agreed with the expert instructed by the opposing side, in which she made a number of concessions that weakened the claim considerably. As a result, according to the injured claimant (Jones), he had to settle the claim for much less than he would have obtained had his expert not been careless. To succeed in the claim, he had to overturn an earlier Court of Appeal decision, which had decided that preparation of a joint statement with the other side's expert was covered by immunity from suit. Kaney therefore succeeded in getting the claim struck out before trial on an application heard by Mr Justice Blake in the High Court of Justice.

The Supreme Court, by a majority of five to two, decided that expert witnesses were not immune in the law of England and Wales from claims in tort or contract for matters connected with their participation in legal proceedings. This reversed a line of authority dating back 400 years. The case considered the narrow issue, namely whether preparation of a joint statement by experts was immune from suit, and the wider public policy issue of whether litigants should be able to sue experts, whom they had instructed, for breach of duty. There was discussion about whether removing the immunity would have a 'chilling effect' on the willingness of experts to participate in court proceedings, although judges on both sides of the decision agreed that there was no empirical evidence on the point.

A litmus test for an expert is to test whether their view is the same regardless of which side (prosecution or defence) has instructed them. The expert may start off as an assessor of the facts and evidence presented to them, but there are pressures exerted as a consequence of the adversarial system that may bring out a partisan view that didn't exist, or worse, that the expert does not know exists.

1.8   Critical Thinking

As vets, we are taught and become immersed in the *clinical* approach to investigating problems in animals. We examine an animal, listen to its history from the owner, order tests, interpret the results, and then diagnose and treat the animal. It is such an ingrained process that we don't even consider that it is the default setting for future exposure to novel situations (including forensics): a trained and learned clinical approach that requires an inquisitive and curious mind. Whenever two vets see an animal with the same history, presenting signs and complaints, there will be two different opinions as to how to treat and what the next step is in the treatment process. This is due in part to the experience and exposure of that vet to that presenting problem. This divergence in opinion between vets has a lot to do with the vying nature of veterinary undergraduate selection. Veterinary science is an ambitious field of study that attracts the most intellectually competitive people.

Critical thinking is a set of skills that vets in the field of forensics are required to have when considering the views of others. This can be problematic when your analysis is confined to animal patients; considerations about them may be replaced by the views of their owners, who are paying you to give them your view. Critical thinking opens up your views and your reasoning to others, and theirs to you. As a result you may change your mind or it may remain unchanged, but it is essential that you are open to this process. Most vets, in my experience, in court and in clinical practice, are lacking

in this skill and it is important to have the humility to expose your views to others and allow those views to be corrected. Vets are, by the nature of their work, unused to patient scrutiny. Vets in a clinical setting are held in high esteem by their clients and so are unaccustomed to having their decisions challenged. It is considered unusual to question vets' views or professional decisions, although this is changing with an explosion of information available through the internet; however, a client pre-armed with more information may not necessarily be more informed.

Critical thinking, as a skill that is differentiated from *clinical* thinking, allows us to become wiser through listening to all that can be said *against* our views by subjecting them to the scrutiny of others. It is a crucial skill to learn, and recognition of the transition from clinical thinking to critical thinking is an important first step in the mindset change that vets entering the adversarial arena would benefit from. It is also a useful life skill.

Critical thinking can also be used as a strategy relating to statements or court reports that others write. Critical thinking is not considered a philosophy or management style; it is a mechanism of problem identification rather than rote solution harvesting and is a key difference between the clinical mindset and the analytical mindset. Clinical thinkers, especially vets, are forced in a clinical consultation setting to provide a solution for each problem they encounter. Critical thinking allows us to identify the problem, not necessarily the solution; to focus relentlessly on the cause and progression of the problem, and to describe the problem as we see it without the added complication of seeking a solution to it (that is the court's role).

This critical thinking ability is not a skill that is lacking in most vets; rather, it is a dormant skill. The vet's strong scientific training in the biological sciences assists in questioning results, and evidence-based decision making is a strong component of undergraduate training; but the clinical thinking ('Let's find a solution') of practice replaces it. This clinical thinking is what many vets take into court with them and they often feel compelled to provide a solution to legal disputes that involve animals, where identification of the problem is required and is often overlooked. This is a key component in vet reports and testimony, where 'Because I say so' is an argument that resists and often rejects any attempt at scrutiny.

One of the key tenets of critical thinking is the difference between *observation* and *interpretation* of events, and then the conclusions drawn from those interpretations.

Each aspect must be independent and a distinction needs to be made between them – critical thinking forces us to do this.

1.8.1   Example

Heavy snow fall in London might provide the following headline:

'Capital paralysed by snow'

While in another publication the headline might read:

'Day off for 30,000 London schools'

Prior to interpreting that information, we need to evaluate it and consequently make inferences from it; inferring requires moving from a known statement to an unknown statement. And all arguments originate from this observation. *How we interpret information* and the inferences we draw are going to be based on our own experiences and observations. When facts are not disputed, then the *interpretation* of the facts always is. In the above example, it is snowing, but what this means to different people is reflected in the disparate headlines.

Analysis leads to interpretation, which leads to an inference or a conclusion. There is usually no dispute with the analysis or evaluation of data (it is snowing in London) – but where critical thinking comes in is to unravel the reasons why we evaluated a particular piece of data or analysis in the way we did. In order to do so, we ask the person to explain the reasons for their interpretation.

Schools off because of snow.

Or

London is paralysed because of snow.

The difference between the two headlines that are describing the same observation is down to the journalist's individual interpretation of what heavy snowfall means to a busy metropolis, based on that journalist's experience and interpretation of the facts. It is also possible that the target audience for that paper could affect the interpretation of the facts and the headline reflects the target audience's interests.

1.9   Conclusion

To be Spock-like in our ability to analyse data is a useful mindset to maintain in forensics. To be *critical* in our ability to interpret data is a crucial mindset to nurture in forensics. Having both aspects in our collective forensic thought process, and combining them with a veterinary clinical mindset, allows a consistent approach to a description of a biological science that is by its nature an inconsistent discipline.

2 Forensic Philosophy

Karl Harrison[1]* and David Bailey[2]*

[1]Cranfield Forensic Institute, Cranfield University, Defence Academy UK, Shrivenham, Wiltshire, UK; [2]Department of Forensic and Crime Science, Staffordshire University, Stoke-on-Trent, Staffordshire, UK

2.1 One of Us Cannot Be Wrong: The Structure of Knowledge and Reasoning in Forensic Science

KARL HARRISON

2.1.1 Introduction

The purpose of this chapter is to consider how the science in forensics is structured. Forensics is a *crossroads discipline*, which encompasses a breadth of skills, from investigative scene examination to analytical chemistry, but despite the vital importance of establishing conclusive facts in a court of law, little has been written about how forensics produces facts or distinguishes them from observations and interpretations.

A scientifically educated professional, such as a veterinarian, considering the further development of their career towards a forensic specialism, might find themselves harbouring a curiosity regarding how forensic science works, how forensic scientists observe salient facts, how those scientists construct interpretations from said observed facts, and how those interpretations might be communicated, either in an academic context or via court testimony. Such curiosity might cause them to seek answers to these questions from either standard synthetic set texts (Lee *et al.*, 2001; James *et al.*, 2009; Pepper, 2010), or from articles in widely read peer-reviewed journals (Inman and Rudin, 2002; Crispino

*Corresponding authors: k.harrison@cranfield.ac.uk; daysbays@yahoo.co.uk

© CAB International 2016. *Practical Veterinary Forensics* (ed. D. Bailey)

et al., 2011). In both instances, a reader new to the field would be forgiven for thinking that forensic science is a discipline solidly based on the quantification of the exchange of material traces, such as cellular DNA (Bond and Hammond, 2008), blood (Sikirzhytskaya *et al.*, 2013), glass (Howes *et al.*, 2014), paint (Wright *et al.*, 2013) or soil (Woods *et al.*, 2014a,b), or on the development of statistically robust techniques for presenting such evidence in court. Synthetic texts repeat some of this material, frequently in the form of introductory discussions of Bayesian statistics (Jackson and Jackson, 2011).

My thesis in this chapter is that, on the whole, this literature reflects the core concerns of a central bloc of laboratory-based forensic biologists, chemists and other scientists focused on trace evidence dynamics, and that these cited publications are primarily concerned with the development and refinement of method, rather than advancing or explaining the theories and concepts that might assist the generalist scientist in developing a clear and comprehensive understanding of what their place in forensic science might be. My intention here is to draw attention to the set of circumstances that has brought about the current theoretical framework in which forensic science resides, and consider it in the light of the discipline's historical roots, as well as to advance a broader discussion about what might be said to constitute science. In providing this discussion, I will also detail why I think this form of consideration is particularly important in the development of specialist forensic disciplines such as veterinary science, and in the professional development of individuals within such specialisms.

2.1.2 Forensics: a plethora of different sciences

Before I begin this discussion, I need to make a number of confessions that help to establish the context within which I have formed these opinions. Rather than coming out of biology or chemistry, my reporting discipline is forensic archaeology.[1]

Prior to becoming a forensic archaeologist, but subsequent to my training in traditional archaeology, I worked as a Crime Scene Investigator and later Scene Manager for two UK police forces. This small piece of personal history is important here for three reasons, I believe: first, forensic archaeology is a niche discipline, somewhat removed from the central pillars of forensic science, biology and chemistry; second, as a science, traditional archaeology has a long history of reflection and conceptualization, which I will argue later that, taken as a whole, forensic science does not; third and finally, the UK's Crime Scene Investigators are primarily employed by police forces, rather than the (now privately run) forensic service providers. While this makes them a part of the wider investigative process, it remains a moot point whether this role is included within broader concepts of forensic science.

My second confession concerns the third point above. Some years ago I wrote a paper entitled 'Is crime scene examination science, and does it matter anyway?' (Harrison, 2006). While this paper drew on the philosophy of science to consider the nature of crime scene examination and, more specifically, the role of crime scene investigators, its main purpose was political, rather than epistemological. I was motivated to write it because of general accounts of forensic science that seemed to gloss over the point of interaction between evidence collection by a CSI and examination by a forensic scientist (cf. Coyle and White, 2010), and was distressed to talk to CSIs content to take a minimal role in the scientific process. I found at the time that models of what constituted science did not adequately encapsulate the forensic process. Crispino (2008) took issue with my conclusions, and offered abductivism, discussed below, as a model of scientific structure that more comfortably accommodated the process of crime scene examination.

Given the fragmentation to which I have eluded within forensic science, the first question I'd like to consider is what level of coherence as a discipline forensic science can be said to possess. In defining this first question, I have used a commonly ascribed definition of forensic science:

> Forensic science is science used for the purpose of the law ... The recently

appointed UK Forensic Science Regulator has further expanded this definition to 'forensic science is any scientific and technical knowledge that is applied to the investigation of a crime and the evaluation of evidence to assist courts in resolving questions of fact in court'.

(Rankin, 2010, p. 2)

By the term coherence, I mean the extent to which a central set of theories or theoretically-defined methods have developed, which identify forensic science to the exclusion of other, non-forensic science disciplines. It is perhaps interesting to note that Brian Rankin, in providing his introduction to forensic practice, regards it as important to specify a number of different roles in the forensic process, separating out forensic scientist from forensic practitioner and forensic medic, but does not consider what points of distinction define the parameters of these terms.

Central to this consideration is the observation that forensic science is defined by its context of application, rather than by any observed or defined boundaries to its subject of study. This is in contrast to a great range of other physical and natural sciences, such as biology, chemistry or crystallography, all of which interact and overlap, but are in some sense defined by their theoretically informed perspective on their subject matter. Perhaps the closest analogue to forensic science would be medical science, in that they are defined by their application, but medical science has perhaps a tighter focus on human biochemical systems. Criminology, a social science interested in concepts of laws versus social codes and morals, the development of legal frameworks over time and the nature of individual and corporate transgressions against laws, has been described in terms that directly parallel the nature of forensic science: criminology brings together psychologists, psychiatrists, sociologists and historians of law and crime into what Downes (1988) described as a 'rendezvous subject'; it being the subject matter that draws together disparate academics, rather than a shared framework of knowledge and methods.

There are areas where coherence can be seen to operate across broad swathes of forensic science. Locard's exchange principle,

as refined by Kirk (1953, p. 4) has provided an overarching theory governing the transmission of trace materials for decades:

Wherever he steps, whatever he touches, whatever he leaves, even unconsciously, will serve as silent witness against him. Not only his fingerprints or his footprints, but his hair, the fibres from his clothing, the glass he breaks, the tool mark he leaves, the paint he scratches, the blood or semen he deposits or collects. All of these and more bear mute witness against him. This is evidence that does not forget.

If there is a point of coherence borne out of theory, then it must be this: while it remains most pertinent to crime scene examiners and particularly examiners of trace materials, the obvious analogue being that the actions of a protagonist may be revealed by traces left on a host. This can be seen in disciplines as diverse as forensic archaeology, bitemark analysis or the study of mobile telephone cell sites. Locard's Theory gives forensic science coherence about how data is created (i.e. by human action on a subject, host or environment), and it defines our scale of interest (we want wherever possible to discuss actions or traces of an individual we might be able to name, identify or characterize in some meaningful way). What Locard's Theory does not do is define a unifying means by which forensic scientists might derive knowledge from this data.

Locard's Theory can be conceived as sitting at the highest level of theory held in common by much of forensic science. Below this it is possible to identify a range of methodological theories that essentially provide quality control and guiding principles across a broad range of forensic disciplines. These lower level theories encompass strategies of optimal searching or evidence recovery (Taupin and Cwiklik, 2011); concepts of primary, secondary and tertiary cross-contamination (Butler, 2011); and improvements to the understanding of trace evidential transfer between actors on a crime scene (Morgan *et al.*, 2010).

As the level of thinking continues to descend towards the application of forensic practice, this high level coherency diminishes. While acquired data is generated and tested against hypotheses, the manner of testing and types of knowledge constructed by different forensic disciplines is different, as each tends to relate back to a distinct 'parent' science. This may seem facile, but it is an important point to stress, as the growth in popularity of Bayesian approaches in forensic science (Taroni *et al.*, 2006), the importance of Daubert criteria in US forensic science (Grivas and Komar, 2008) and the development of specific guidance for Forensic Service Providers related to ISO accreditation standards (ISO/IEC, 2005) together provide a tension which uncomfortably pulls forensic science towards an agreed mechanism of data interpretation.

That scientific knowledge is in some ways more valuable than other forms of knowledge is a commonly held belief from which the philosophy of science sets out its stall (Bird, 1998; Chalmers, 1999). In this regard, science presented in the courtroom is no different. While 'normal' witnesses of fact might be asked to comment in court on what they saw, what happened to them, or on the character of a defendant, they are generally limited in their responses to their own experiences or perceptions (Wall, 2009). By contrast, the forensic scientist, while giving evidence within their area of expertise, is an expert witness, able to give evidence of opinion based on their findings on examination and their professional experience. As a professional expert operating in England and Wales, such a scientist would be expected to by familiar with and abide by the Crown Prosecution Service's guidance to experts (ACPO/CPS, 2010).

Forensic scientists are by no means the only experts recognized under this system; indeed, the system of classification is purposefully flexible to allow the broadest range of professional experience to qualify as an expertise. As forensic science has continued to develop and become ever more specialized, however, the notion that scientific reasoning might be able to provide a sound basis for expert opinion in the courtroom has become ever more commonplace.

2.1.3 The philosophy of science

Philosophy of science recognizes a number of schools of thought regarding structures of scientific reasoning: deduction, induction and abduction (Jackson and Jackson, 2011). Deduction outlines knowledge contained within logical statements, but in order to retain the integrity of these statements, the knowledge they shed light on must already be entailed within the structure of the premises of the prior statements, thus:

> Forensic evidence is recognized by the careful attention to detail at crime scenes.
>
> Forensic scientists pay careful attention to detail at crime scenes.
>
> *Therefore*
>
> Forensic scientists identify forensic evidence at crime scenes.

This statement makes logical sense, but the conclusion cannot give us any further information than that which is already entailed in the prior statements. While some forensic disciplines may rely heavily on aspects of deductive logic, particularly where they have a mathematical or geometric aspect to their functioning, such as angle calculation in blood pattern analysis (Bevel and Gardner, 2001), the structure of most forensic interpretation is not based upon deduction from logically entailed statements.

Induction, by contrast, attempts to derive scientific knowledge about universal criteria from the careful observation of smaller samples of relevant data. Observations are made via the senses and general patterns can be suggested in the form of hypotheses, and tested via experiment or further observation. Abductive reasoning combines elements of deduction and induction in order to fashion 'likely explanations', but it remains unclear what this process of generation exactly is (Jackson and Jackson, 2011).

Philosophers of science have noted limitations with the inductive model that are directly pertinent to forensic practice. In the Empiricist view of Locke and Hume (Carlin, 2009), facts exist as external things to be observed; they are fundamentally a priori, in that their existence is entirely independent from the observer, and precedes the act of observation. In the courtroom, the forensic scientist will report on and explain observations that form the basis of their interpretations; such explanations are vital, as without them, the observed facts alone might appear to be entirely incidental, or even invisible, to an untrained jury. Furthermore, even when a forensic scientist explains their observations, these may very well not be something a jury can see with their own eyes in a direct fashion; a DNA profile might be rendered as a series of numbers representative of allelic characteristics expressed at particular loci of the DNA molecule, or a trace of petrol detected in a sample of fire scene debris as a series of peaks on a chromatogram. Even with seemingly more obviously intuitive evidence types, such as the presence of toolmarks in the side of a grave revealed on a Crime Scene Investigator's photograph, the forensic scientist may ultimately describe diagnostic features of importance either not perceptible to an untrained eye, or not distinguishable as being any more valuable than any of the associated background 'noise', whether that noise be formed from other confounding peaks on the chromatogram, or natural variation in the soil that comprises the grave side.

The philosophical problem that is intrinsic to arguments based on induction is one regarding the weight of evidence placed on inference: to what extent is it possible to rely on or defend knowledge gained when it is based on reference to observations taken from a small sample, when ultimately it is being asked to apply to a much larger – or even universal – population? Such samples might be found in the small control DNA sample populations from which are derived the specific frequencies of different allelic characteristics, which in turn form the basis of match probabilities stated in court, or a software library of different accelerants from which a petrol sample might be identified. Falsificationism takes a sceptical view of this practice (Rosende, 2009), claiming that such observations can only establish a 'hypothetically adequate' conclusion, ra-

ther than advancing on a more conclusive truth. Any knowledge supported by such inductive observations only holds true until the first recorded observation of variance to the proposed rule; such as the discovery of a group of people possessing similar allelic characteristics that might alter our understanding of the frequency of such characteristics in a large unknown population.

In direct contrast with this sceptical view, abductivism (Crispino et al., 2011) holds that structured inference to a best estimate is a satisfactory means of establishing scientific knowledge in a forensic context; although the notions of structured enquiry proposed by abductivists are in places so general that it becomes hard to distinguish between scientific observation and a rigorous, systematic but fundamentally non-scientific investigation.

Bayes' Thoerem has enjoyed considerable attention from forensic scientists and associated academics in the past 10 years (Taroni et al., 2006), as it offers a means of providing a quantified probability of the occurrence of a given set of circumstances, based on an assessment of available evidence. This represents a very powerful tool for forensic scientists, as it offers a mechanism for the communication of technical interpretations to a jury of non-scientists. This power is balanced with a set of concomitant risks according to some critics (Kruse, 2013); the prior probabilities that define the preliminary calculations of Bayes' Theorem require fundamental scientific research in order to establish their values – such as in the shattering of glass from a window pane (Curran et al., 2000). But these fundamental researches cannot account for the hypervariability of real-life scenarios. It is also possible that in attempting to assist a jury by providing them with a Likelihood Ratio, the forensic scientist might cause them to place more weight on the evidence, because it appears to offer a quantified, rather than qualified opinion (Anon., 2010).

There is a further distinction to be drawn between central tenets of Bayes' Theorem and its application in the context of forensic science. Bayes' Theorem offers an alternative means of supporting inferential arguments by turning qualitative observations into clearly defined quantified probabilities. Forensic scientists, by contrast, have applied Bayes primarily to express quantified opinions in court. While ambitious plans have been mooted to try to broadly quantify common variables (Gee, 1995), this has not occurred wholesale across forensic science.

It should be remembered that these theoretical discussions about what constitutes knowledge and science in a forensic context rarely impinge directly on the working life of the vast majority of forensic scientists, but rather present a broader background against which their methods of examination and parameters of interpretation develop. Legislative controls on forensic expert opinion in US courts under the Daubert criteria, and in the UK under Crown Prosecution Service Guidance to Experts, as well as the establishment of the role of the Forensic Regulator, and the growth in importance of International Standards (ISO 17020 for scene examination and ISO 17025 for laboratory examination) have all acted to provide a framework for the manner in which credible forensic science should be seen to operate.

2.1.4   Conclusion

The nature of what constitutes credible scientific knowledge in forensics cuts across a range of key debates that have a direct effect on the nature of practice, interpretation and dissemination in court: considerations of what are the distinctions between police investigation, crime scene examination and forensic analysis; conceptualization of what features are common and definitive across forensic science; and what constitutes a legitimate balance between qualitative and quantitative interpretation. There are no simple answers to these questions, but awareness of their existence clarifies the nature of forensic science to newcomer and established practitioner alike. In specialist fields such as forensic veterinary science, where practitioners move out of a strong

parent discipline and into the 'rendezvous subject' of forensic science, these discussions are even more important, as they assist in providing an overarching framework of the discipline for scientists new to the field.

2.2   Junk Science

David Bailey

Seeing is believing.

2.2.1   Pseudoscience

Definition:
Any of various methods, theories, or systems, as astrology, psychokinesis, or clairvoyance, considered as having no scientific basis.

2.2.2   Junk science

Definition:
Faulty scientific information or research, especially when used to advance special interests.

One would not normally associate declining quality with increasing demand for a service. In court, however, in a feature of the adversarial system, what is bad for one side is almost invariably good for the other. Viewed from the right side of the aisle, bad expert testimony looks excellent and, while the views of opposing expert witnesses cannot be excluded from a legal dispute, there are problems for experts when they rely upon science that is just plain wrong. While some examples provided here are historical, the case study provided in Appendix 2.1 occurred in Northern Ireland as recently as 2007.

2.2.3   Conclusion bias

In 1895 W.C. Röntgen discovered X-rays; eight years later N-rays were identified and were named after the University of Nancy in France. Their discoverer, Monsieur René Blondlot, was a distinguished French physicist and a member of the French academy of sciences. He had detected N-rays by observing their ability to brighten an electric spark through which they were beamed. More than 20 other French physicists soon confirmed the discovery of N-rays and interest in this exciting development even surpassed the interest in X-rays.

In the 18 months following Blondlot's announcement, the number of publications on the newly discovered N-rays proliferated rapidly. In 1904 the French journal *Comptes Rendus* published three papers on X-rays but 54 on N-rays. A century later in 2015, we utilize X-rays in diagnostic imaging; however, after 1904, no one published anything further on N-rays. N-rays do not exist; they have never existed and are remembered chiefly for the insights they can provide into the fringe sociology of the competitive academic world of research. N-rays were discovered and subsequently rediscovered on more than 54 occasions because people *wanted* to see them. The methodology used in the experiments to describe them was flawed; yet so anxious were the scientists to declare the existence of N-rays that they chose results over methodology (Huber, 1991).

In another example, Anita Menarde had an accident on the morning of 16 May 1949. While alighting from a Philadelphia streetcar, she was slightly injured as she stumbled and later sued the providers of the streetcar service after developing breast cancer. Immediately after her fall she was treated at her local hospital for minor scrapes and abrasions to her left ankle, right knee and both hands. Upon undressing that evening she had noticed a discolouration on her right side and breast. She called her doctor about her bruised breast; he examined it, found no lumps and prescribed hot compresses. He examined her periodically for the next two months – the breast seemed normal.

At the end of July (ten weeks after her accident) she detected a lump in her breast at the same place as her earlier bruise. She was diagnosed with breast cancer and had a mastectomy. She was awarded $50,000 in damages from the streetcar service providers, having successfully argued that trauma causes cancer. By the time of her court case, this medical theory was almost three centuries old and about to be debunked as a cause of cancer. In 1676, an eminent English surgeon, Richard Wiseman, had reported two interesting cases of cancer. Both patients, he observed 'thought the cancer came from an accidental bruise' (Stoll and Crissey, 1962); Wiseman thought so too and he proceeded to identify bruises, errors in diet and 'ill handling' (Huber, 1991) as among the causes of cancer. By the late 17th century, many doctors had come to believe that simple trauma could trigger a malignant tumour in a human patient.

Yet, by the mid-19th century, the traumatic cancer theory was in decline. Most physicians were beginning to understand that among the causes of cancer, many as there were – simple trauma was not one of them. Like the discovery of N-rays, it was another hypothesis *on its way* to the museum of scientific curiosities. Then suddenly and without any scientific reason, there was a rapid shift in attitude among doctors in Germany and the US in the late 19th and early 20th centuries. In 1875 the scientific literature suggested that one in eight cancers were now caused by trauma. In 1897 nearly half of all bone cancers were now *caused* by trauma and in 1932 it was determined that two in five brain tumours (40%) were traumatic in origin or caused by simply being upset.

Whereas the N-ray was discovered to not exist by the one, singular correctly identified methodology and test experiment, there was no similar research carried out to disprove a traumatic cause of cancer. In fact there were now many scientific references designed to demonstrate that a traumatic cause of cancer could be demonstrated reliably. So what had changed?

In the late 19th century in Germany and the USA, *the laws had changed* and Germany had introduced the world's first workers' compensation programme. Combined with the introduction of health insurance for workers, a race began to determining the cause for the traumatic cause of cancers – any cancers, all cancers, including testicular cancer.

Over the next 16 years more than 2000 books and papers on traumatic cancer were published and republished in Germany and the USA. A phantom risk existed between cancer and trauma and, importantly, it couldn't be proved to be false. When in doubt, the courts favoured the injured: doctors, medics and researchers were all called to provide expert witness testimony and insurance companies bore the brunt of claims. It is a cardinal rule of science that statistics alone cannot prove causation. It is very highly unlikely that a traumatic cause of cancer exists. The research hadn't changed, but the law had changed, and so too did the opinions of those experts who would in the past have sought compensation for clients apparently stricken by traumatic cancer.

Note

[1] Forensic archaeology has been variously defined as 'the potential application of archaeological theory to scenes of crime' (Hunter and Cox, 2005, p. 2) and 'the application of mapping and excavation skills … to recent death scenes or places where bodies have been disposed' (Skinner and Sterenberg, 2005, p. 223), and has been most commonly applied in aspects of search, location, excavation, recovery and interpretation of human remains concealed by acts of burial.

References

ACPO/CPS (2010) Guidance Booklet for Experts. Disclosure: Experts' Evidence, Case Management and Unused Material. Available online at: https://www.cps.gov.uk/legal/assets/uploads/files/Guidance_for_Experts_-_2010_edition.pdf (accessed 16 September 2015).

Anon. (2010) R. v. T [2010] All ER (D) 240 (Oct); [2010] EWCA Crim 2439. Available online at: http://www.criminallawandjustice.co.uk/clj-reporter/R-v-T-2010-All-ER-D-240-Oct-2010-EWCA-Crim-2439 (accessed 15 December 2014).

Bevel, T. and Gardner, R.M. (2001) Blood Pattern Analysis: With an Introduction to Crime Scene Reconstruction. CRC Press, Boca Raton, Florida, USA.

Bird, A. (1998) Philosophy of Science. McGill Queens University Press, Montreal, Quebec, Canada.

Bond, J. and Hammond, C. (2008) The value of DNA material recovered from crime scenes. Journal of Forensic Sciences 53(4), 797–801.

Butler, J. (2011) Advanced Topics in Forensic DNA Typing: Methodology. Elsevier Academic Press, Waltham, Massachusetts, USA.

Carlin, L. (2009) The Empiricists: A Guide for the Perplexed. Continuum, London, UK.

Chalmers, A.F. (1999) What Is This Thing Called Science? 3rd edn. Open University Press, Maidenhead, UK.

Coyle, T. and White, P. (2010) Crime Scene to Court, 3rd edn. Royal Society of Chemistry, Cambridge, UK.

Crispino, F. (2008) Nature and place of crime scene management within forensic sciences. Science & Justice 48, 24–28.

Crispino, F., Ribaux, O., Houck, M. and Margot, P. (2011) Forensic science – a true science? Australian Journal of Forensic Sciences 43(2–3), 157–176.

Curran, J.M., Hicks, T.N. and Buckleton, J.S. (2000) Forensic Interpretation of Glass Evidence. CRC Press, Boca Raton, Florida, USA.

Downes, D. (1988) The sociology of crime and social control in Britain, 1960–1987. British Journal of Criminology 28(2), 175–187.

Gee, D.J. (1995) Reaching conclusions in forensic pathology. Medicine, Science and the Law 35(1), 12–16.

Grivas, C.R. and Komar, D.A. (2008) Kumho, Daubert, and the nature of scientific enquiry: implications for forensic anthropology. Journal of Forensic Sciences 53(4), 771–776.

Harrison, K. (2006) Is crime scene examination science, and does it matter anyway? Science & Justice 46(2), 65–68.

Howes, L.M., Kirkbride, K.P., Kelty, S.F., Julian, R. and Kemp, N. (2014) The readability of expert reports for non-scientist report-users: reports of forensic comparison of glass. *Forensic Science International* 236, 54–66.

Huber, P.W. (1991) The Midas touch: how money causes disease. In: Huber, P.W. *Gallileo's Revenge: Junk Science in the Courtroom*. Basic Books, New York, USA, p. 41.

Hunter, J. and Cox, M. (2005) *Forensic Archaeology: Advanced in Theory and Practice*. Routledge, Abingdon, UK.

Inman, K. and Rudin, N. (2002) The origin of evidence. *Forensic Science International* 126(1), 11–16.

ISO/IEC 17025 (2005) General Requirements for the Competence of Testing and Calibration Laboratories. Available online at: http://www.iso.org/iso/catalogue_detail.htm?csnumber=39883 (accessed 13 October 2015).

Jackson, A. and Jackson, J. (2011) *Forensic Science*, 3rd edn. Prentice-Hall, Harlow, UK.

James, S.H., Nordby, J.J. and Bell, S. (eds) (2009) *Forensic Science: An Introduction to Scientific and Investigative Techniques*, 3rd edn. CRC Press, Boca Raton, Florida, USA.

Kirk, P. (1953) *Crime Investigation*. Interscience, New York, USA.

Kruse, C. (2013) The Bayesian approach to forensic evidence: evaluating, communicating and distributing responsibility. *Social Studies of Science* 43(5), 657–680.

Lee, H., Palmbach, T. and Miller, M.T. (2001) *Henry Lee's Crime Scene Handbook*. Academic Press, Waltham, Massachusetts, USA.

Morgan, R., French, J., O'Donnell, L. and Bull, P. (2010) The reincorporation and redistribution of trace geoforensic particulates on clothing: an introductory study. *Science & Justice* 50(4), 195–199.

Pepper, I. (2010) *Crime Scene Investigation: Methods and Procedures*, 2nd edn. Oxford University Press, Oxford, UK.

Rankin, B. (2010) Forensic practice. In: Coyle, T. and White, P. (eds), *Crime Scene to Court: The Essentials of Forensic Science*, 3rd edn. Royal Society of Chemistry, Cambridge, UK, pp. 1–24.

Rosende, D.L. (2009) Popper on refutability: some philosophical and historical questions. In: Parusniková, Z. and Cohen, R. (eds) *Rethinking Popper*. Springer, Dordrecht, The Netherlands, pp. 135–154.

Sikirzhytskaya, A., Sikirzhytski, V., McLaughlin, G. and Lednev, I.K. (2013) Forensic identification of blood in the presence of contaminations using Raman microspectroscopy coupled with advanced statistics: effect of sand, dust and soil. *Journal of Forensic Sciences* 58(5), 1141–1148.

Skinner, M. and Sterenberg, J. (2005) Turf wars: authority and responsibility for the investigation of mass graves. *Forensic Science International* 151, 221–232.

Stoll, H.L. and Crissey, J.T. (1962) Epithelioma from single trauma. *New York State Journal of Medicine* 62, 496–500.

Taroni, F., Aitken, C., Garbolino, P. and Biedermann, A. (2006) *Bayesian Networks and Probabilistic Inference in Forensic Science*. Wiley, Oxford, UK.

Taupin, J.M. and Cwiklik, C. (2011) *Scientific Protocols for Forensic Examination of Clothing*. CRC Press, Boca Raton, Florida, USA.

Wall, W. (2009) *Forensic Science in Court: The Role of the Expert Witness*. Wiley, Oxford, UK.

Woods, B., Lennard, C., Kirkbride, K.P. and Robertson, J. (2014a) Soil examination for a forensic trace evidence laboratory – Part 1: spectroscopic techniques. *Forensic Science International* 245, 187–194.

Woods, B., Lennard, C., Kirkbride, K.P. and Robertson, J. (2014b) Soil examination for a forensic trace evidence laboratory – Part 2: elemental techniques. *Forensic Science International* 245, 195–201.

Wright, D.M., Bradley, M.J. and Hobbs Mehltretter, A. (2013) Analysis and discrimination of single-layer white architectural paint samples. *Journal of Forensic Sciences* 58(2), 358–364.

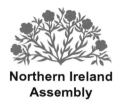

**Northern Ireland
Assembly**

RESEARCH AND LIBRARY
SERVICES

BRIEFING PAPER 09/07

ALPHA NORTESTOSTERONE

BACKGROUND

In 1988 the EU introduced a prohibition on the use of hormonal substances for animal growth production. Legislation prescribing the measures to monitor for residues and the actions to be taken on the finding of positive results was introduced (96/22/EU, 96/23/EU/, 2003/74/EC and 2005/34/EC). The use of anabolic agents is prohibited for a variety of reasons including possible adverse human health effects, consumer resistance, negative effects on animal welfare and the impact of residues in the environment[1].

Nortestosterone is a well known anabolic-androgenic steroid. It was first synthesised in the 1950s and initially it was believed to have no natural source. However, it was subsequently shown to occur naturally in boars, stallions, pregnant cows and veal calves[1].
Its presence in adult male bovines is currently deemed illegal under EU law.

ALPHA NORTESTOSTERONE IN NORTHERN IRELAND

Occurrences

On two occasions since January 2004 the hormone, nortestosterone, was identified in bottles, or syringes, on two separate farms in Northern Ireland.

On 10 March 2006 a urine sample was collected from an "On Farm Emergency Slaughter" (OFES) steer presented to ABP Newry, and it screened positive for Alpha Nortestosterone at a low level (1.05ppb).

---

[1] Professor Patrick Wall report http://www.dardni.gov.uk/wall_report.pdf

ALPHA NORTESTOSTERONE

In the light of these findings all Official Veterinary Surgeons (OVSs) were instructed to take samples for hormone testing from OFES animals.

DARD Response

Between April 2006 and March 2007 the Department of Agriculture and Rural Development (DARD) tested all male OFES cattle presented at meat plants for growth hormone Alpha Nortestosterone. More than 150 cattle tested positive for the hormone and were condemned, with the farmer incurring the financial loss. However, no evidence of illegal administration was found following on-farm investigations. Scientific evidence now supports the view that the hormone can occur naturally in male cattle[2].

The Minister for Agriculture and Rural Development, Michelle Gildernew MP MLA, met the farmers associated with the cases in June 2007 and said:

> *"The Department is required by law to remove any male bovine from the food chain that tests positive for alpha nortestosterone, regardless of whether evidence of illegal administration has been found, and it is permitted to do so without incurring legal liability to pay compensation".*

However, in recognition of the fact that farmers have lost animals without any evidence of wrongdoing on their part, she announced that farmers who have had OFES male cattle will be offered a goodwill payment[3].

The full cost of these payments will be around £80,000[4]. These payments cover the value of the cattle removed from the food chain when the farmers were being investigated by the DARD, and do not take account of loss of earnings when herd sales were suspended nor a potential loss of reputation. DARD insists it is under no obligation to offer compensation.

---

[2] Houghton, E., Teale, P. and Dumasia, M.C. (2006) "Studies related to the origin of C18 neutral steroids isolated from extracts of urine from the male horse" Analytica Chimica Acta 586: 196-207.

[3] Source from Northern Ireland Assembly Oral Answers to Question 11th June, 2007. http://www.northernireland.gov.uk/news/news-dard/news-dard-070607-cattle-harmone-residues.htm

[4] "Agri-Business – Cattle farmers to be reimbursed" Irish News 12th June, 2007.

ALPHA NORTESTOSTERONE

Ulster Farmers Union Response

The Ulster Farmers Union has welcomed the way the Minister has dealt with the issue swiftly after entering office but has urged DARD to deal with each case on an individual basis. Some farmers who were investigated at an early stage still have grievances over their treatment and the money they lost.

Some suffered financially because cattle prices dropped while herd sales were suspended. They had to pay feed costs for cattle they had been intending to sell, plus some animals passed the 30-months mark, dropping in price. No compensation has been offered for any of these costs.

> "Our big issue is that it is all too easy for people to jump to the wrong conclusion. It just goes to prove that science can be wrong. A lot of people suffered traumatic episodes and stress over the head of this" Wesley Aston of the Ulster Farmers Union[5].

On 11th June 2007, the Minister promised to undertake a review of the handling of the alpha nortestosterone issue and to consider what lessons can be learned. The outcome of that review is likely to be made public[6] in autumn 2007.

---

[5] "Poor cows and innocent farmers are pilloried" Belfast Telegraph 15 June 2007.
[6] Source from Northern Ireland Assembly Oral Answers to Question 11th June, 2007. http://www.northernireland.gov.uk/news/news-dard/news-dard-070607-cattle-harmone-residues.htm

3 Law and Animals

Deborah Rook[1]* and Pippa Swan[2]*

[1]*Northumbria Law School, Northumbria University, Newcastle-upon-Tyne, UK;*
[2]*Clare Veterinary Group, Ballyclare, Co. Antrim, Northern Ireland, UK*

3.1 Challenges to the Legal Status of Domestic and Captive Animals

Deborah Rook

3.1.1 The property status of domestic and captive animals

The law distinguishes between 'persons' and 'things'. Human beings are legal persons and in consequence enjoy certain fundamental

---

*Corresponding authors: debbie.rook@northumbria.ac.uk; pippaswan@gmail.com

rights, such as freedom from torture and slavery. Domestic and captive animals are legal things and in consequence lack the capacity to possess legal rights. Legal personhood is not synonymous with human beings; it identifies those entities that are capable of having legal rights. Legal personhood can be a more restrictive category than 'humans' and has sometimes been denied to certain humans; for example, slaves, women, indigenous peoples. In other instances it can be a wider category, which allows non-human entities to enjoy legal personhood. For example, a private company is a legal person and, under English Law, enjoys a right to the protection of its property under the Human Rights Act (HRA) 1998. The question that has been asked recently in a number of courts across the globe is whether a captive animal such as an adult chimpanzee or orang-utan can be classed as a legal person. This is clearly a direct challenge to the current legal status of animals.

There are also more indirect challenges arising in the courts: cases which highlight the fact that the current property status of domestic animals is inadequate to resolve certain disputes. Pet custody cases, to decide the residency of a family dog or cat following the breakdown of a relationship between a married or co-habiting couple, are an example of this. Using pure property law principles to decide the question of where the dog or cat lives is often inappropriate. Increasingly civil courts are being asked to recognize dogs and cats as a unique form of living and sentient property, different from inanimate property, and to thereby take the interests of the animal (not just the owners) into account. This also constitutes a challenge to the current legal status of domestic animals, but it is a more subtle and indirect challenge.

3.1.2 Pet custody cases

Cases to decide the residency of family pets, following the breakdown in a couple's relationship, have been reported in a number of countries, including the USA and Israel (Rook, 2014). What is so interesting about these cases is that they highlight the difficulty in applying pure property law to determine the question of a pet's residency. Since the pet is property, the question of who gets to keep the pet will be decided on the same principles as who gets to keep the family TV or kitchen table. In some cases the courts have done this, but in other cases the courts have recognized the unique nature of this living and sentient property and have taken other considerations into account. For example, in the case of *Raymond versus Lachman* in 1999 the appeal court in New York reversed the earlier decision of the trial court, which had awarded custody of a pet cat to the person with the better claim to property title, the cat's owner. Instead the appeal court took into consideration the age and life expectancy of the ten-year-old cat and allowed it to 'remain where he has lived, prospered, loved and been loved for the past four years' (695 N.Y.S.2d 308, 309 (N.Y, App.Div. 1999)). This case appears to take into account the interests of the animal itself and not merely the status of the animal as property. Although the outcome of the case may seem reasonable and just to a layperson, the case has significant implications at law because of its challenge to the pure property status of domestic animals. There have been a number of cases since 1999 adopting a similar approach, and Switzerland has even gone so far as to amend its Civil Code to provide a test that takes the interests of the animal into account in pet custody cases (Michel and Schneider Kayasseh, 2011).

3.1.3 Direct legal challenges to the property status of animals

Law, ethics and science are intricately linked in the question of the legal status of animals. The law reflects, or in some cases helps to lead, changes in moral thinking about animals. Changes in moral thinking can arise from our greater understanding of animal behaviour and welfare through scientific discovery. For example, science has given humans a greater understanding of the cognitive and behavioural characteristics of chimpanzees, which in turn led to concerns over whether the use of great apes in research was ethical.

In 2010 the EU banned the use of great apes in scientific research (Directive 2010/63/EU).

Progress in scientific research has led to calls for a change in the legal status of some animals, such as great apes, from property to persons (Rook, 2009). However, others call for caution as the ramifications of granting some animals legal personhood will be significant. Wise (2000) supports a change in legal status and advocates that any being with mental abilities adding up to what he calls 'practical autonomy' should be entitled to the basic legal rights of bodily integrity and bodily liberty (freedom from torture and slavery). A legal thing does not enjoy rights so this change would involve granting legal personhood to the relevant being so that they become a legal person.

Wise defines practical autonomy as evident where a being 'can desire; and can intentionally try to fulfil her desires; and possesses a sense of self-sufficiency to allow her to understand, even dimly, that it is she who wants something and it is she who is trying to get it' (Wise, 2000). He examines scientific research findings in relation to the cognitive abilities of great apes (chimpanzee, bonobo, gorilla and orang-utan) as well as Atlantic bottle-nosed dolphins and discovers that they are self-conscious, possess some of, or all, the elements required for a theory of mind and can solve complex problems (Wise, 2002). He concludes that these animals possess sufficient practical autonomy to be entitled to basic legal rights of bodily integrity and bodily liberty. Wise has put his theory into practice and in 2013 the Nonhuman Rights Project (a group founded by Wise) filed three lawsuits in the USA in relation to four captive adult chimpanzees in the hope that the courts will recognize the chimpanzees as legal persons. The case of *Nonhuman Rights Project versus Lavery* concerns a chimpanzee called Tommy who is privately owned by Mr Lavery and lives alone in a cage at a used trailer lot. The Project seeks a court order to have him removed to a sanctuary where chimpanzees live in groups on a number of islands in an artificial lake. To be able to remove Tommy from his owner (who is not in breach of any state

or federal laws) requires the court to grant a writ of habeas corpus. This court order can only be given in relation to a legal person and is not available for a legal thing. We should remember that in law a 'person' is not synonymous with a human being; it is a legal concept, not a biological one. Under English law a private company is a legal person and enjoys a right to the protection of its property under the HRA 1998.

The case was rejected at trial, but went on appeal to the Supreme Court, Appellate Division, which in 2014 also declined to grant a habeas corpus in respect of Tommy. The Supreme Court adopted a Contractualist approach, which explains rights in terms of a social contract; a person enjoys the benefit of rights in return for submitting to societally imposed responsibilities. Relying on the work of Cupp, the court held that 'unlike human beings, chimpanzees cannot bear any legal duties, submit to societal responsibilities or be held legally accountable for their actions' (Cupp, 2013). This is only one interpretation of legal rights and other theories do not rely on the reciprocity of rights and responsibilities. The Nonhuman Rights Project is pursuing an appeal to New York's highest court – the Court of Appeals. Wise draws hope from historical cases on the African slave trade to demonstrate how judges can make a decision to break the mould and permit the law to adapt to changing moral climates.

Tilikum is a bull orca whale who was captured off the East coast of Iceland in 1983. He was born wild and therefore was not property at birth; however, he became someone's property when he was captured by humans for the purpose of providing entertainment in captivity. Tilikum has lived in captivity for over 30 years and in 2012, when living at SeaWorld Orlando in Florida, he became the subject of a court case. The case alleged that five wild-captured orcas, including Tilikum, were being held by SeaWorld in violation of the Thirteenth Amendment to the Constitution of the USA, which prohibits slavery and involuntary servitude. It was argued that orca whales engage in complex social, communicative and cognitive behaviours and that their confinement in unnatural conditions at SeaWorld negatively impacts on their welfare. The court examined the wording of the Constitution in its historical setting to ascertain the purpose of those who drafted it. On this basis the court rejected the plaintiff's argument and stated that the Thirteenth Amendment only applies to humans because 'slavery' and 'involuntary servitude' are uniquely human activities, which do not apply to nonhumans (*Tilikum, Katina, Corky, Kasatka and Ulises, five orcas by their Next Friends, People for the Ethical Treatment of Animals, Inc. versus Sea World Parks & Entertainment Inc.* (2012) 842 F.Supp. 2d.1259).

The recent proliferation of cases making a direct challenge to the current legal status of captive animals demonstrates the strength of feeling driving this debate, and indicates that there are interesting times ahead in deciding whether an animal can ever be a legal person.

3.1.4 The basis of a challenge to the legal status of animals – autonomy versus sentiency

The USA is not the only country in which there have been legal challenges to the property status of animals. There have also been significant cases in Brazil, Argentina and Austria. Interestingly, the cases so far have all been in relation to animals that possess what Wise calls 'practical autonomy' (Wise, 2000). It seems that the complex cognitive abilities of these animals may engender stronger feelings in humans of the need to ensure justice for these intelligent animals. Wise takes a pragmatic approach and argues that we are more likely to dismantle the thick legal wall that separates humans and animals if the animal has practical autonomy. For Wise, it is the cognitive abilities of the animal that are crucial. Whereas for others, sentiency is enough. For Singer it is the sentiency of the animal, the fact that it can experience pleasure and pain, which is crucial (Singer, 1995). According to Singer, sentiency is sufficient to require a rethink of how we treat animals. He develops the work of the famous 18th-century philosopher, Jeremy

Bentham, who advocated the better treatment of animals and wrote: 'the question is not, Can they reason? Nor, Can they talk? But, Can they suffer?' (Burns and Hart, 1970, p. 283). Like Bentham before him, Singer is a utilitarian. In simple terms, a utilitarian makes moral decisions by weighing the costs of a particular action against the benefits or satisfactions, and then takes the option which brings the best balance of total benefits over total costs. The principle of equal consideration is an important concept for utilitarians. It requires that the interests of everyone affected by an action are taken into account and given the same weight as the *like interests* of any other being. This principle of equality prescribes how we should treat each other; it is a moral idea, not a factual occurrence. Singer applies the principle of equal consideration to animals. Just as a person's IQ is irrelevant to their moral treatment – we don't give less consideration to the interests of those with a low IQ compared to those with a higher IQ – Singer argues that the cognitive abilities of animals should also be irrelevant to how we treat them. It doesn't matter whether an animal has complex intellectual abilities or not, what matters is whether it can suffer pain. Sentiency is a prerequisite to having interests; if a being suffers, Singer argues that 'there can be no moral justification for refusing to take any suffering into consideration'.

3.1.5 Utilitarianism in practice

Let's consider a simple practical example to illustrate this theory. Should someone living in the affluent West eat pig meat? This is a moral decision because the pig is sentient and has interests that can be harmed by being raised for meat, killed and eaten. For a utilitarian, making the decision of whether or not to eat pig meat involves weighing up the costs against the benefits to see if the benefits outweigh the costs. A difficulty soon becomes apparent: which costs and benefits are considered? The suffering of the pig is relevant; there is evidence that pigs suffer due to intensive farming practices, transport and pre-slaughter handling at the abattoir.

But are there wider considerations, such as the significant environmental costs of eating meat highlighted in the United Nations' report, *Livestock's Long Shadow* (Steinfeld *et al.*, 2006)? Is this a relevant factor to be weighed in the balance when someone is deciding whether or not to eat meat, or is this cost too far removed? What are the benefits of eating the pig? Where there are healthy alternatives to meat, as in the West, thereby removing the need to eat meat for a balanced diet, then the benefits appear to be taste and cost; a person enjoys the taste of meat and, where it is produced by intensive farming methods, it is relatively cheap. For Singer the suffering of the pig in terms of physical pain, stress and the frustration of not being able to display natural behaviours all outweigh the benefit to the human and consequently a utilitarian will be likely to decide not to eat pig meat. For Singer, the sentiency of the pig is sufficient to require equal consideration to be given to the suffering of the pig as would be given to the suffering of a person. Wise, however, would focus on the cognitive capacity of the pig and examine scientific research findings to ascertain whether a pig has practical autonomy deserving of the rights to freedom from torture and slavery.

Singer and Wise have their critics, and one of the arguments against their theories is the idea that humans and animals are different and we are justified in treating animals differently and favouring our own kind (Posner, 2004). Imagine seeing a polar bear in Alaska about to kill a young seal. If we had the means to do so, would we intervene to save the seal? Most people would not intervene but would accept it as a natural event. The polar bear must eat the seal to survive. But what would happen if we saw a polar bear about to kill a human child? Now our response is likely to be very different. We would intervene to save the child, even though polar bears must eat meat to survive. What accounts for this different response? This scenario illustrates the extent to which we favour our own species and will act to prevent harm to other humans, even at the expense of animal suffering.

3.1.6 The concept of unnecessary suffering

The law faces a dilemma. How to deal with what Francione calls our 'moral schizophrenia' (Francione, 2004). On the one hand, humans now recognize the sentiency of animals and there is a desire to protect animals from pain and suffering. But on the other hand, humans feel justified to use animals for our own benefit, and as a consequence we accept what Francione calls 'the institutionalized exploitation' of millions of animals; for example, in factory farms, entertainment and scientific procedures. The law has developed a clever concept to deal with this dilemma; a concept whose success is demonstrated by the fact that it spans international boundaries. It is the concept of 'unnecessary suffering' and it is a pivotal concept in animal protection law across the world. Many countries have criminalized cruelty to animals, making it an offence to cause domestic and captive animals unnecessary suffering. The concept of 'unnecessary suffering' prohibits suffering that is unnecessary but permits necessary suffering. Thus the test of necessity is crucial, as it determines whether an offence has been committed. The act of hitting an animal may be an offence if it is unnecessary but a legal act if it is necessary; for example, in the English case in 1999 in which it was alleged that Mary Chipperfield (of the then-famous Chipperfield's Circus) had caused cruelty to a camel by hitting it with a broom handle, the Magistrate said that the force Mary had used was necessary to train the camel to perform. Notably, in assessing necessity the Magistrate was not prepared to consider whether it was necessary for the camel to perform in a circus in the first place. It was held that no offence was committed on the facts because the suffering caused to the camel was deemed necessary to train it to perform.

3.1.6.1 *Necessity as a balancing exercise*

In England and Wales, the Animal Welfare Act 2006 governs the offence of cruelty to domestic animals. Under Section 4 a person is guilty of the criminal offence of cruelty if their act (or failure to act) causes a protected animal to suffer unnecessarily and he/she knew or ought reasonably to have known that it would have that effect. Vets and lawyers both have a part to play in the concept of unnecessary suffering; it is for the vet to decide whether suffering has occurred and it is for the judge to determine the question of necessity. Suffering is a prerequisite to the offence; without it there can be no offence, so the role of the vet is crucial. Once suffering has been established by the vet, there are a number of statutory considerations set out in the Act for the court to consider, such as whether the suffering could reasonably have been avoided or reduced and whether the conduct was that of a reasonably competent and humane person. These statutory considerations encapsulate a test that had been developed through case law under the Protection of Animals Act 1911, which preceded the Animal Welfare Act 2006. Case law established that there must be a legitimate purpose for the act which caused the animal suffering, but a purpose on its own was not sufficient. There must also be proportionality between the purpose to be achieved and the means of achieving it. Proportionality is an important legal concept used in human rights law which involves a balancing exercise. In the case of *Ford versus Wiley* in 1889 a farmer was alleged to have been cruel to his young cattle by cutting off their horns, close to the head, with a common saw. It was accepted by the court that the cattle suffered extreme and prolonged pain as a result of this procedure. The farmer justified his actions on the basis of cost and convenience. The court accepted that there was a legitimate purpose, but nevertheless cruelty was established because the purpose did not justify the means of achieving it. The court held that the suffering was completely disproportionate to the purpose and the practice was consequently found to be cruel and illegal. The problem with the concept of necessity is that it is subjective; it is for the court to decide on the respective weight to attach to the conflicting interests of humans and animals. In most cases a court is likely to give greater weight to the interests of humans.

The Israeli case in 2002 of *Noah versus The Attorney General et al.* is an excellent example of the subjectivity involved in assessing necessity (HCJ 9232/01, 215 Israeli Supreme Court). This case is unusual because, in the balancing exercise to decide necessity, the interests of the animals ultimately outweighed those of the humans; in practice this is rare. The case concerned the practice of producing foie gras by inserting a tube into the oesophagus of geese and force-feeding them until their livers become abnormally large and fatty. The court had to consider whether this caused unnecessary suffering. Interestingly, in reaching its decision the court was willing to examine the literature on the ethical theories applied to our treatment of animals, and referred to the work of Singer and Francione. The court weighed in the balance the suffering caused to the geese by the method of force-feeding against the benefit to humans of a food delicacy. The majority view of the court was that the suffering was not justifiable for a delicacy and therefore the suffering outweighed the benefit. The minority of the court felt that the suffering was necessary because of the suffering that any ban on foie gras production would cause to the farmers who would lose their livelihoods. More than 500 t of foie gras was produced in Israel every year at that time and hundreds of farmers were dependent on the industry. This is a significant case for the promotion of animal welfare in agriculture. The English courts have been less willing to attach weight to the suffering of the animal. The case of *Roberts versus Ruggerio* in 1985 concerned the use of the veal calf crate system. Under this system of intensive farming, calves were individually confined in a narrow stall, chained at the neck and denied access to roughage in their diet. Roberts was the director of Compassion in World Farming, which advocated that the use of veal crates caused the animals' unnecessary suffering and consequently the farmer was guilty of the offence of cruelty. The court took the view that it would only consider suffering beyond that which is to be expected from the use of the veal crate. It would not challenge the use of the veal crate itself, even though there was evidence that it caused the calves suffering, and that alternative practices were available to produce veal that caused the animals less suffering. Fortunately, the veal crate has since been banned as being cruel, first in England and Wales, and more recently in Europe.

3.1.6.2 Property status and proportionality

For Francione, the property status of animals is the root of the problem. He advocates that the concept of unnecessary suffering does not protect animals because the weighting to be attached to the respective interests of the animals and humans has already been predetermined by the property status of the animals. He states that:

> The property status of animals renders meaningless any balancing that is supposedly required under the humane treatment principle or animal welfare laws, because what we really balance are the interests of property owners against the interests of their animal property.
>
> (Francione, 2004)

Therefore, for Francione, the dilemma can only be solved by giving animals the right not to be treated as our property. The Israeli foie gras case shows that the interests of animals can sometimes trump humans; however, this is relatively rare.

3.1.7 Conclusion

Law, ethics and science are intricately linked in the debate surrounding the legal status of domestic and captive animals, especially in relation to animals with higher cognitive abilities, such as the great apes. There has been a wealth of scientific discovery about the cognitive and social abilities of great apes since the pioneering work of Jane Goodall in the 1960s in the Gombe National Park, Tanzania (Goodall, 2010). And, since Singer's groundbreaking book, *Animal Liberation* (Singer, 1995), there has been an explosion of ethical theories relating to our treatment of animals. The recent appearance and growth of legal challenges in the courts, both direct and indirect, to the property status of domestic and captive animals suggests that it is time for the law to respond and adapt to the developments in science and philosophy. It would seem that exciting times lie ahead for animal law.

References

Burns, J.H. and Hart, H.L.A. (eds) (1970) *Jeremy Bentham, An Introduction to the Principles of Morals and Legislation*. Athlone Press, London, UK.

Cupp, R. (2013) Children, chimps and rights: arguments from 'marginal' cases. *Arizona State Law Journal* 45, 1–50.

Francione, G. (2004) Animals – property or persons? In: Sunstein, C. and Nussbaum, M. (eds) *Animal Rights*. Oxford University Press, New York, USA, pp. 108–142.

Goodall, J. (2010) *In the Shadow of Man*, 50th Anniversary of Gombe edn. Mariner Books, New York, USA (first published in 1971).

Michel, M. and Schneider Kayasseh, E. (2011) The legal situation of animals in Switzerland: two steps forward, one step back – many steps to go. *Journal of Animal Law* 7, 1–42.

Posner, R. (2004) Animal rights: legal, philosophical, and pragmatic perspectives. In: Sunstein, C. and Nussbaum, M. (eds) *Animal Rights*. Oxford University Press, New York, USA, pp. 51–77.

Rook, D. (2009) Should great apes have 'human rights'? *Web Journal of Current Legal Issues*. Available online at: http://nrl.northumbria.ac.uk/2816/1/Should%20great%20apes%20have%20human%20rights%20-%20full%20text.pdf (accessed 2 November 2015).

Rook, D. (2014) Who gets Charlie? The emergence of pet custody disputes in family law: adapting theoretical tools from Child Law. *International Journal of Law, Policy and the Family* 28(2), 177–193.

Singer, P. (1995) *Animal Liberation*, 2nd edn. Pimlico, London, UK.

Steinfeld, H., Gerber, P., Wassenaar, T., Castel, V., Rosales, M. and de Haan, C. (2006) *Livestock's Long Shadow: Environmental Issues and Options*. Food and Agriculture Organization of the United Nations, Rome, Italy. Available online at: http://www.fao.org/docrep/010/a0701e/a0701e00.htm (accessed 8 January 2016).

Wise, S. (2000) *Rattling the Cage: Toward Legal Rights for Animals*. Perseus Publishing, Cambridge, Massachusetts, USA.

Wise, S. (2002) *Drawing the Line: Science and the Case for Animal Rights*. Perseus Publishing, Cambridge, Massachusetts, USA.

3.2 Unnecessary Suffering

PIPPA SWAN

3.2.1 Introduction

The term 'unnecessary suffering' has long been used to define the legally unacceptable ways in which animals are treated. Its evolution and use in law are described in this chapter.

3.2.2 A legal definition

For nearly 200 years in the UK there existed an offence of cruelty to animals. When the legislation was first enacted, the idea that men be prohibited from treating animals in any way they chose, and that any treatment they meted out could be labelled 'cruel', had little sympathy in many quarters. By contrast, the correctness of such a prohibition is now widespread. Although the relevant legal offence in most jurisdictions has changed to one of 'causing unnecessary suffering', many people, including the media, still refer to this offence as 'cruelty to animals'. Some organizations with the aim of promoting animal welfare still contain the word cruelty in their title. Cruelty is defined in the *Oxford English Dictionary* as 'a cruel act or attitude; indifference to another's suffering'. In laws relating to animals it has been defined in reference to the necessity of any pain or suffering caused. The Royal Society for the Prevention of Cruelty to Animals and the Royal Commission publication on regulating vivisection in 1876 makes the point that under statute 'man may not *cruelly* inflict pain – that is, he may not cause unnecessary pain; for cruelty is the infliction of *unnecessary* pain' (RSPCA and Royal Commission, 1876). The accusation of cruelty carries with it emotive images and assumptions, both historical and cultural, and is largely subjective, depending on the viewpoint of the accuser. While the concept of cruelty to animals is still widely used in popular culture, the legal offence has been replaced by one which is capable of better and more precise definition by the courts.

Using the term 'unnecessary suffering' rather than 'cruelty' to define what constitutes unacceptable and criminal behaviour means that two important aspects of the offence must be proven. First, it must be established that an animal has been caused to suffer by an act, or failure to act, of somebody. Unless it can be demonstrated that suffering has occurred, then no offence has been committed. In the UK there are separate offences to cover circumstances in which animals are likely to suffer unless steps are taken to improve their situation. Second, the issue of necessity must be addressed. Before the UK Animal Welfare Act of 2006 the 'necessity' of any suffering caused was the subject of some debate within courts. Given the varied and complicated position of animals within society, what people consider necessary in pursuance of their aims or that which is required by their responsibilities can vary greatly. The result of much legal argument has been distilled into five main considerations:

(a) whether the suffering could reasonably have been avoided or reduced;
(b) whether the conduct which caused the suffering was in compliance with [any other legislation];
(c) whether the conduct which caused the suffering was for a legitimate purpose, such as – (i) the purpose of benefiting the animal, or (ii) the purpose of protecting a person, property or another animal;
(d) whether the suffering was proportionate to the purpose of the conduct concerned;
(e) whether the conduct concerned was in all the circumstances that of a reasonably competent and humane person.[i]

Use of the terms 'reasonably avoided', 'legitimate purpose' and 'proportionate' all serve to demonstrate the intended meaning of the term 'unnecessary' when linked to animal suffering. A motorist who injures an animal because it runs out in front of their car could

---

[i] Animal Welfare Act 2006. Section 4(3).

not reasonably have avoided causing the injury. Choking a dog who is attacking a child would be legitimate to protect the child. Failing to seek veterinary attention for a seriously sick animal because of concerns about fees or euthanasia would not be considered the conduct of a reasonably humane person.

In some cases there will clearly be a balancing act between the intentions of someone in relation to an animal and the actual outcome. How much chastisement is acceptable, for example, when trying to train an animal in desisting from unwanted, potentially dangerous, behaviour? At what point do the initial good intentions of an animal hoarder become unacceptably lacking in insight? There also exist certain, somewhat anomalous, situations, which permit treatment of animals in one set of circumstances and prohibit them in another. Despite a specific prohibition on the administration of poisonous substances to all 'protected' vertebrates, there is lawful authority to poison animals which are seen as pests. The humaneness of the destruction for rats and mice living as 'pests', for example, is not required to be of the same standard as that required for those living under the control of man.

3.2.3   The legal test

Because a person's intentions can sometimes be key in deciding how to judge their actions, the law considers intent in certain types of offence. With some offences, such as speeding in a car, the motivations or attitude of the person responsible are irrelevant. The deed was done and penalties are issued. This is known as strict liability. In other situations the state of mind of an accused is crucial in deciding their culpability, in law this is known as *mens rea* (meaning 'a guilty mind'). When proving that someone is guilty of murder, the proof must include evidence that they knew what they were doing would bring about the death or serious injury of another person. Since there is no way to measure or directly observe the state of someone's mind, this is known as a subjective test, since it requires interpretation and subjective judgement by the court.

A third type of test has also been used when judging defendants, which takes into account the circumstances of the accused, but compares their actions with that of a reasonable person in the same situation. This is known as an objective test. When using an objective test a person's behaviour is judged not by what they know but what they *ought* to know, using the 'reasonable' person as a benchmark. Ignorance or extreme beliefs cannot be used as a defence in these situations, since stupidity or wilful disregard for the consequences of one's actions should not be rewarded by impunity.

The offence of causing unnecessary suffering has generally been viewed as one which requires an objective test. The application of strict liability would be inappropriate since, as outlined above, the infliction of suffering on an animal may in some circumstances be caused by people who are not blameworthy and so would not deserve prosecution or censure. The use of a subjective test would potentially make the case extremely difficult to prove, since assumptions would have to be made about the defendant's knowledge and beliefs and the defence could more easily argue that lack of insight or education were relevant mitigating factors. Any further discussion about the nature of the test to be applied to offences of causing animals unnecessary suffering has been clarified in the UK by the wording of the legislation 'he knew, or ought reasonably to have known, that the act, or failure to act, would have that effect or be likely to do so'.[ii] In addition, the explanatory notes issued by the government which accompany the Act state that: 'The effect of [paragraph (b) above] is to introduce an objective mental element. It will not be necessary to prove that a defendant actually knew his act or failure to act would cause suffering'.[iii] The word 'humane' is also used in the legislation and implies that some degree of compassion or sensitive feeling towards animals is expected when measuring the behaviour of the 'reasonable' person.

[ii] Animal Welfare Act 2006. Section 4(1)b.
[iii] Explanatory Notes on Animal Welfare Act 2006. 2007, p. 4, para 19.

3.2.4 Animal suffering

Identifying animal suffering can, at times, be a slippery task and lacking in an overall consensus. Again, precise definitions of a word can become imprecise when tested against the reality of animal existence. Human suffering is incapable of direct observation or measurement, even given our abilities for language and shared experiences; animal suffering is even more complicated. There are scientific definitions of animal suffering, for example: 'Suffering should not be equated with stress. Suffering occurs when the intensity or complexity of stresses exceeds or exhausts the capacity of the animal to cope, or when the animal is prevented from taking constructive action' (Webster, 1994, p. 38). Numerous attempts have been made to define and assess the welfare of animals scientifically, and many would place suffering at the negative end of a spectrum of welfare states. When that line, between poor welfare and suffering, is crossed, however, is still a matter for conjecture in each situation. Some scientists have simplified the nature of suffering by just associating it with feelings and emotional states: 'a set of negative emotions such as fear, pain and boredom, and recognized operationally as states caused by negative reinforcers. It may or may not be accompanied by subjective experiences similar to our own' (Dawkins, 2008). Similarly, it is 'an unpleasant state of mind that disrupts the quality of life. It is the mental state associated with unpleasant experiences such as pain, malaise, distress, injury and emotional numbness (e.g. extreme boredom)' (Gregory, 2004, p. 1).

In whichever way suffering in animals is described, their feelings and emotional state are the ultimate issue. That pain, hunger or thirst can cause suffering would rarely be in dispute, but the law is clear that mental distress will also qualify as suffering. When providing information to a court about whether suffering has occurred, there may be demonstrable physical evidence of a painful condition, disease or malnutrition. On the basis of the physical evidence, a logical inference of unpleasant feelings can be made. Where the evidence is based on more anthropomorphic

assumptions of an animal's mental state, given its situation or behaviour, some more subjective interpretation for the court, or argument by analogy, is required from an expert witness. This person is usually a veterinary surgeon, but other experts with relevant training or experience may also be qualified to give an opinion to the court.

> Science can never 'prove' that an animal is or is not suffering, because we can never really access the private world of another's mind. But what science can be used for is the collection of evidence from which to make inferences (much like those made by the clinician who uses symptoms to make a judgement about a disease).
> (Mason and Mendl, 1993, p. 312)

When considering whether an animal's condition or situation has caused it to suffer, there is often some discussion about whether severity or duration are instrumental to the conclusion. It should be remembered that 'such criteria do not apply to offences based on causing an animal unnecessary suffering, where *any* unpleasant emotional response may amount to suffering'. And that 'factors such as severity and duration *are* taken into account, but in relation to the question of necessity rather than suffering' (Radford, 2001, p. 272). Ultimately, it is for the court to decide, not experts or advocates, whether suffering has occurred and whether that suffering is considered to be unnecessary.

3.2.5 Animal killing

Another important dimension of unnecessary suffering is a specific exemption for killing animals. Provided that animals are destroyed in 'an appropriate and humane manner',[iv] there is no offence caused under animal welfare legislation. Because animals have a legal status as property, there may be an offence of killing an animal which belongs to someone else without their permission. But owners are entitled to kill, or cause to be killed, their

---

[iv] Animal Welfare Act 2006. Section 4(4).

own animals, whatever other parties might
perceive to be the potential 'cruelty' of the act.
The catchphrase 'death is not a welfare issue'
is borne out by the law and it then remains
a matter of ethical and physiological debate,
dependent on the situation and method of
killing used.

3.2.6 Conclusion

Personal interpretations and opinions of
what constitutes unnecessary suffering will
vary widely. The aim of the legal process is to
examine the detail of each case and apply
tests as objectively and uniformly as possible.

References

Dawkins, M.S. (2008) The science of animal suffering. *Ethology* 111(10), 937–945.
Gregory, N. (2004) *Physiology and Behaviour of Animal Suffering*. Blackwell, Oxford, UK.
Mason, G. and Mendl, M. (1993) Why is there no simple way of measuring animal welfare? *Animal Welfare* 2, 312.
Radford, M. (2001) *Animal Welfare Law in Britain*. Oxford University Press, Oxford, UK.
RSPCA and Royal Commission (1876) *Vivisection*, 2nd edn. Smith, Elder & Co., London, UK. Introduction, p. iii. Available online at: https://ia600302.us.archive.org/18/items/vivisection00unkngoog/vivisection00unkngoog.pdf (accessed 8 January 2016).
Webster, J. (1994) *Animal Welfare: A Cool Eye towards Eden*. Blackwell Science, Oxford, UK.

4 Forensic Science and Applications to One Health

Lloyd Reeve-Johnson[1]* and David Bailey[2]*

[1]*Institute of Health and BioMedical Innovation, Queensland University of Technology, Brisbane, Australia and Principal Research Fellow, Translational Research Institute, Brisbane, Australia; [2]Department of Forensic and Crime Science, Staffordshire University, Stoke-on-Trent, Staffordshire, UK*

4.1 Introduction

DAVID BAILEY

Currently (in 2015) in the UK there are scientific databases being constructed and built for the use and application of evidence-based veterinary medicine. But while the hierarchy of evidence for evidence-based medicine leaves expert opinion as the lowest-ranked in terms of quality, it does not provide any criteria to define the term 'quality' of evidence. The pyramid in Fig. 4.1 is widely used as an accepted tool to rank the *quality and strength* of evidence used to base clinical decisions upon in veterinary science, yet it is a tool that demonstrates caution in the over-use of personal experience in the application of evidence-based medicine and the construction of an evidence-based medicine tool.

---

*Corresponding authors: lloyd@goydpark.com; daysbays@yahoo.co.uk

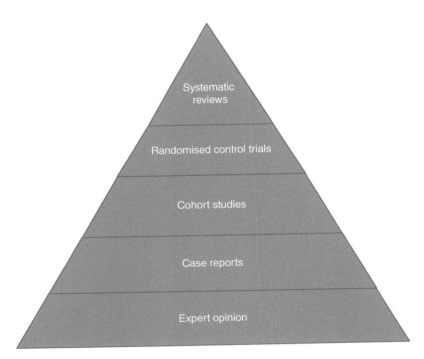

Fig. 4.1. Schematic representation of the 'hierarchy of evidence'.

In contrast, the use and application of expert opinion is the preferred method of dealing with disputes as they arrive and progress through the judicial process, and the use and reliance of meta-analyses and other higher 'quality' indicators are not the preferred tools for use in a legal dispute. The hierarchy of 'quality' of evidence is flipped upside down in a legal dispute, with professional opinion being the preferred tool on top of this judicial pyramid of strength and quality of evidence. Here is an important difference in the acceptance of forensic science into the scientific world. The higher 'quality' indicators reserved for non-legal academic disputes are fixed in dried ink and are set like concrete, unable to answer, bend, yield or provide answers to that single inevitable marginal example query that is asked of an opposing barrister, that a person can process, analyse and construct the appropriate answer to only under oath. Courts prefer scientists, and not science, to answer questions. Evidence-based medicine is very good at telling you what would have happened and what has happened, but very poor at predicting what is going to happen in biological systems. Evidence-based medicine will tell you what *should* happen, but it is precise at telling you exactly what *has* happened and therefore what you should expect to happen if you follow the same process, conditions and methodology. A scientist should be able to tell you the outcome under different processes, dates, times and places based on the available evidence, and the available evidence cannot do this. Only the scientist can.

Personal opinion can be stress-tested under examination-in-chief and cross-examination, and all the randomized controlled trials and meta-analyses cannot do what an expert can do under questioning – that is, to change its mind and deliver a different possible outcome, result, interpretation or conclusion under appropriate adversarial questioning. This is a major difference between evidence-based medicine and evidence-based testimony. In evidence-based medicine, one allows the findings of the studies and trials to navigate our opinion toward a reliable, accepted and verifiable outcome and conclusion. It is safe, but sometimes narrow in application. In evidence-based testimony, one reads the appropriate studies, literature and available material and provides another layer of reliability that science despises: we allow our interpretation and our own experiences and application of this material to cover areas which may not be presented in the available literature. It is not as safe, but has a wider application. In the former, you have your opinion handed to you and it is flanked by descriptors such as 'best practice', 'gold standard' and 'good guidance', along with the inevitable inclusion 'the available evidence leads us to conclude … '. In the latter, you seek your own interpretation and opinion from your own analysis of the available evidence as it applies to the dispute, the material and the questions in front of you.

And while the use of the word 'evidence' is being used in both evidence-based medicine and evidence-based legal disputes, a translation is required of what the two uses of the word 'evidence' mean; this translation can be summed up visually by inverting the pyramid of evidence hierarchy.

Translational research is the term adapted to explain the difference between evidence-based medicine and bridging the research results between species, pathogens and situations. And while One Health can be used as a descriptor to bridge the research results between human and non-human species, the use and application of forensic science to research of the species is also a translational research relationship that requires an inverting of the hierarchy of quality evidence that is used in all research. You need to know the subject, know it well and provide interpretation to the relevant questions; and while your opinion is of little value in evidence-based medicine, it is of the highest value in a legal dispute of evidence-based medicine.

This translational research requires the hierarchy of 'quality' evidence to be flipped upside down when making the transition from evidence-based medicine to evidence-based legal disputes. The two are not the same, and an understanding of the concept

is required before an understanding of translational research can be enjoyed.

While One Health can be used to describe a world with no boundaries between species in terms of disease, health and welfare, the understanding of the One Health concept requires an understanding of the scientific evidence-based medicine process. Any potential application of legal issues that can potentially stem from One Health issues require a translation and transition away from how we understand and apply science to One Health research and how we again apply this science differently to legal disputes. The science doesn't change between evidence-based clinical science on the one hand and forensic science on the other, but the application and understanding of how it is applied between clinical science and forensic science does change.

An understanding of science allows us the tools to evaluate the scientific use of certain advances, methods and research. The forensic application of science allows us to apply what we know to a legal arena. Translational science is a descriptor which allows us to understand the journey through scientific research into legal application, when the science has not changed but the application has. Problems can arise when one person has the ability or power to evaluate all of the available material, and make a decision based on his or her translation and interpretation of that material into practice. Politicians are usually best placed to make these decisions, and errors in translation are often seen at this political level. Where there are political factors involved in any scientific process, then the hierarchy pyramid is not inverted; it may be replaced with other non-scientific factors that reinforce the political stance on a certain scientific argument. It is at this level, where scientific process is no longer useful and forensic opinion hierarchies are not required, that the scientist in us is allowed to be removed from the decision-making process. Thus there is the emergence and translation of pure science through the forensic application into a tool of the political process; understanding this limit of our input is as important as the understanding of how we input into decisions and findings as scientists, and how we alter our application of science as legal scientists.

LLOYD REEVE-JOHNSON

The majority of the world's population live in urban or semi-urbanized environments. In the 21st century, humans tend to perceive the world around them as being shaped more by culture, industry and themselves than by natural history. Vital to understanding, controlling or eradicating disease is a sound understanding of the origins, evolution and reservoirs of infection, and interactions between different species and potential pathogens. Translational research implies understanding the health, husbandry and physiology of different species, as well as the influence of their local environment, before findings can be applied to different situations. This increases the chances of achieving medical research outcomes that are sustainable, effective in practical situations, and attuned to the impact on other species and the environment. Incorporating a broad perspective of the epidemiology of diseases results in improvements in research quality and efficiency. Consideration of multiple dimensions of host–pathogen interactions and the physiology of health greatly strengthens the objectivity of evidence upon which medical decisions are ultimately made.

Research in humans is constrained by personal preferences, lifestyle, religion, culture and ethical boundaries. These factors limit enrolment, restrict randomization, decrease experimental control, confound results and slow progress in comparison to the experimental study conditions typical of animal science research. Evidence-based medicine has been strongly advocated for many years, yet human studies used to generate medical evidence are undermined by the above factors and rely on sample populations that differ from patient populations in health-status, age, race and multiple other ways, due to unavoidable sources of study bias. This was highlighted in a review of 49 of the most-cited papers on the effectiveness of medical interventions in highly visible journals between 1990 and 2004. It was found that by 2005 a quarter of the randomized study trials and five out of six non-randomized studies had already been contradicted (Young et al., 2008).

Human health care is transforming, largely to seek more cost efficiency. Funding is increasingly linked to superior societal outcomes. Technology is necessary, but not sufficient, and is constantly adapting to the reality of competing for resources and optimizing resource reallocation. The true value of time, knowledge and insight of translational approaches to societal goals, including preclinical phases of human health care and the innovation that underpins incremental food production, remains to be fully captured. Animals suffer from many of the same chronic diseases as humans, including heart disease, cancer, diabetes, asthma and arthritis. Sometimes a disease entity is recognized in animals long before it is recognized in humans. The concept of comparative medicine was understood by the ancient Greeks and dissection and studying of animals has long been used to understand human diseases (Olsson, 1969). Comparative anatomical and physiological studies have been responsible for significant advances in medicine: Banting and Best discovered insulin through such work, and Edward Jenner developed the smallpox vaccination based upon observations of cow pox.

While translational research considers issues of bridging research results between species, pathogens or situations, the macroview of interconnectedness between all health issues has been branded with titles such as World Health, One Medicine, Global Health and more recently One Health. Definitions embrace a common theme of collaboration between multiple disciplines, working locally, nationally and globally to attain optimal health for people, animals and the environment (American Veterinary Medical Association, 2008). In an era of specialization, the alarming breadth of this definition should not detract from the importance of communicating collaborative cross-disciplinary approaches to medical research, and of stimulating funding bodies to provide necessary incentives for collaboration to occur. As illustrated in the list below, the importance of collaborations has been formally accepted by many international organizations.

What remains to be seen is how effectively these collaborations will be organized, which ultimately determines whether they will fulfil their potential.

Examples of major organizations which have formally adopted One Health in their formal agendas include the following.

1. USA: American Medical Association, American Veterinary Medical Association, American Academy of Pediatrics, American Nurses Association, American Association of Public Health Physicians, American Society of Tropical Medicine and Hygiene, Centers for Disease Control and Prevention (CDC), United States Department of Agriculture (USDA), US National Environmental Health Association (NEHA), and a number of university centres focused on One Health research.
2. European Union: Belgium: Institute of Tropical Medicine, Antwerp. Sweden: Department of Animal Health; The Infection, Ecology and Epidemiology Network, University of Uppsala, founded an inaugural Chair in 2012 in Integrative Biology. UK: British Veterinary Association; a new Veterinary School at the University of Surrey has pledged to differentiate by making One Health central to their teaching of veterinary students; the Royal Veterinary College in London and the Royal (Dick) School of Veterinary Studies of Edinburgh University recently established new academic staff positions in One Health. The European Association for Veterinary Pharmacology and Toxicology held its first session on the topic in Amsterdam in 2012.
3. Other global organizations: The World Bank, World Health Organization, Food and Agriculture Organization, World Organization for Animal Health, Global Alliance for Rabies Control and The Gates Foundation.

4.2   The Need for Translational Research and One Health Collaborations

In 2010, the human population surpassed 7 billion and is set to reach 9 billion by 2050. Four billion people earn less than US$3000 per year (the majority of the world's population). The world's poorest have the greatest potential to benefit from health care, nutritional and other medical innovations. They are also likely to live in closest proximity to animals often to the point of interdependence for economic, nutritional and health goals. Besides ethical imperatives there are commercial opportunities to offer health solutions to this population. Empirical measures of the behaviour of the world's poorest consumers 'and their aggregate purchasing power suggest significant opportunities for market-based approaches to better meet their needs, increase their productivity and incomes, and empower their entry into the formal economy' (Hammond *et al.*, 2007, p. 3). Besides altruistic motives, eradicating infection among the poorest makes disease transfer to others less likely. Increasing occurrence of viral and bacterial resistance to treatments that are only affordable in affluent communities, provides motivation to minimize reservoirs of infection elsewhere. Translational approaches to health care are highly relevant to many macro-economic challenges of the future including: food production, poverty, disease spread, disaster relief, sustainability, affordable health care provision, antimicrobial resistance and psychosocial issues.

In 2010 global GDP approached US$70 trillion with human health care expenditure of US$5.95 trillion (pharmaceuticals accounted for US$850 billion) and human retail food expenditure $4 trillion. The capitalized value of animal health delivery was tiny in comparison at US$20 billion. The point is that animal health is substantially undervalued in terms of market capitalization when the value added to other industries is taken into account. Animal research has a vastly disproportionate influence on other markets. It is firmly placed at the meeting point of two dominant markets: human health and nutrition, and impacts other major markets including energy production (see Fig. 4.2). Animals provide: the test-bed for mammalian genetic research into food productivity and reproduction; testing of human medical and surgical innovations; pre-clinical pharmacology and toxicology; and function as sentinels in disease surveillance. Pharmaceutical companies recoup development costs of products which fail regulatory scrutiny for human use,

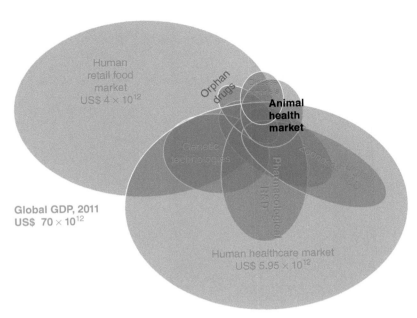

Human
retail food
market
US$ 4×10^{12}

Orphan
drugs

Animal
health
market

Genetic
technologies

Pharmacological
R&D

Global GDP, 2011
US$ 70×10^{12}

Human healthcare market
US$ 5.95×10^{12}

Fig. 4.2. Schematic diagram of approximate market sizes and the interrelationship between expenditure on human health care, human food, animal health care and subsidiary markets.

and commercialize related molecules in animal health that were developed alongside lead candidates for human use. When patent protection in humans expires the animal health market provides additional patent opportunities against generic competition. There is huge value remaining to be captured through improving our ability to 'translate' animal physiology to relevant human contexts and vice versa. Animal models are much more flexible, scientifically controllable, repeatable, less costly and results can generally be obtained much more rapidly with shorter generation times than in human research (Reeve-Johnson, 1998).

Medical and surgical interventions pioneered in animals contribute greatly to the quality of life and longevity of humans. There is a traditional 'linear' view of pre-clinical testing from animals to humans which loses sight of the continuum of results relevant to multiple health issues that can be interpreted across species. No animal is an exact replica of another, yet each animal species provides a new window of enlightenment – each a different perspective of an incomplete picture into potential applications for products, adaptation

of physiology, possible toxic reactions, or different ways to harness biological systems. Participants in animal aspects of comparative medicine have for many years failed to adopt a macro-economic approach to quantify their societal impact and ensure this is valued as effectively as contributions by medical professionals. This includes knowledge management and the downstream impact of information and subsequent technological development.

The majority of the world's population still lives in close proximity to animals, and control of zoonotic disease remains vital to public health. The propensity to travel internationally extends the risk of pandemic infection to all communities. Despite this, clinical veterinary and medical research have remained remarkably independent with significant lag-time in adopting innovation between professions. The musculoskeletal system is well suited to comparative medicine. Information gained from one species can be translated to others, advancing diagnosis and treatment.

Since the early 1930s, comparative orthopaedic research has incorporated the One Health concept. Otto Stader, a veterinarian, used a comparative medicine approach and developed the first form of external skeletal fixation, the Stader splint to stabilize fractures in dogs. During the Second World War, Navy surgeons improved the treatment of fractures in sailors by incorporating Stader's advances. During the 1940s and 1950s, another veterinarian, Jacques Jenny, performed one of the first intra-medullary pinning procedures in animals and significantly advanced fracture repair strategies in horses and humans. In 1966, Sten-Erik Olsson and John L. Marshall, both of whom had medical and veterinary medical degrees, founded the first laboratory dedicated to comparative orthopaedic research at the Hospital for Special Surgery in New York. In the 21st century, comparative orthopaedic laboratories are located throughout the world and use both comparative and translational research approaches in an effort to improve diagnostic capabilities, enhance preventive and therapeutic strategies, and advance the understanding of disease mechanisms. Advances in fracture fixation, total joint replacement, and cartilage repair are examples of how knowledge flows in both directions, to benefit both human and animal health (Cook and Arnoczky, 2009).

4.3   Why Interest in One Health Now?

The cost of human health care coupled with ageing populations is a major economic burden to developed countries. Diseases such as diabetes mellitus and dementia represent a growing threat, not only to patients, but to our ability to keep human health care affordable. A critical role for new medicines will be prevention, treatment and management of diseases suffered by an increasingly ageing population. There are animal models for many 'human' diseases. What is often lacking is relating clinical reference points and applying these across species. As one example, research into the objectivity of using traditional clinical signs to measure disease severity in animals with respiratory infections showed poor correlation between three species, yet these measures are routinely used to justify regulatory approval of new antibiotics and other therapeutic products

for use in animals (Reeve-Johnson, 1999). Given that it was possible to gain elective necropsy comparisons at each stage of the disease in these animals to compare clinical and pathological measures directly (which clearly could not be done in humans), this highlights the importance of understanding differences in the way diseases manifest in different species. It also raises the question of validity of a variety of traditional clinical signs used in humans as prognostic indicators.

Changes in antimicrobial resistance patterns have been highlighted as a serious threat to global public health. The World Health Organization raises the possibility of a post-antibiotic era in the 21st century where common infections and minor injuries are fatal (World Health Organization, 2014). This is an area of mutual concern to both human and veterinary health. However, the answer is not as simple as restricting antibiotic use. Treatment and prevention strategies differ between species and this relates to husbandry as much as to pathogenesis. Hospital antibiotic use poses the highest risk of selecting for resistant pathogens in human populations. The practicalities of entire flock medication in feed or watering systems for animals dismay medics; however, repeated studies generally fail to show a link to human health. Although initially counter-intuitive, this is better understood in the context of strictly enforced antibiotic withdrawal periods before slaughter and food-chain entry, competitive exclusion of human pathogens by natural flora better suited to the gut of healthy animals, lack of contact on commercial farms with typical human pathogens, the lack of viable human pathogens in situations that antibiotics are used on farms, and even the potential for benefit through use due to a decrease in bio-burden (e.g. *Salmonellae* and coliform bacteria) that may become pathogenic if allowed to persist to the time of meat processing.

Advances in health-oriented telecommunications, medical imaging, massive database capacity, memory miniaturization, satellite technology, and other information systems are all fundamentally changing the organization of health care. These technologies allow doctors to communicate more easily and quickly and facilitate multidiscipline collaboration.

Health care managers can drive systems in real time. Consumer awareness about health is better than ever before and through the use of interactive cable systems, online forums, and personal health information systems, this can occur easily in remote locations, as occurs with the Telehealth and e-Health initiatives, such as that run by the Australian College of Rural and Remote Medicine (ACRRM). Between 2000 and 2005 the number of mobile phone subscribers globally grew more than fivefold to 1.4 billion. The greatest growth is now in developing countries. This provides massive opportunities for outreach, training and remote medical access in disadvantaged communities.

Electronic medical records, once developed into national databases, have the ability to radically change the way patients interact with health professionals and provide patients with the ability to engage more fully in their own health care. They allow costs to be monitored and more cost-efficient ways of allocating public funding to be derived. Patients can schedule appointments, receive reminders or review test results. The explanation of medical terminology can be included, taking cost out of the system and allowing the savings to be reallocated to areas of need. This is already in place with current software for veterinary patient care which provides a useful prototype with less concern on potential privacy issues and an ability to make refinements before application in human medicine. Algorithms, predictive modelling to draw on billions of specific health indicators, outcomes from laboratory data and clinical information, and even insurance claim history can comprehensively describe an individual patient's health status. Using the rules of probability, a computer can weigh the data against a patient's particular needs and help the clinician determine which treatment option is most likely to work. Other algorithms take sets of rules for how to treat a disease or condition and translate them into formulae derived by a peer-reviewed system within each health speciality, which generates a comprehensive list of treatment options useful for remote diagnosis and treatment. Using a computer or handheld device, the physician can use an algorithm to get a treatment plan that is based on best practices and the patient's

unique needs. The capability is already available in the databases of the largest veterinary practices, yet this prototype for much larger and more costly human versions has not been fully leveraged.

The expectation of 'personalized medicine' is that screening will reveal whether an individual is likely to respond well to a drug, highlight risk factors and avoid toxic side effects. A targeted approach to treatment can ensure that each patient receives the right medicine at the right time. One example is screening for Human Estrogen Receptor (HER) display to determine treatment and prognosis in the management of breast cancer. Since molecular diagnostic tests can reveal a patient's susceptibility to disease, they can also guide preventive treatment before symptoms arise. The emergence of personalized medicine will shift the focus of medical care from 'disease treatment' to 'health care management'. Many animal genomes were mapped before the human genome. The use of genetic markers to screen populations for risk factors are being developed. Increasingly, therapeutics will be guided by predictive evidence from genetic and other molecular tests. Safety evaluations will continue to use animal toxicology as a final screen, and disease models in animals will continue to play a role in the evaluation of the safety and efficacy of new pharmaceuticals in the future.

New modes of pharmaceutical research go beyond high throughput screening trial-and-error approaches to molecular design: microorganisms may be genetically modified to carry out specific tasks, lock onto specific receptor sites in the body, or target pathogens. Nanotechnology, the science of building molecular-scale machines, also holds the promise of a completely new type of treatment, from a translational science approach between engineering and medicine. Tiny machines with the tools and intelligence to perform specific tasks are being developed to kill viruses, repair cells, and manufacture proteins or enzymes.

The biggest immediate impact of health care innovation is likely to be more effective use of the techniques that we already have. Improvements in efficiency require integrating our understanding across different paradigms and the willingness to implement changes to current practice. This includes better pharmaco-vigilance data, leading to changes to dosage regimens, management of external sources of infection, and immune modulation of patients. There is still much progress to be made in refining the use of existing treatment options. In developing countries, many easily solvable health problems require improved access to treatment and innovative ways of providing cheap and locally available preventive measures rather than new technology per se. Approaches that also incorporate the interdependent health status of humans who live in close proximity with animals (including vectors) will have most effect. In human medicine, despite huge budgets, reducing cost is a major driver for change. In contrast, veterinary medicine has always been cost-constrained and has evolved with a culture of seeking cost-efficiency, limiting diagnostic testing to the essential, and the ability to demonstrate return on investment to a full fee-paying clientele (akin to countries where there is no social security safety net). There are also differences in diagnostic tradition, where human medicine prioritizes clinical history above the physical examination, while veterinarians have been shown to minimize collateral history-taking from owners and rely predominantly on physical examination of patients to form initial diagnoses (Reeve-Johnson, 2012). There are still huge amounts that each medical discipline can learn from the other.

4.4 Macro-economic Issues of the 21st Century Where Animal Health-based Innovation is Integral to Human Survival

4.4.1 Food production and security

Food and Agricultural Organization figures indicate that total demand for food will rise 70% in the 44 years from 2006 to 2050. Meat demand in particular is predicted to increase strongly and it is forecast that, by 2050, double the current level will need to be produced (The Economist, 2011, p. 6).

The scale of problems that can arise when an integrated approach is not taken to either biological or chemical contamination is vast. Many cooked meat factories can process in excess of 1000 t of meat each week (approximately 20 million individual servings). These meat products move rapidly into a very diverse range of products distributed internationally, e.g. sandwiches, tinned foods, pizza toppings. In 2008 a product from a cooked meat factory in Canada became contaminated with *Listeria monocytogenes* and resulted in 26 deaths (Attaran *et al.*, 2008). The same year in China, contamination of dairy products with melamine caused over 300,000 babies to fall ill, with 53,000 being hospitalized, six deaths, and mass product withdrawals in many countries (Wall, 2014).

4.4.2 Energy demands

The only market that exceeds human food sales or health care in size is the consumption of energy. In 2008 global energy use was 11.29 billion t of oil equivalent, at 7.33 billion barrels/t. This equates to 82.8 billion barrels (bbl). Multiplied by US$85–100/bbl = US$7.0–8.3 trillion, or 10–12% of global GDP. This is relevant to food production because in 2011 it was reported that 40% of America's wheat crop was being used to provide just 8% of their fuel needs for vehicles (The Economist, 2011, p. 4). The European Union has a target of 10% biofuel. This has a substantial effect by pushing up the price of food for humans and animal production. Veterinary drugs used to alter fermentation in the rumen have been applied to selectively enhance fermentative ethanol production, decreasing the amount of wheat diverted to the biofuel market. This market is sustained by the world's developed economies, but results in increases in the price of food, causing a disproportionate burden on the world's poorest.

4.4.3 Poverty

Four billion low-income people, the majority of the world's population, constitute the base of the economic pyramid. However, their aggregate purchasing power suggests significant opportunities for market-based approaches to better meet their needs, increase their productivity and incomes, and to empower their entry into the formal economy. Their purchasing power constitutes US$5 trillion (over 7% of the global economy (Hammond *et al.*, 2007). They need cheap food, have the lowest life expectancies and would benefit disproportionately from breakthrough innovations in malaria and tuberculosis prevention. Furthermore, these people represent nearly 60% of our population and ethically deserve to have better lives as a consequence of innovations that result from those with adequate funding, time and facilities to undertake research. Figure 4.3 shows the predominant expenditure of this sector of our population on food.

This sector of the human population is predominantly rural, depends directly on agriculture for their food sources and has a greater likelihood of living in close proximity with animals, sharing their diseases or starving if their animals die. The impact of animal health care is not recognized by formal accounting measures to quantify human disease prevention or nutritional benefits to the majority of the human population. Although Africa has made the first progress in early adoption of One Health approaches, Fig. 4.4 illustrates that the majority of health care expenditure by the world's poorest communities at the Base of the Economic Pyramid is in Asia.

4.4.4   Zoonotic disease

Management in humans tends to fall into the sphere of human health specialists. General practitioners in human health in developed economies have less daily contact with endo and ecto parasites than veterinarians in routine practice. The expertise in managing populations gained by poultry and swine specialists is especially relevant to containing and preventing viral pandemics, and is underutilized outside the field. The epidemiology of many of the world's major diseases (tuberculosis, malaria, gastro-enteric infections, influenza virus or other blood and vector-borne viral diseases) involve animal reservoirs of infection. Tangible savings in human health costs, human morbidity and mortality can be attributed directly to implementation of animal health measures. The vector-borne disease accounting for the highest mortality is malaria, thought to kill over 1.2 million people each year, mostly African children under the age of five. Dengue fever is also rapidly re-emerging as a major threat, along with the chikungunya virus (CKV), now spreading through the Americas and Caribbean.

Graphic examples of vector-borne viruses that have recently 'jumped' large distances include West Nile Virus in the USA, African Swine Fever in the European Caucasus, and Bluetongue in Benelux (Oura, 2014). A recent report also demonstrated an increase in the altitude of malaria distribution in warmer years (Siraj *et al.*, 2014), which implies potential for increased malarial infections in the densely populated highlands of Africa and South America.

In 2000 Saudi Arabia experienced an outbreak of Rift Valley Fever, which not only resulted in abortions in 60–90% of infected animals, but it was estimated that 40,000 sheep, goats and camels died (Al-Afaleo and Hussein, 2001). In addition, Rift Valley Fever cases in people, manifesting as unexplained haemorrhagic fever, were reported in people living in close proximity to affected animals: 883 human cases were reported, resulting in 124 human deaths (Balkhy and Memish, 2003).

The ability to promptly diagnose outbreaks in animals and humans, understand vector biology and the epidemiology of pathogen interactions in different environments, manage water and other environment-based control measures, as well as treat and prevent disease in humans and animals, illustrates the need for collaboration of multiple disciplines to achieve cost-effective, sustainable outcomes. This is particularly important in developing countries, where financial and technological hurdles are greatest, and when responding to bioterrorism, where animals may be early-warning sentinels and need to be managed as part of containment strategies.

Estimated BOP market by sector
$5 trillion

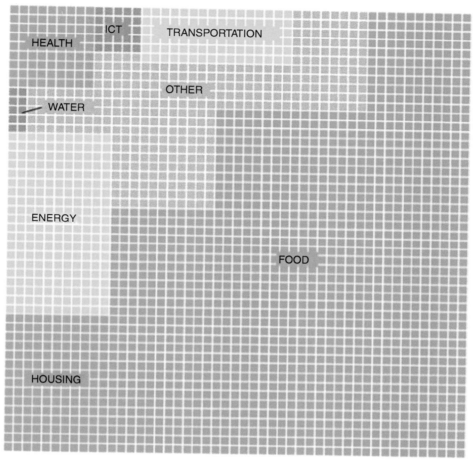

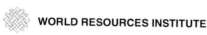 **WORLD RESOURCES INSTITUTE**

Fig. 4.3. Estimated Base of Economic Pyramid (BOP) market by sector.

4.4.5 Environmental disaster relief

Shortage of food supplies around the world causes increasing concern. Adverse climatic conditions have brought famine to areas of the world not suited to crop production. The most sustainable food source remains animals converting the sparse vegetation to protein in the form of meat, milk or eggs. Disaster relief has repeatedly focused on humanitarian aid, temporary supplies of imported food and medical aid; this has not solved the problems of sustainability. Veterinary insight into animal production, zoonotic disease control, animal pathology, sanitation, public health and developing sustainable solutions has not assumed a position of leadership. The skills imparted by a quality veterinary education closely match the range of skills needed to attain sustainable human solutions in these situations.

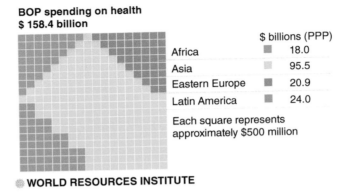

Fig. 4.4. Base of Economic Pyramid (BOP) spending on health.

4.4.5.1 Ethical use of animals

The measurement and quantification of pain in animals and humans has long presented problems. Anthropomorphic approaches to animal pain assessment, although widely used, are of limited use because human responses to pain are influenced by the ability to communicate, dependence on social groups, learned social behaviour, and have variable individual psychological dimensions (Livingston, 2002). Our research indicated that 80% of veterinarians diagnose pain via a clinical examination of the patient and titrate treatment accordingly. In contrast, medical general practitioners relied 95% of the time on the patient's description of pain in the clinical history and 70% of patients with pain lasting over 60 days were referred for specialist opinion. Less than 10% of veterinary patients were referred for specialist treatment (Reeve-Johnson, 2012).

4.4.6 Mental health

There is a large body of often unstructured and anecdotal literature on animal–human relationships, with claims of improvements of various medical conditions, including neurological rehabilitation or epilepsy (Latter, 1995). Yet, we understand almost nothing of the psychology of animals. Even human psychology is one of the more recent medical disciplines. To objectivize psychological diagnoses, criterion referenced databases comparable to the Diagnostic and Statistical Manual (DSM) is needed for animals. Veterinary specialists with a good understanding of human psychology are best placed to do this and this is likely to enhance our understanding of human psychology. Many of the sentinel experiments done in previous centuries (e.g. by Skinner on operant conditioning and learning, or imprinting and attachment theory by Douglas Spalding and Konrad Lorenz, or Ivan Pavlov with conditioned responses and the ethology of aggression and 'flight or fight' survival responses) were done on animals and still form the basis of our understanding of human conditions and therapy. Yet, veterinary and medical disciplines continue to diverge as each becomes more specialized.

4.4.7 Cloning, embryo research and genetic manipulation

Therapeutic cloning, reproductive cloning and replacement cloning have the potential to change medical and surgical treatment for hitherto untreatable inherited conditions as well as acquired ones. Research is usually restricted to animals until the later stages of development. Food production through increased fecundity, disease resistance, improved growth and production, represents a fundamental hope for producing greater amounts of food for the world's population at lower cost.

4.4.8 Toxicology

Toxicology will continue to diversify and, regardless of whether from a veterinary or medical background, will increasingly involve integrating computational and synthetic chemistry, proteomics, metabolomics, bioinformatics and molecular epidemiology. Toxicogenomics and nanotoxicology will become increasingly mainstream, while environmental toxicology will continue to be an area of increasing concern, to limit the effects of the dwindling natural resources. In forensic toxicology and medical toxicology, there is great scope for more interprofessional interaction. Animal studies still form the basis of carcinogenicity testing, residue depletion and degradation studies, where conditions can be replicated in ways that could not be done in humans.

4.4.9 In summary

One Health is nothing new. Comparative medicine has been with us from the beginning. The sheer breadth of the definition, however, presents a paradox in an age where the quest for specialization in medical research has made us increasingly myopic with regard to implementation of global solutions. One Health was reinvigorated as a concept by the threat of pandemic disease at the beginning of the 21st century. Most notably the threat of Avian Influenza HPAI H5N1 in 2004, where the potential for up to 50 million human deaths was raised, and the problem was clearly both a human and animal health issue (Gibbs, 2014). The global society in which we live provides greater opportunity for pathogen distribution and health threats than the capacity of the health system of any single nation or international organization. Efficiency, economics and sustainability of responses strongly suggest there is much to be gained from stepping back from the minutiae of hyper-specialized medical research, to consider wider macroeconomic impact and the practicalities of affordable implementation. In practice, global responses need to be implemented in diverse environments, including conflict zones or poverty-stricken regions with little access to technology, as well as major economies with socialized medicine. Our interdependence is greater than ever before. While conflict zones may represent reservoirs of infection which lack infrastructure, developed countries contribute to bacterial and viral resistance to treatment through overuse of medicines. Global markets, travel and animal movement can distribute contamination rapidly, while climate changes alter vector habitats, and national boundaries rapidly become irrelevant. To succeed, One Health advocates the need to be mindful of a few core objectives.

4.5 Core Objectives for Successful One Health Collaborations

- There should be no hierarchy between contributors: doctors, veterinarians, engineers, economists and others all meet on an equal footing, as specialists in narrow fields collaborating to create broad solutions that are practical and sustainable. None should be viewed in the One Health group as having ownership, as this quickly undermines motivation of others.
- One Health agendas should be driven by agreed measurable clinical end points.
- Business administration, cost management and commercialization are vital skill components to ensure sustainability.
- The human may be the most valued species to some, but vectors, pathogens and climatic conditions have no such pretensions. Knowledge of host–pathogen interactions within each species provides new perspectives, and possibilities for comprehensive solutions.
- Accurate joint communication endeavours in journals, at conferences, with news media and with policy makers, is more helpful than segregating research into 'human versus animal' components.
- Multi-species epidemiological and disease transmission studies are more likely to lead to a sustainable solution than focusing on the human component alone.

- Joint development, evaluation and utilization of new diagnostic methods, medicines and vaccines will lead to better prevention and control of diseases if applied across multiple species.

4.6   Conclusions

The veterinary specialities are in a prime position to increase collaboration and cross-fertilization of knowledge with human medical and food production sectors. Indeed it is from the veterinary specialities that impetus must come. They have the breadth of knowledge and are accustomed to working across species and scientific disciplines. The veterinary sector has become the poor relation to its human medical counterpart in terms of research funding because of the lack of recognition of the importance of a much broader approach to solving global health problems than focusing on studies designed to extract statistical evidence from subsets of human patients.

Human health care is transforming, largely to seek more cost efficiency. This is a time of particular importance to ensure that the perception of the role of veterinary pharmacologists, toxicologists and practitioners is wider than securing the health of animals.

The participants in animal aspects of comparative medicine need to adopt an economist's approach to quantify the wider societal value of their activities, and ensure that these are valued as highly as the contributions of the medical professions. This includes knowledge management and valuing the downstream impact of information and technological development. Investment needs to be linked to new technology to ensure that health care systems reward superior societal outcomes, not just local service or streamlining existing practice. Technology is necessary but is not a sufficient response – it is only one aspect of a complex society that needs to constantly adapt to the reality of competing for resources and optimizing resource reallocation. Clear data sets and economic analyses are the basis of securing future funding. The vast majority of funding will always be dedicated to human issues. It is vital that those from a veterinary or animal science background involved in translational research recognize the true value of their time, knowledge, insight and career development to societal goals beyond the animal health market, including pre-clinical phases of human health care and the innovation that underpins incremental food production, and provide economic justifications to support this.

References

Al-Afaleo, A.I. and Hussein, M.F. (2001) The status of Rift Valley fever in animals in Saudi Arabia: a mini review. *Vector-Borne and Zoonotic Diseases* 11, 1513–1520.

American Veterinary Medical Association (2008) *One Health: A New Professional Imperative*. One Health Initiative Task Force: final report. Available online at: https://www.avma.org/KB/Resources/Reports/Documents/onehealth_final.pdf (accessed 18 September 2015).

Attaran, A., MacDonald, N., Stanbrook, N.B., Sibbald, B.B.J. and Flegel, K. (2008) Listeriosis is the least of it. *Canadian Medical Association Journal* 179, 739–740.

Balkhy, H.H. and Memish, Z.A. (2003) Rift valley fever: an uninvited zoonosis on the Arabian Peninsular. *International Journal of Antimicrobial Agents* 21, 153–157.

Cook, J.L. and Arnoczky, S.P. (2009) The One Health concept in comparative orthopaedics. One Health Newsletter Florida Department of Health. Summer 2(3), 11–13. Available online at: http://www.floridahealth.gov/diseases-and-conditions/diseases-from-animals/one-health-newsletter/_documents/summer2009.pdf#search="one health concept in comparative orthopaedics" (accessed 13 September 2015).

Economist, The (2011) Plagued by politics. In: *The 9 Billion-people Question: A Special Report on Feeding the World*. 26 February, 4–6. Available online at: http://www.economist.com/sites/default/files/special-reports-pdfs/18205243.pdf (accessed 13 October 2015).

Gibbs, E.P.J. (2014) The evolution of One Health: a decade of progress and challenges for the future. *Veterinary Record* 174(4), 85–91.

Hammond, A., Kramer, W.J., Tran, J., Katz, R. and Walker, C. (2007) *The Next 4 billion: Market Size and Business Strategy at the Base of the Pyramid* (World Resources Institute). Available online at: http://www.wri.org/publication/next-4-billion (accessed 18 September 2015).

Latter, L. (1995) *Article: Human Pet Bonding.* Animal Welfare Society of Southeastern Michigan, Madison Heights, Michigan, USA.

Livingston, A. (2002) Ethical issues regarding pain in animals. *Journal of the American Veterinary Medical Association* 221, 229–233.

Olsson, S.-E. (1969) Comparative orthopaedics. *Clinical Orthopaedics and Related Research* 62, 3–5.

Oura, C. (2014) A One Health approach to the control of zoonotic vectorborne pathogens. *Veterinary Record* 174(16), 398–402.

Reeve-Johnson, L. (1998) Use of experimentally induced diseases in the development and evaluation of therapeutic agents. *Veterinary Record* 142, 638–642.

Reeve-Johnson, L. (1999) The use of experimental infection models to investigate the correlation between clinical and pathological measures of the severity of respiratory disease in three species. DVMS thesis, University of Edinburgh, Edinburgh, UK.

Reeve-Johnson, L. (2012) The medical consultation: comparing the diagnostic process between human and veterinary patients. *Proceedings of the 12th EAVPT Congress.* Amsterdam, Netherlands.

Siraj, A.S., Santos-Vega, M., Bouma, M.J., Yadeta, D., Ruiz Carrascal, D. and Pascual, M. (2014) Altitudinal changes in malaria incidence in highlands of Ethiopia and Colombia. *Science* 7, 1154–1158.

Wall, P. (2014) One Health and the food chain: maintaining safety in a globalised industry. *Veterinary Record* 174(8), 189–192.

World Health Organization (2014) *Antimicrobial Resistance: Global Report on Surveillance.* Available online at: http://www.who.int/drugresistance/documents/surveillancereport/en (accessed 13 October 2015).

Young, N.S., Ioannidis, J.P.A. and Al-Ubaydli, O. (2008) Why current publication practices may distort science. *PLoS Medicine* 5(10), e201. DOI: 10.1371/journal.pmed.0050201.

5 Evidence Collection and Gathering: The Living Evidence

David Bailey*

Department of Forensic and Crime Science, Staffordshire University, Stoke-on-Trent, Staffordshire, UK

'The cat had fleas.'

           Prosection Expert

'Prove it.'

           Defence Expert

5.1 Introduction

There are many texts and much guidance relating to the successful gathering of evidence from a crime scene. Many principles, theories and concepts have been copied from our forensic scientist counterparts in the non-animal lead disciplines and are often successfully utilized in the emerging field of veterinary forensics. While the successful retrieval of evidence from a crime scene is well documented for almost all items of putative evidence, there is one aspect of veterinary

*Corresponding author: daysbays@yahoo.co.uk

evidence that separates it from all others, and this fact is reflected by an absence of literature or text material for guidance in this area. Veterinary evidence, it would seem, is often living.

In a dispute that involves the seizure of living animals, this attribute makes it difficult for even the most competent authority to mount a successful prosecution, and provides the defence with a great deal of material with which to mount a successful challenge. Living evidence creates a unique set of challenges: it usually belongs to someone else and so is the responsibility of authorities that do not own it. It is often the single determinant in any legal dispute involving living animals – how was it looked after or examined after it was seized? How was it stored prior to trial and what evidence was retrieved from it after seizure? As I have already observed, a living animal cannot be sealed in a bag and placed on a shelf in an evidence locker. It costs a large sum of money to board and keep a living animal for a prolonged period prior to trial.

5.2   Animals as Property

Legally classed as property, there are no forensic protocols for dealing with sick, injured or healthy living property that is deemed to belong to someone else, to be labelled, packaged and stored as evidence attributable to allegations of cruelty against that owner. While there are protocols for the storage of evidence and the continuity of evidence and prevention of contamination of evidence, it has not been established in any jurisdiction what an agreed protocol is for the seizing, storage and examination of *living evidence* that is classed as property.

A living human involved as a *victim* in an assault case can provide evidence of the assault through verbal testimony as a witness. Photographs and examinations of injuries in a human can be documented, and following crimes visited upon human *victims* it is normal for the *victim* to be examined by a medical (or other) specialist. These *victims*

are then allowed to go home to await a trial and, when required, they provide oral testimony as to the nature of the assault, and the court determines, as best it can, what had actually occurred. If necessary, it will punish the guilty party with the powers afforded to it through the relevant legislation.

A living animal can also provide testimony to the court as evidence, but only as a silent witness. They are property, alive and, though able to communicate non-verbally, they cannot speak. The language of forensics becomes their tool for communication, and the ability to interpret that language is the role of the forensic veterinarian. These animals are seized, examined, photographed and clinically examined and, instead of being sent home, they are kennelled, euthanized, taken into possession, signed over or simply stored until trial, during which period they can lose or gain weight, become pregnant, die, fight or become ill.

Living evidence needs to be weighed regularly, kept healthy and have its needs met while still being the property of the owner from whom it was seized. In any legal investigation involving the seizure of living animals, it is always the storage of these living animals that is the area of most concern. There is the potential for exposure of a weak chain of custody by the prosecuting authority, an area of exploitation by the defence expert, who is entitled to ask how the evidence was stored and what condition that evidence is in now.

A lot of probative and relevant information that is crucial to a successful prosecution or defence of a dispute involving living animals is often harnessed in the period immediately post-seizure and during storage, when the living evidence is waiting for trial. It is, however, the experience of this author that when dealing with cases as both a prosecution and defence expert, the area of the storage of the living evidence immediately post-seizure is the evidentially most yielding, and also the aspect least utilized by many seizing authorities. There are unlikely to be any references to the storage of living evidence in the human forensic literature, and this is where the field of veterinary forensics differentiates itself from that of non-veterinary forensics.

Animals are unusual in this respect, as they have, under the law, the legal status of property that is living. Depending on the jurisdiction and the alleged act, animals can be classed as property, as evidence or, in the case of sexual assault, as a victim. This victim status of animals that have been sexually assaulted temporarily elevates their legal classification to that of personhood status (in some jurisdictions), and therefore obliges anyone found guilty of committing a sexually motivated act against an animal to be placed on a sexual offenders' list. A sexual offender must commit an offence against a *victim*, not *property*. An animal as property cannot be classed as a victim, so some jurisdictions class animals as persons for the duration of the alleged offence, to ensure that a legal victim (and a temporary person) has been created and that sexual offenders against animals are appropriately placed on a sexual offenders' list. Some jurisdictions regard any elevation of an animal to personhood status, no matter how temporary, as a precedent for giving all animals greater rights as legal persons. For this reason, many jurisdictions actively choose to not address the issues of sexual assault against animals and do not class animals as victims of any assault, preferring not to class it as a criminal act. In many countries, there is no specific offence of sexual assault of an animal, in order to avoid this legal anomaly. Those animals that are protected by relevant animal-related legislation against human sexual contact are legally classed as property, and so can be bought, sold, owned and traded, creating an anomaly in society's expectation of what is normal treatment of animals. An ability of an animal to suffer doesn't change, but the tolerance of that suffering by others is what animal welfare and cruelty laws are designed to confront.

5.3 Living Evidence

This issue of living evidence makes it difficult for seizing authorities to appropriate and maintain this property alive for a prolonged period prior to a court contest. This difficulty and expense then has an impact on the appetite for many authorities to investigate, prioritize or enforce crimes against animals. While there may be existing legislation that is appropriate for resolving disputes involving animals, it is a lack of ability or motivation to enforce the existing legislation that is, in this author's experience, the weak point in any investigation involving animals and animal derivatives.

As a rule, when investigating a claim of cruelty to an animal at a crime scene, there must be a demonstration of pain and suffering that has occurred. The goal of the forensic evidence collector is to present material to a court so that the court may be equipped with the necessary tools to establish that pain or suffering had occurred; in addition there must also be evidence that indicates that this pain and suffering was *unnecessary*. Therefore there are two conditions of unnecessary suffering that are required to be satisfied by the Court:

1. a demonstration of the existence of pain and/or suffering; *and*
2. the simultaneous demonstration of the necessity of that suffering.

Evidence can also be used to establish contact, ownership, negligence or welfare offences; however, this chapter will focus on the general forensic principles of collection of living and dead evidence.

Vets may be able to provide expert opinion to a court as to whether pain or suffering had occurred. Where there are conflicting views on the occurrence, demonstration or manifestation of pain or suffering in an adversarial system (and there usually are), then the court will determine, after considering the conflicting views, if pain and/or suffering has occurred or, more realistically, if pain and/or suffering has been demonstrated to have occurred. Vets are usually very good at providing an opinion as to whether pain and suffering had occurred but are usually poor at *demonstrating* that pain and suffering had occurred in any animal. If there is one word that can replace the word *forensics* in this book, it is the word demonstrate.

5.4   Necessity

Many vets and animal welfare officers seem to focus only on signs of pain or suffering in animals during the investigation of a crime scene – they need to slightly adjust their approach to look also for evidence that *unnecessary* pain or suffering occurred. And while the courts will determine a conviction on the necessity of the pain and suffering, many attempts at prosecution will fail because the focus has been on the demonstration of pain only or the demonstration of suffering only. Animals are not guaranteed an existence free from all pain and suffering, just unnecessary pain and suffering. This *unavoidable or avoidable* suffering needs to be approached as an obtainable piece of evidence, like all evidence which can be gathered, collected, stored and released, and if it isn't, then it will be the first question asked by a reasonable defence.

5.4.1   What is the necessity for this suffering?

Suffering and cruelty are not synonyms for veterinary pathology and, while pathology can assist to determine whether suffering did or did not occur, it is the evidence surrounding the event at the crime scene that can determine the necessity, or not, of that suffering to the satisfaction of the court. Determination of the *necessity* for pain and suffering is the ultimate issue for the courts to decide.

A crime scene investigator is looking for evidence of needless pain and suffering or for evidence of the *necessity* of this pain or suffering. This evidence can be collected in the form of photos, dead animals, dying animals, living animals, gunshot residue, bruising, blood sample analysis, pathology, hair collection, blood pattern analysis, bitemark analysis and also in the discovery of documentation, trophies and, more increasingly, the habit of individuals to take 'selfies' on their mobile phones, or to video an act of cruelty to replay to interested onlookers. Evidence can occur and be gathered outside of the singular specialism of veterinary pathology and a good crime scene examiner needs to be aware

of this. The most useful piece of evidence in cases like this is documentary evidence. Receipts, log books, menus, diaries and laptops can provide more evidence at a crime scene than all pieces of other evidence combined; yet they are often overlooked by forensic vets, who are zealously looking for evidence of animal origin, smell or appearance. Scenes of animal abuse and cruelty often involve human mental health issues, and they can be dangerous places for attending responders. Individuals suspected of animal abuse should be regarded as unsafe to accompany unattended. At a crime scene involving allegations of animal abuse, a vet may unwittingly become a de facto social worker, engaged in very deep and prolonged discussions with suspects – this should not be at the expense of collecting evidence for court.

5.5   What Is a Crime Scene?

A crime scene is not defined as a place where a crime occurred. A crime scene is a location where evidence of a crime can be found. It is for the courts to determine whether a crime has or has not occurred.

A crime scene can be declared by a statutory enforcement officer – usually a police officer or local council officer. A vet or a local charity inspector cannot declare a crime scene. Allow those with the statutory responsibility to declare and take charge of a crime scene. As a veterinarian, you are there to advise and assist: a vet is a small element of a crime scene investigation and of a subsequent trial involving allegations of animal welfare shortcomings or animal cruelty claims.

Once a crime scene has been declared, it (and the potential evidence within it) needs to be protected. Protection may be necessary from the external weather, individuals inside the crime scene (suspects), police, other animals or accompanying animal welfare officers.

5.5.1   Arrival on scene

On arriving at a crime scene, a veterinarian should do the following:

1. Attend and define who is in charge (usually the police or local council).

2. Take a note of the time you arrived and the names of the people you are speaking to.

3. Ask whether the suspect has been read their rights.

4. Explain who you are, your qualifications and your aim, and then walk through the scene with police initially to get an overview of the scene.

5. Try to speak with the suspect, but be aware that they may have a right to remain silent.

6. Be aware that if any animals are near death, it is important that you attempt to save life before you gather evidence. If it is raining or the suspects are disposing of evidence, then it is for others to prevent this. An attempt to save the animal's life is a professional obligation and, regardless of how much evidence is lost or destroyed, it is a priority for a veterinarian attending at a crime scene.

7. Do not allow an animal to die in order to preserve evidence. You must treat the animal and prevent suffering even if this means destruction of evidence. However, if a suffering animal is part of a crime scene in which a serious crime has been committed, then you may not be allowed to enter to treat that animal. These crime scenes usually involve the injury and death of humans, with animals as secondary victims who are also a part of the crime scene. It is an example of necessary suffering, in order to preserve and avoid contamination of a crime scene that is focused on a human crime.

8. If it isn't safe, don't do it. If the scene cannot be controlled, then it is important to state your reasons for leaving and document these reasons prior to departure.

9. Your professionalism, approach and demeanour will determine whether the suspect(s) at the scene will seek to resolve or to contest any charges or allegations made against them. It will also determine whether they choose to fight the matter on principle, or accept advice and voluntarily surrender any animals that concerns have been expressed about. Suspects at scenes of animal cruelty who show animal welfare concerns are often receptive to the idea of seeking some type of counselling and support. While some express relief at your visit, others may respond angrily. There are different ways to deal with each response, but the overriding principle remains the same – process the scene as if you intend to prosecute. Outcomes such as seeking counselling or voluntarily surrendering animals cannot be imposed by a court and, while some issues can be resolved by a stern or a soft tone, it isn't the social worker approach that makes individual suspects receptive to changing their questionable animal-keeping habits. All scenes should be processed with a view and an intention to prosecute. Nearly all of these scenes will fail to make it to court; it is likely that, with the benefit of legal representation and prior intervention by others, pleas will be entered before any likely court contest, or the matter will be resolved amicably. On the other hand, if a crime scene involving animals is processed with the assistance of a vet who holds the view that *no* prosecution is going to follow, then, with the benefit of the defendant receiving sound legal advice, these crime scenes almost always end up in court. Nineteen out of 20 disputes involving the collection or seizure of animals will end at the crime scene, but a good forensic examiner will *always* be prepared to go to court and gather evidence from all 20 crime scenes. When you stop approaching all crime scenes as places to articulate and reason your input to a court, then, paradoxically, you will find that you will end up in court on a more frequent basis. A solicitor for the suspect will become involved and questions of a relaxed attitude to crime scene processing and evidence collection and gathering become apparent.

5.6 The Five Cardinal Rules for Examining a Crime Scene

I use the mnemonic PREGS when collecting evidence from a crime scene involving living animals. The PREGS protocol must be applied in a cyclical loop manner when dealing with living evidence.

P. Protect
R. Record
E. Evaluate
G. Gather
S. Store

These five steps should be performed in this order, as each one has an effect on the continuity and viability of the next and/or preceding step. It is a circular chain for gathering *living* evidence and non-circular when dealing with *non-living* evidence (see Fig. 5.1). When dealing with living animals, the five aspects of evidence gathering should be repeated until the animals are disposed of post-trial, or a resolution is agreed with the animal owners. During a court contest, the chain of custody that has been built around the PREGS protocol may be appropriately stretched to breaking point by an experienced defence team. This ability to be stretched and stress-tested is one of the features of the adversarial system.

This continuous cycle includes the weighing of animals, the repeat body condition scoring of animals, blood sampling and analysis, documentation of the treatments given, and the response to treatment. It is relevant and probative to a court case, as the

animals are alive; they are also the property of their owners and any deterioration in their condition after seizure will invite justifiable criticism of the care of the animal and the continuity of the evidence in an adversarial legal system. Conversely, any improvement in their condition could attract criticism of the owner by the courts.

5.7 PREGS

5.7.1 Protect

A crime scene needs to be protected. Evidence that can be gathered can be transient in nature and may need protection from the elements or from suspects at the scene. The alleged offenders may be affected by mental illness or chronic substance abuse, in which case responders at that scene need to take steps to distance or protect themselves. As a vet, it is often your responsibility to protect others at that scene from any injury they may sustain from animals. You are protecting animals, evidence and personnel. And when you gather evidence and write and sign a report, you need to protect yourself in the face of scrutiny by an inquisitive, informed and adversarial-by-nature barrister.

Take control of the scene immediately, particularly if there are living animals. As a vet, upon arrival you may be responsible for the injuries others could sustain from the animals at the scene. Keep out unauthorized or uninvited personnel and utilize any available police to assist with this. Determine the extent to which the scene has been protected. Obtain information from personnel who have knowledge of the original condition of the scene.

Initiate a logbook and record those who enter and leave, the names of the personnel involved, the address and the time. You may need to take charge of personnel and, importantly, develop the skill to control personalities at a crime scene who can evoke strong emotional responses in attendees and interested onlookers, in order to fulfil your aim of protecting the scene, animals, evidence and others.

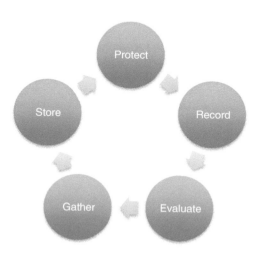

Fig. 5.1. Circular PREGS protocol. It is circular and linear to reflect that veterinary forensics deals with living evidence and to reinforce that this evidence must be protected after it has been seized and can yield useful probative material after seizure.

5.7.2 Recording the crime scene – measuring and sketching

5.7.2.1 Photography

Photography can accurately record the scene as it appeared at the time the vet arrived. It is the most common piece of evidence, and is relied upon in animal cruelty investigations. Many vets make the error of photographing the animal without attributing an evidence marker in the image and without correlating this image to an evidence log. Don't take a photo unless you have a pen and a piece of paper to log the image and create a descriptor in the image. All close-up images of an animal that would otherwise demonstrate injury or cruelty may not be reliable if these images cannot be attributed to a particular animal and a corresponding entry in an evidence log, with an accurate evidence descriptor within the image.

Each item of interest requires at least three images:

1. An overview shot.
2. An approach shot.
3. A close-up of each individual item of evidence.

The easiest method is to use numbered placards in each image you take. I was once involved in a dispute that had more than 1000 images taken of equines, that demonstrated overgrown hooves, close-ups of emaciated animals, serious rain scald and mud fever. Much of this evidence was dismissed, as the defence argued (successfully) that the images had no evidence markers and no evidence log to match the images with the horses. Suffering was demonstrated in the images, but it could not be attributed to the very specific charges relating to individual horses. The evidence was admissible, but did not carry the appropriate weight – the images were taken so close to the animal that identification of the animal (or even species) was not possible.

Still photography is one of the four principal means of providing courtroom participants with visual evidence of what took place/existed at a crime scene (the others are sketches, videos and animated movies).

The photography rule is a rule of threes: as there are three approaches used to create an image of an item of interest (overview, approach and close-up), there are also three elements to a close-up image:

1. A scale.
2. An evidence descriptor.
3. The item of interest.

Sketches, videos and still photos all complement and support one another in the preservation of evidence and one should not be afraid to produce all three from any crime scene.

It is common for photographs depicting deceased and/or mutilated animals to draw vigorous objections from the defence. Defence barristers can successfully argue that such grim images are more prejudicial than probative, will probably inflame the jury or court, and are therefore inadmissible.

The use of animated movies can be used to reconstruct such photos or images, eliciting a non-emotional response and leading to a decision based on practicalities rather than emotion. These movies or virtual reconstructions can also be used to take the observer on a virtual tour of the now digitally sterilized crime scene. In the past I have asked a graphic designer with forensic experience to produce digitized images of small children who have been killed or severely injured by dog attacks.

Videos allow a complete and continuous unbroken view of a crime scene. They provide panoramic views, but lack definition, light and dark contrast, positional context and the higher resolution that can be obtained with still photos.

5.7.2.2 Sketching

While photos can be digitally altered, sketches have three advantages: (i) they provide greater width and depth of field of view (a sketch can give an overhead view of a scene inaccessible to video or still photography); (ii) they can eliminate distortion caused by perspective; and (iii) they can allow the important features to be shown without the unnecessary distraction of detail.

The purpose of a sketch is to help to clarify what is relevant at a crime scene. It also depicts things that are important at the time it is made. It gives the relative positions of all items; this can be more useful than a photograph as it gives basic information about the scene and its contents at a glance, where a photograph may appear under- or overexposed or too cluttered. Importantly, a sketch also depicts the relative positions of items, and with measurements it can be a helpful adjunct to a photographic image.

I will sketch at most crime scenes I attend, to record an overview and/or fine detail (see Fig. 5.2).

Initial sketches should be drawn in ink (not pencil) and include all relevant measurements. It is acceptable to redraw your sketches at a later date, either by hand or computer-aided design (CAD).

A sketch should include the following:

1. Directional orientation – which way is north?
2. Name and signature – print your name and sign (these form part of your contemporaneous notes).
3. Date of scene processing, and possibly the time.
4. Case number (if applicable).
5. Relevant labels – these must be appropriate and unambiguous, i.e. the address of the property and which room it is. For vehicles this should include number plate information and/or Vehicle Identification Number (VIN code), make, model and colour.
6. Scale (if used); and
7. Evidence items – these would normally be represented by a number on the sketch in the relevant position in the room (the number is then related to the evidence log – see below).

Measuring of a crime scene (if required) satisfies two main needs:

1. To allow accurate sketching of the evidence in its found position.
2. To determine critical distances between objects.

It is claimed that it is not possible to accurately document a crime scene without measuring; however, though I have measured some crime scenes, I do not measure all of them –

the decision whether or not to do so is dictated by the evidence that one encounters. Any measurement of heights or distances should be demonstrated in a report by a sketch that need not be to scale. When measuring items in a scene on a sketch, you should use two points of reference from which you have measured. Simply providing information on heights and measurements without a sketch to refer to can make interpretation of any scene processing more cumbersome. The two reference points used in a sketch must be distinct and permanent. If measuring an indoor crime scene I tend to use walls at 90° to each other as my fixed point of measurement although I have been tasked to investigate in some Eastern European countries where this isn't always a reliable assumption.

5.7.2.3   Evidence logs

At the crime scene, an evidence log must be kept, recording information such as who seized the item, a description of the item, the location of the item, etc. At non-animal crime scenes, a scene manager will be in control of the evidence log. In scenes involving animals, the vet may be expected to do this. But vets tend to focus and manage their skills at a crime scene in a vertical manner, focusing upon any available evidence of animal origin, while an evidence log manager needs to link up all the discrete and independent items seized and retrieved from a crime scene. Due to the horizontal nature of this management process and the importance of the evidence log to the dispute, it is preferable for a person other than the vet to assume this role. The forensic vet needs to focus on the living animals or the evidence of animal origin and not initially on crime scene log-book management.

Utilizing an evidence log to record the location measurements of the evidence items means that only the number of the item need be recorded on the sketch, so avoiding sketch cluttering.

The evidence log, like the sketch, is part of your notes made at the scene and therefore requires appropriate and unambiguous labels that link it to the sketch and any photographs taken with evidence markers.

(a)

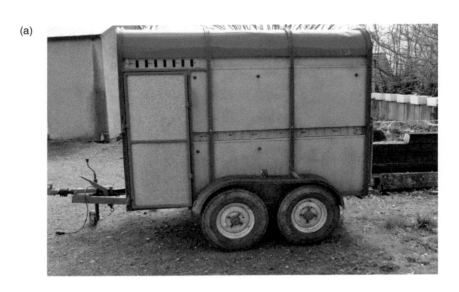

(b)

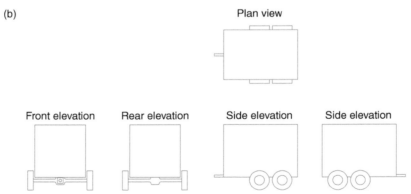

Fig. 5.2. A photograph (a) and a sketch (b) of a trailer used to cart a stag for hunting purposes.

Evidence logs should indicate the following:

1. Who is there?
2. The location you are attending.
3. What time and date you entered and left, who declared the crime scene, and who has overall responsibility for the scene.
4. What evidence you have gathered, linking it to the sketch and an itemised legend that links that evidence to the evidence log; e.g. A. Dead Dog, B. Living Dog – Jack Russell microchip number 123456.
5. Who is responsible for that evidence and where is it going?
6. What injuries the animal had at seizure.
7. What injuries the animal had upon arrival at boarding destination.
8. What was the weight and accurate body condition of the animal.

5.7.3 Evaluate physical evidence possibilities

This evaluation begins upon arrival at the scene and becomes detailed in the preliminary survey stage. Once you have established that aspects of the scene are safe to proceed with, move on to your recording of evidence through sketching and imaging while creating an evidence log. Then stop and evaluate. Consider what evidence is there to be collected and examined away from the scene. If in doubt, then seize and collect it. Do not start to consider what the defence position will be. Focus on your role, which is to provide the court with evidence to enable it to arrive at a safe decision. This step of the protocol is an evaluation of your own personal safety and the organization of the scene, which can be quite complex, and lays the groundwork for any subsequent seizure.

- Ensure that the collection and packaging materials and equipment are sufficient and that a logistical infrastructure is in place to collect living animals if required.
- Focus first on evidence that could be lost. Leave the least transient evidence to last.
- Ensure that personnel consider the variety of possible evidence, not only evidence within the specialism of veterinary science

that is of animal origin. Documentary evidence is often overlooked at a crime scene involving animals.

- Search the easily accessible areas and progress to out-of-view locations. Look for hidden items.
- Evaluate whether evidence appears to have been moved inadvertently.
- Evaluate whether the scene appears contrived.

5.7.4 Gathering of evidence

Evidence gathered needs to be logged in your evidence log. Living animals should be weighed and body condition scored, and checked for a microchip prior to being seized. They should be examined by a vet to ensure they are fit for removal and transport. They need to be examined again after transport and prior to boarding, to document any injuries they may have received during transit. A seizing authority is always responsible for a seized animal and it always remains the property of the owner until this has been relinquished by the owner or surrendered by a court direction. Dead animals can be packaged in a body bag and frozen and treated as an individual crime scene at a later post-mortem examination in a different location, where a pathologist may then assume responsibility for that crime scene to protect, record, evaluate, gather and store.

Living animals should not be transported together or stored together in order to save costs. They fight and they impregnate; both of these have happened to evidence I have seized, which curtails the ability of the prosecution to successfully prove a lack of care on the part of the defendant. The gathering, documenting, subsequent storage of evidence and re-evaluation of the animal as it remains in storage is the most evidentially yielding period in the chain of custody, which non-living items of evidence cannot provide. It is also the area of weakness in any prosecution authority and is prone to challenge by a defence team who will seek out and discover weaknesses in this area of your crime scene processing protocol first.

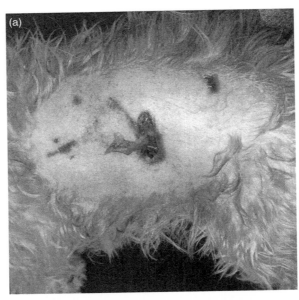

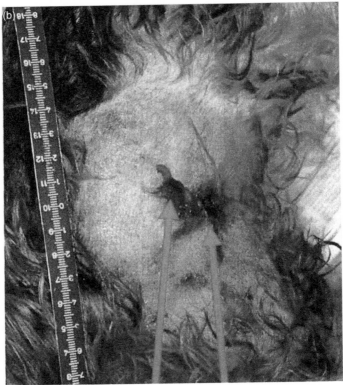

Fig. 5.3. (a) Before: a dog that was euthanized after being bitten by another dog. This image was taken immediately after euthanasia. (b) After: the same dog after being stored in a sealed plastic bag in warm conditions. The post-mortem changes in wound appearance were attributed to ante-mortem conditions and impacted on the ability of the magistrate to reach a reliable conclusion in this dispute.

5.7.4.1   Final survey

The final survey is another opportunity to review all aspects of the PREGS protocol followed so far. The search should be discussed with all remaining personnel and you must ensure that all documentation, in particular the evidence log, is correct and complete.

A photograph of the scene showing the final condition is necessary to avoid claims of damage or destruction. Ensure that all seized evidence is secured and alive before leaving the premises. Avoid leaving behind contaminated equipment, and ensure that hiding places or difficult-to-access areas have not been overlooked. It is a feature of crime scenes involving animals that some target species are seized, while others animals of a different species are allowed to remain behind. A claim that the suspect was causing unnecessary suffering to the seized animals can be compromised if other animals were left under the care of the same owner.

5.7.5   Storage

Animals being legally classified as property that is living is the largest issue for vets to deal with at a crime scene while gathering evidence. These items of evidence need to be stored in conditions that are specific only to this field of forensics.

Living animals get sick and die – because they are evidence, all these changes need to be documented. The facility where animals are stored must be considered as an extended and de facto continuation of the crime scene. At suitable intervals following seizure, animals need to be weighed, examined, inspected and blood-sampled. Vets need to ensure that the animals' needs are met and they are not living in conditions that could be worse than those from where they were removed. The PREGS cycle continues at Storage by examining the animals once they have been off-loaded and the Protect element starts again. The conditions of the new premises must also be recorded and evaluation of the animals must occur regularly, particularly at the start of any boarding of living evidence. Further evidence, such as weight gain or loss, must be gathered and this information stored in a relevant log. The PREGS cycle should be repeated until the dispute has ended, including any legal appeals.

5.7.5.1   Dead animals

Animals that die during evidence storage or at the crime scene can be taken away for further examination. They should be photographed *in situ* and then placed in a bag, sealed, labelled, entered into an evidence log, and taken away and frozen for later examination as necessary. There is plenty of debate as to what type of bag is appropriate for dead animals; I have been involved in a case where the storage of evidence in a dispute was central to the evidence presented (see Fig. 5.3). To avoid any post-mortem changes occurring in dead animal storage, as a result of being placed in sealed plastic bags, I use human body bags to store and transport dead animals to cold storage.

6 Forensic Examination of Animal Hair

Claire Gwinnett*

*Department of Forensic and Crime Science, Staffordshire University,
Stoke-on-Trent, Staffordshire, UK*

*Corresponding author: c.gwinnett@staffs.ac.uk

6.1   Introduction

The use of hair as evidence in criminal casework is well established, with hair being a common type of trace evidence retrieved from crime scenes (Petraco, 1987; Robertson, 1999). Hairs are readily lost from individuals, whether human or animal, and these hairs may be transferred during a crime, helping to link suspects to scenes, suspects to victims, objects to scenes or animals to individuals (to name but a few possible permutations). Edmond Locard's Exchange Principle (Locard, 1930), 'every contact leaves a trace', explains the mechanisms for trace evidence transfer at crime scenes. It is a fundamental principle that whenever objects, people or animals come in contact with each other, an exchange in material will occur. This includes hairs, fibres, glass, paint and any other particulate evidence. In the past, animal hair was disregarded as forensic evidence and not frequently analysed in forensic laboratories, but now animal hair is commonplace in forensic hair analysis (Petraco, 1987), partly due to development in identification schemes and research outlined in this chapter.

This chapter aims to provide to veterinarians, personnel who work in animal welfare (e.g. RSPCA officers), forensic scientists, police officers and anybody who may be tasked to analyse animal hair for criminal casework, an overview of forensic hair analysis. The focus of this chapter is to provide an insight into how animal hair evidence should be reliably recovered, documented, analysed and interpreted for criminal cases.

Human hair analysis will not be detailed in this chapter, but interpretation methods used when analysing human hair that are also applicable for animal hair will be introduced. Similarly, textile fibres evidence will not be focused upon, but as animal hair may be defined as a type of 'fibre', and are used abundantly in textiles such as clothing (Wildman, 1961), many of the underlying principles of recovery, documentation and interpretation are comparable and will therefore be described where appropriate.

6.2   Hair as Evidence

Hair can be defined as 'any of the fine thread-like strands growing from the skin of humans, mammals, and some other animals' (Oxford Dictionaries, 2014). Composed of the protein keratin, hairs are generally stable in nature, hence forensic scientists are able to use this type of evidence more readily in environments which have degraded other biological matter (Taupin, 2004). Hair evidence has been used in all types of criminal cases, including, but not limited to: murder, sexual assault, burglaries, abuse cases, arson and terrorist incidents (Robertson, 1999). This breadth of use is partially due to the ease of transfer of hairs between individuals, individuals and crime scenes and individuals and objects. Hairs transferred to highly important objects from a crime, e.g. a balaclava identified as being used in an armed robbery, enables the wearer to be identified and linked to the scene.

Hairs used in the analysis of a criminal investigation are defined as either questioned (aka target) or control samples. Target hairs are the extraneous hairs that have been transferred during contact and are the evidential hairs that will provide information about the case.

Hair evidence can provide a large range of different information beyond associations between suspects, victims, places and objects depending on the type and quantity of hair available. Hair evidence can provide intelligence information in the form of suspect descriptions, i.e. hair colour and type, as well as information regarding how the person treats their hair (for example, the use of styling products and dyes) and any diseases present in the hair. Examination of the hair can identify whether it is human or animal and the body area from which it has been shed. In the case of human hair, the ethnic origin of the individual the hair has been shed from may also be determined. If nuclear material is present on the root, then the potential for DNA profiling can allow for a more conclusive identification of the individual, beyond just microscopical analysis.

Hair evidence is a transient evidence and due to this the evidence will transfer and persist depending on certain factors (discussed in Section 6.8.2 below). By understanding transfer and persistence, timeframes of when certain contact occurred can help to reconstruct a crime scene and understand whether the evidence has been transferred at the time of the crime, thus making it evidentially useful. Hair evidence can also provide information about any drug use of an individual. Any damage to the hair can also provide the investigator with information about the crime and potential suspect(s); this includes heat, decomposition and fungal damage.

Hair evidence, like other evidence, has limitations. The lack of acknowledgement of these limitations in the past has led to miscarriages of justice and led to investigators overstating the value of the evidence (Taupin, 2004). The main limitations include the subjectivity involved in the microscopical analysis of hairs and the intra-variation in hair characteristics seen in individuals; this will be discussed later in the chapter. Knowledge of these limitations does not undermine hair evidence, but enables investigators to correctly interpret it.

6.3 The Use of Animal Hair in Criminal Casework

Hair evidence from animals has been used successfully in the solving of many human crimes; for example, when domestic dog hair

has been transferred from the dog owner's clothes to a victim of a crime during an assault. The information that can be obtained from an animal hair is the same as in human hair, although some information is not applicable, such as ethnic origin. Animal hair analysis in criminal cases primarily focuses upon the species identification of the animal it originated from, although identification of a particular individual has been carried out. In terms of animal-related crimes, including wildlife crimes, hair analysis can be widely used: for example, illegal fighting involving dogs, cockerels or hogs (USA); intentional poisonings; poaching; carting of deer; ritualistic crimes; hit and runs; cruelty cases; badger baiting; import/export of endangered animals; and animal products and bush meat. In rare cases, animal hair may be utilized as the primary source of evidence, but more commonly it is used as corroborative evidence, analysed initially to obtain intelligence information or to justify further, more costly analysis (as a screening tool). Following are examples of the types of cases that utilize animal hairs as evidence (Case Studies 6.1, 6.2 and 6.3).

6.4 Recovery, Documentation, Packaging and Storage Methods for Animal Hair Evidence

It is important for anyone attempting to locate and retrieve animal hair evidence to be aware of the three Rs of evidence; Recognition, Recording and Recovery (Robertson and Roux,

Case Study 6.1.

A farmer had a prolonged problem with sheep worrying, culminating in one of her livestock being killed and mutilated. Veterinary examinations indicated that the wounds were probably caused by a dog, but this was not conclusive because of potential interference from scavengers. Hairs found in the wound of the sheep were retrieved and analysed and identified as being of canine origin, leading to further investigation, including DNA analysis, of the hairs. The owner of a local dog that was

regularly walked in the area and whose dog had been seen chasing the sheep previously was questioned regarding the case, but refused to allow control samples to be taken from his dog for comparison. The information gathered in the analysis of the hairs was presented in court in order to obtain sufficient control samples and allowed a conclusion that the hairs from the wound and the dog could be associated, linking the dog to the sheep carcass.

Case Study 6.2.

Meat from a London market had been seized by the police as it was suspected to be illegally imported bush meat (described as gorilla meat). The meat appeared to have been treated (smoked and charred) but hair was still present on the skin (this is common with bush meat).

Before testing of the meat, police wished to ascertain whether it was from an endangered animal or legal livestock such as bovine. Hairs taken from the skin were identified as being from sheep origin, thus eliminating the need for further analysis.

Case Study 6.3.

It was suspected that a racehorse was wrongly administered a drug over a lengthy time period; however, because the dose terminated one month earlier, removing the opportunity for blood and urine tests. Hair can provide information regarding type of drugs administered and drug use history, and, although hair is not as accurate in determining concentrations of drugs at a particular point in time (e.g. at the time of a crime or just before death), it can provide a profile of drug use over a long time period. Consequently, hairs were obtained from different

clean locations on the racehorse, where there is low variability in growth rate and hairs had grown to sufficient length to span the suspected timeframe of the dosing. Segmental hair analysis was carried out. This is where the hair is cut into segments and analysed using a suitable technique, such as gas chromatography, to allow the time of administration to be identified by locating the position of the drug along the hair shaft. The results indicated the presence of clenbuterol hydrochloride in mane hairs extending back in time by 8 months.

2010). As evidential animal hairs are not necessarily easily seen when examining exhibits or animals, they may not be recognized without appropriate search techniques. Systematic searching of objects and animals for hair evidence should include looking for areas where hair transfer is most likely to have occurred during the incident rather than through innocent means, e.g. hairs found in a wound of an animal suspected of being involved in dog fighting is more evidentially valuable than if found just on the collar of the dog. To identify whether any hairs found are evidentially valuable, information such as whether the animal or object could have come in contact with any other animal should be sought, and if hairs have been taken from a scene, e.g. trailer or house, knowledge of animal access since the crime is required. Without correct recording of any animal hair evidence, then the evidential value may not be fully realized and, in the worst case, may not be admissible in court. Finally, without appropriate recovery methods, potential hair evidence will be left behind.

6.4.1 Recovery of questioned aka target animal hairs

Veterinarians and other individuals encountering live animals, carcasses or other objects potentially containing animal hair evidence need to know how to retrieve these transient samples reliably and efficiently before they are lost. The acronym GIFT (Get It First Time) is a principle that anyone attempting to retrieve evidence should abide by and an appropriate method must be chosen for the recovery of any questioned hairs (Robertson and Roux, 2010). The retrieval method used must allow all target hairs to be recovered, without loss or contamination. The recovery method chosen depends on a number of factors: surface type, surface area, presence of debris and whether the hairs are loose or embedded in the surface in which they are found. Table 6.1 outlines the seven methods that are accepted techniques for the retrieval of hairs.

Table 6.1. Methods for the retrieval of animal hairs.

Retrieval Method	Description of Use	Preferred Surfaces	Advantages	Disadvantages
Tape lifting	Sticky tape is gently placed on the surface, removing any surface hairs. Tape is then placed upon an acetate sheet to preserve the evidence and allow for searching (Choudhry, 1988).	Any dry porous or non-porous surface, especially useful for smaller surface areas, e.g. inside of pet carrier.	Able to capture multiple hairs at a time and also know from which part of an object the hairs have been retrieved from.	Hairs must be dissected from the tape to allow for further examination due to the need to encapsulate hair in a medium of similar refractive index (RI). This is time-consuming. A new tape, called Easylift, has been introduced that removes the need for dissection (Jackson and Gwinnett, 2013).
Tweezering	Use of clean tweezers to remove obvious hair evidence from surfaces.	All surfaces but usually only when hairs are found in prominent positions, could otherwise be easily lost and/or when the exact location of the hair is required to be known.	Good for when hairs are embedded within a substance or object, e.g. mud or a wound.	Time-consuming for large areas.
Vacuuming	Use of vacuum filters which attach to a vacuum cleaner and use suction to remove hairs.	Dry, large surface areas, e.g. pet bedding, large pet carriers.	Quick for retrieving large amounts of hair. Vacuum filters can be individually sealed.	More time-consuming than other methods when searching for target hairs, as there is usually a lot of 'background' information gathered in the form of debris and material from the surface itself.
Shaking	The object is shaken over a large collection funnel and any evidence collected in a Petri dish.	Fabric type objects, e.g. pet rugs.	Very quick method for retrieving loose evidence.	May miss evidence that is stuck in the weave of the fabric. Does not allow the exact location of the evidence to be identified.
Scraping	Use of a scalpel to remove very embedded hairs.	Any surface which has hairs embedded in it, e.g. painted surfaces.	Enables quick retrieval of hairs from situations that other methods would not be able to remove.	May damage hair during removal.
Combing	Use of a seeded comb (a comb in which cotton wool has been pressed into the base of the teeth or brush which removes and retains extraneous target hairs (McKenna and Sherwin, 1975).	Pelage of an animal.	Gently removes surface hairs without pulling out hairs from the animal.	Sampling a moulting animal may cause problems when trying to identify any target hairs present on the comb.
Filtering	Uncommon technique involving the use of different solvents to remove debris and extract hairs from contaminated samples.	Samples which are heavily contaminated with soil and other debris, e.g. buried samples.	Allows large numbers of hairs to be quickly extracted from soil.	Care is required to ensure that the solvents do not alter the hair evidence in any way.

6.4.2 Recovery of control aka known hair samples

Control samples are hairs that have been taken as reference hairs from any animal that could be involved with the crime or could have transferred hairs to any other animal, object or person linked to the crime. The taking of control samples from animals is usually undertaken after a police or court request. If possible, 20–30 hairs should be taken from different points on the animal, ensuring that all hair types have been retrieved and the samples represent the different lengths and colours present on the pelage. It has been suggested that a total of 400–500 hairs should be retrieved for comparison purposes (Suzanski, 1988). Control samples from animals should ideally be taken from a clean uncontaminated area and depending on the purpose of the analysis, for example, whether the hairs are for comparison only or for the analysis of the presence of drugs, additional considerations may be needed. Ideally hairs should be gently combed from the body, so as to allow the full hair to be collected (Wildman, 1961), but if this is not possible, hairs can be removed by cutting them close to the skin.

6.4.3 Packaging and storage

Prior to packaging, certain anti-tampering and anti-contamination procedures may be required. If a tape lift has been created, the edges of tape need to be sealed with additional tape. The evidence tape also must be scored with a scalpel so that it marks the acetate backing, but avoids damaging any evidence, protecting against fraudulent replacement. The type of evidence bag used for hair evidence depends on the police force and available equipment, but there are recognized procedures for the packaging and storing of such evidence. Loose hairs should be stored first in a labelled paper wrap, sometimes referred to as 'drug wraps' and then placed in a plastic evidence bag. Tape lifts and vacuum filters should be fully sealed and also placed in plastic evidence

bags. If the hairs are wet with body fluids that are to be analysed for DNA, then the hairs should be packaged in a paper evidence bag and stored in a freezer.

6.4.4 Documentation of evidence

Normal documentation of evidence applies with animal hair, including the need to photograph evidence *in situ* and fully document when, where and who obtained it, along with a unique identifying number (Lenertz, 2001). Additional information is required for animal hair evidence when retrieving control hairs either for comparison to a questioned hair or for a reference collection. This may include the following:

- Known species and sub-species.
- Gender.
- Age (Wildman, 1961).
- Any known hair or skin diseases.
- Body area sampled (Wildman, 1961).
- Method of hair removal.

6.5 General Structure of Hair

Hairs consist of three regions; the root (proximal end), the shaft, and the tip – also known as the shield region in animal hairs (distal end).

In addition to this, hairs are composed of three main types of cell: cuticle, cortical and medulla. If a hair is envisaged as a pencil, the central graphite column of the pencil is the medulla, the wood surrounding the graphite is the cortex, and the paint on the outside is the cuticle. Figure 6.1 demonstrates the basic structure of an animal hair. Each area provides information about the hair and can contain distinguishing features. The cuticle is made up of overlapping scales that usually do not contain pigment (Partin, 2003). The cortex, consisting of spindle-shaped cells, makes up the main component of the hair, contains pigment granules and may also include small irregular-shaped air spaces called cortical fusi and larger solid oval structures called ovoid

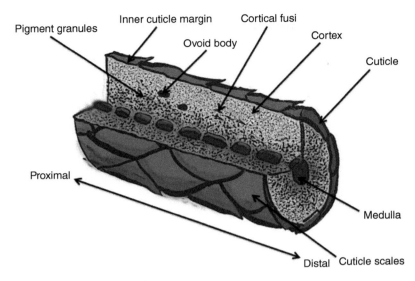

Fig. 6.1. Basic structure of an animal hair.

bodies. The medulla is a central core of shrunken cells with the spaces between the cells filled with air, and whose structure can vary dramatically in animal hair (Deedrick and Koch, 2004).

6.5.1 Types of hair

The complete covering of hair over a mammal is called the pelage. There are five main hair types that cover a mammal's body, serving particular functions such as heat preservation and sensory aids. Table 6.2 describes these five hairs and their general features.

6.6 Forensic Animal Hair Analysis

Forensic animal hair analysis focuses most commonly upon species identification, but may also include comparisons between target samples and controls, the latter being much more difficult. In addition to this, analytical techniques may be employed to ask specific questions about the hair, e.g. about the presence or absence of drugs. This chapter will concentrate on the microscopy of animal hair, as this is the most versatile and common technique

used. A variety of questions beyond the species of the hair may be asked of the forensic hair analyst regarding a case, either by the police or in court. These may include the following:

- Do all species of animal have a combination of unique hair characteristics?
- How confident are you that the hair has originated from the particular animal in question?
- How and when did the hair evidence transfer to the scene/victim?
- Could the hair have been transferred innocently?

These questions need further work beyond the use of analytical techniques and need to take into account processes such as transfer and persistence and commonality of different characteristics, covered in Section 6.8 below.

6.6.1 Stages of hair analysis

Analysis of hair evidence usually starts with general observations about the number, condition and position of the hairs found. Analysis will also include some macroscopic observations, where the hairs

Table 6.2. Animal hair types.

Hair Type	Found?	General Characteristics	Evidential Value
Vibrissae (whiskers)	Nostrils and muzzle	Generally coarser than other hairs and are thickest at the root end.	Low Limited variations in this hair type between species mean limited value for identification and comparison (Teerink, 1991). There are some exceptions, such as tiger and leopard vibrissae, which exhibit differences in cross-sectional shape (Partin, 2003).
Over-hairs	Main pelage	Longer than other hairs present on the pelage. Generally coarse, straight with elongated tips.	Low, limited value for identification and comparison.
Under-hairs	Main pelage	Usually shorter and finer than the other hairs and show uniform thickness from the root to tip ends.	Medium Can aid species identification, but do not hold the same value as guard hairs.
Guard hairs	Main pelage	Commonly make the bulk of the pelage; coarser and longer than under-hairs but shorter than over-hairs.	High Have the greatest significance in species identification due to the interspecies variation present and the most useful when undertaking a comparison between a control and target hair (Suzanski, 1988).
Bristle	Found on the body of animals such as domestic and wild pigs and boar	Generally thick hairs with forked tips and with either absent, narrow or intruding medullas (Deedrick and Koch, 2004). Cross-sections are usually oval, circular or oblong.	Low

are placed upon a contrasting backing to allow general features such as colour, length, shaft profile and condition to be observed and can allow samples to be divided into smaller groups, e.g. under hairs and guard hairs. Shaft profile can sometimes be particularly useful when identifying species; for example, deer hairs have a distinctive crimped appearance (Deedrick and Koch, 2004).

The next stage of analysis is the use of high-powered microscopes in the form of a compound microscope (for the use of bright field microscopy) or a comparison microscope. Comparison microscopes are particularly popular, as they comprise two high-powered microscopes connected by a bridge which allows two samples, i.e. the control and the target sample, to be viewed at the same time under the same conditions.

Microscopy is debatably the most important stage of analysis and its advantages include the following: being a non-destructive technique; relative speed (important for timeliness of analysis, case throughput and if repeat measurements are needed); and its inexpensiveness, after the initial outlay (very few consumables). Sample preparation for fibres to be used for using brightfield microscopy is very simple, typically involving only placing the hair in a mounting medium between a glass slide and cover slip.

In some situations a polarized light microscope may be used; this allows the same observations as a compound microscope, but also allows qualitative and quantitative measurements using plane polarized light and between crossed polars (where the sample is placed between two polaroid films). Although not regularly used by animal hair analysts, it does provide additional information about the hairs' optical properties, such as their interference colours seen under crossed polars. This property has been used in the analysis of exotic animal hairs (Partin, 2003).

Scanning Electron Microscopes (SEM) utilize high-energy electrons to scan the surface of the hair and may be used after compound microscopy to create high resolution, three-dimensional images at very high magnifications, allowing characteristics such as the scale pattern to be more clearly viewed, this can be seen in Bahuguna and Mukherjee's (2000) work on identifying Tibetan antelope hairs.

Finally, further analytical techniques may be utilized if additional information is required, such as dye analysis or drug analysis. Common techniques are High Performance Liquid Chromatography (HPLC) and Thin Layer Chromatography (TLC) for extracted dyes, and radioimmunoassays (RIA) and chromatography techniques, such as Gas Chromatography (GC), for the analysis of extracted drugs (Gratacos-Cubarsi et al., 2006).

6.6.2 Microscopy preparation of animal hairs

Any target samples, or even control samples, which are covered in debris or body fluid must be cleaned prior to analysis. This can be completed by gently washing with distilled water and a mild detergent if necessary. Organic solvents such as isopropyl alcohol or acetone can be used to remove grease and other surface impurities (Ogle and Mitosinka, 1973).

If DNA analysis is possible, hairs should initially be mounted in distilled water so as to prevent any nuclear DNA being destroyed by a mounting medium.

6.6.2.1   Creating a whole mount

Mounting mediums such as Entellan® (Refractive Index (RI) = 1.49–1.51), DPX (RI = 1.52) or Meltmount® (RI = 1.539) are required for microscopical analysis. Refractive Index is the measure of the bending of light when passing from one medium to another. Generally, mounting mediums are thought to be best when they have a similar RI to the hair (keratin RI = 1.548) so as to allow a clear view of the internal characteristics of the hair (Petraco, 1987). Wildman (1961) describes the use of liquid paraffin (RI = 1.47) as a useful mountant, which is somewhat lower in RI than keratin, but allows both the internal features and surface characteristics to be viewed adequately. If the hair needs to be removed from the microscope slide and mountant, then this is possible by cracking the glass cover slip and applying a few drops of Tissue-Tek® Tissue-Clear®or xylene and then gently removing the loosened hair.

6.6.2.2   Scale casts and impressions of the animal hair surface

Prior to mounting on a microscope slide, a scale cast (or cuticle slide) can be produced to allow the outer scale profile to be determined. To do this, a thin layer of gelatine (10%–20%) (Teerink, 1991), polyvinyl acetate, Meltmount® (Petraco, 1987), or clear nail polish can be painted on to a microscope slide in a uniform thickness. The hair sample can then be placed gently into the substrate, leaving the end of the hair out of casting material for easier removal, and allowed to dry. If PVA is used, an additional slide can be placed on top of the hair and the slide gently heated to the melting point of the PVA and then allowed to cool before removal of the hair (Wildman, 1961). The hair can be rolled if a full impression is required as described by Wildman (1954), although this may damage the shaft and is not always appropriate, as the shield of the animal hair is normally slightly flattened in cross-section (Huffman and Wallace, 2012). When the substrate is fully dry, the hair can be carefully removed and the resultant cast can be viewed under a high-power light microscope.

6.6.2.3   Medulla slides

When the formation of medulla is difficult to visualize, a medulla slide may be produced, which removes the air present in the medulla to allow for a detailed view of the structure. This is achieved by infiltrating the medulla with xylene or paraffin oil, which makes it transparent when viewed under a microscope (Teerink, 1991; Linacre, 2009). To do this, the hair is cut at various positions using a razor blade, such that the xylene can seep into the medulla. This process can take up to three hours. To make these permanent, the oil can be replaced with a medium such as Canada balsam (Teerink, 1991). The production of these slides is particularly useful for lightly pigmented hairs, but with some highly pigmented hairs, such as some primates and black bears, there must be additional treatment of the cortex to make it transparent. This can be achieved by submerging dry hairs in hydrogen peroxide and a few drops of ammonia solution until the desired lightness is achieved (Linacre, 2009).

6.6.3 Microscopical analysis of animal hairs

In microscopical analysis of hairs, a balance exists between observing the whole hair to identify species and/or any similarities and differences between control and target hairs. To achieve this, a systematic approach is required. Analysis evidence sheets can be used that provide a systematic method for noting down relevant characteristics, sketches and comments using standardized terminology; these analysis sheets simplify comparison

and interpretation of the evidence. In an investigation, an analyst may be expected to analyse a few hairs, partial or complete hides, an object from a crime scene or a finished product such as a fur coat or hat (Linacre, 2009); therefore analysis methods must be adaptable but still recorded in a robust and reliable manner.

It is also beneficial to provide sketches and/or photomicrographs of the hairs. Sketches should include all three areas of the hair (root, shaft and tip) and be large, in ink, annotated, and signed and dated.

It is logical for an analyst to start at the root end, move through to the shaft area and then to the tip to identify any variation in characteristics and to view the whole hair. Each area can provide information specific to that region; for example, the root can provide information about the growth stage of the hair, the shaft can provide information about the pigment and medulla and the tip can provide information about damage and whether a fork or split is present.

For each of the cortex, medulla and cuticle regions, there are particular observations that are deemed useful for the analysis of hairs; these are listed in Table 6.3.

Figures 6.2 and 6.3 demonstrate examples of standard animal hair analysis forms and the categories used to describe the observations stated in Table 6.3. Further descriptions of the key observations can be found in Section 6.7, 'Species Identification from Animal Hair', below.

Table 6.3. Microscopical observations for the cortex, medulla and cuticle.

Hair Region	Characteristic
Cortex	Commonly noted: colour/hue, pigment density, pigment distribution, presence/absence of ovoid bodies.
	Additional observations: pigment granule shape, pigment granule size, texture of cortex, presence/absence of cortical fusi.
Medulla	Commonly noted: medulla distribution/type, medulla opacity, Medullary Index (MI) (Medulla diameter/shaft diameter).
	Additional observations: form of the medulla margins (straight, fringed, scalloped) (Teerink, 1991).
Cuticle	Commonly noted: cuticle thickness, scale pattern, scale position in relation to longitudinal direction of the hair, scale edge shape, distance between scale edges.
	Additional observations: distinctness of the inner cuticle margin.

ANIMAL HAIR EXAMINATION – SHEET 1						

Case reference:

Page   of

Macroscopic characteristics

Hair evidence number						
Length (cm)						
Shaft profile						
Colour						
Presence of banding						

General description:

Examined by:

Notes by: Day: Date: Time:

Fig. 6.2. Example of a standard animal hair form: Part 1 (macroscopic observations and sketches).

In addition to these observations, the root growth stage may be noted: this can be categorized into anagen (active growth stage with the presence of nuclear material), catagen (transitional growth stage with limited nuclear material) or telogen (dormant stage where hairs are readily shed and no nuclear material present) (Robertson, 1999). The diameter of the shaft should be measured in micrometres using a calibrated eye-piece scale, and variation along the length of the hair should be noted.

Depending upon the particular crime, and when and where the hair was found, animal hair evidence may have been subject to external influences such as weathering

ANIMAL HAIR EXAMINATION – SHEET 2									
Case reference:									
Page of									
Microscopic characteristics									
Hair evidence number									
Pigment density	None								
	Light								
	Medium								
	Heavy								
Pigment distribution	Even								
	Central								
	Peripheral								
	One-sided								
Medulla distribution/ type	None								
	Broken (fragmented/interrupted)								
	Unbroken/continuous (lattice/aeriform lattice/simple/vacuolated)								
	Ladder (uniserial/multiserial)								
	Miscellaneous (globular/stellate/intruding)								
Scale edges shape	Smooth								
	Crenate								
	Rippled								
	Scalloped								
	Dentate								
Distance between scales	Close								
	Near								
	Distant								
Scale pattern	Mosaic (regular/irregular)								
	Wave (regular/irregular/single chevron/double chevron/streaked)								
	Petal (broad/elongate/diamond*)								
	Transitional								
Ovoid bodies (Y/N)									
Shaft diameter (µm)									
Root shape									
Tip shape									
Medullary Index (MI) = Medulla diameter/shaft diameter									
Other									
Examined by:									
Notes by: Day: Date: Time:									

* note whether narrow or broad diamond

Fig. 6.3. Example of a standard animal hair form: Part 2 (microscopic observations).

(Chang, 2005), causing change in the morphological features, but nevertheless providing additional information about the case. In certain cruelty cases, animals may have been exposed to heat sources such as cigarette burns, irons or complete burning of the hair with accelerants. Hair samples found in bedding, discarded collars and at crime scenes can indicate the temperatures that hair has been exposed to.

When hairs are exposed to heat, changes in colour, swelling and bubbling of the hair may occur. Research conducted by Pangerl and Igowsky (2007) on human hairs indicated that variables such as temperature, exposure time, and how the heat is applied to the hair must be considered to fully interpret this type of damage. Research conducted by Ayres (1985) identified that colour changes occurred in hairs when exposed to a hot plate, but when exposed directly to flame, colour changes were absent; however, the presence of charring and bubbling was observed. Work conducted at Staffordshire University has shown that it is also possible to identify the presence of accelerants on even a few strands of hairs that have been in close range of an accelerated fire, using headspace gas chromatography.

Other environmental factors that cause damage to the hair, such as crushing, insect damage and fungal damage, can alter the appearance of the hair, but also potentially provides an evidentially useful characteristic. For example, hair from a decomposing body may exhibit a decomposition band, i.e. the section of hair lying below the skin surface has darkened in colour due to the decomposition process (Linch and Prahlow, 2001).

6.7   Species Identification from Animal Hair

It has been noted by Petraco (1987) and Moore (1988), that with use of their schemes of identification, even inexperienced examiners can accurately identify the species of an animal from its hair, albeit with use of other resources, such as reference materials (Moore, 1988). This comment should be taken with caution, as it is recognized that animal hair identification is one of the more difficult analyses attempted by forensic scientists (Wildman, 1961; Moore 1988). Possible explanations for this include: the variation that can exist within a species (Moore, 1988); the variation in terminology used in species identification keys; the subjective nature of the analysis (no single characteristic will allow identification of a species); and the fact that hairs from closely related species can show similar characteristics (Wildman, 1961).

For species and sub-species identification, there are five main characteristics: scale morphology; medulla type; medullary fraction (MF); colour banding; and root shape. The nomenclature for the different characteristics differs between ID keys and guides, but the following categories for each characteristic primarily combines the terminology and species examples used by Appleyard (1960), Wildman (1961), Petraco (1987), Moore (1988), Teerink (1991), Partin (2003), Deedrick and Koch (2004) and Linacre (2009). All examples are for guard hairs unless otherwise stated.

6.7.1   Scale morphology

Broadly the scale pattern of animal hairs can be classified into two main groups: coronal (where the scales go around the entire shaft, completely encircling it); and imbricate (where there are multiple scales encircling the shaft). Further classifications can be made of the scales on the cuticle by observing four main characteristics.

1. Scale position in relation to the longitudinal axis: this can be categorized as transversal (where the scales are at right angles to the longitudinal axis and appear to have a greater width than length – seen in Fig. 6.4f); longitudinal (where the scales are aligned with the length of the hair and are longer than they are wide – seen in Fig. 6.4b); or intermediate (where the width of the scales is the same as the length – seen in Fig. 6.4a).
2. Shape of the scale margin: this is the shape of the distal end of the scale, which can be smooth, crenate (shallow and relatively pointed indentations), rippled, frilled, scalloped or dentate (pointed, like teeth).
3. Distance between the external margins of the scales: this is usually categorized as close (as seen in Fig. 6.4g); near (as seen in Fig. 6.4a); or distant (as seen in Fig. 6.4b). Sometimes scale count is also completed, which counts the number of scales per unit of measure, e.g. 40µm (Rosen, 1974).

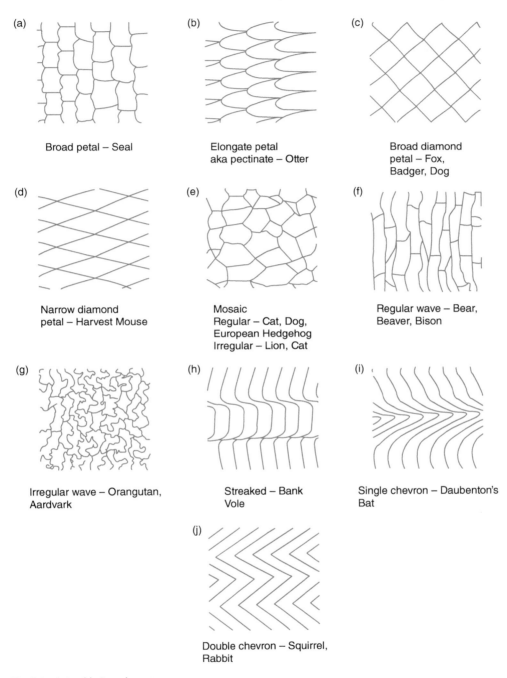

(a) Broad petal – Seal

(b) Elongate petal aka pectinate – Otter

(c) Broad diamond petal – Fox, Badger, Dog

(d) Narrow diamond petal – Harvest Mouse

(e) Mosaic Regular – Cat, Dog, European Hedgehog Irregular – Lion, Cat

(f) Regular wave – Bear, Beaver, Bison

(g) Irregular wave – Orangutan, Aardvark

(h) Streaked – Bank Vole

(i) Single chevron – Daubenton's Bat

(j) Double chevron – Squirrel, Rabbit

Fig. 6.4. Animal hair scale patterns.

4. Scale pattern: this describes the overall shape and regularity of the outer scales. Figure 6.4 demonstrates the most common patterns seen in animal hair, with some examples of animals that exhibit these. In addition to these, a pattern may also be transitional, which is the presence of more than one pattern along the length of the hair.

6.7.2 Medulla types

The medulla can vary dramatically between species and even subtle differences can be seen between sub-species. First, medullas can be categorized by their distribution as being unbroken, broken (e.g. interrupted and fragmented which is also seen in human hair), laddered, or miscellaneous; and then further categorized by their structure (and width, for certain types). Teerink (1991) also further categorized medulla by the form of the medulla margin, i.e. the silhouette of the medulla's edges, as straight, fringed or scalloped. Figure 6.5 demonstrates the most common medulla structures seen in animal hair, with some examples of animals that exhibit these.

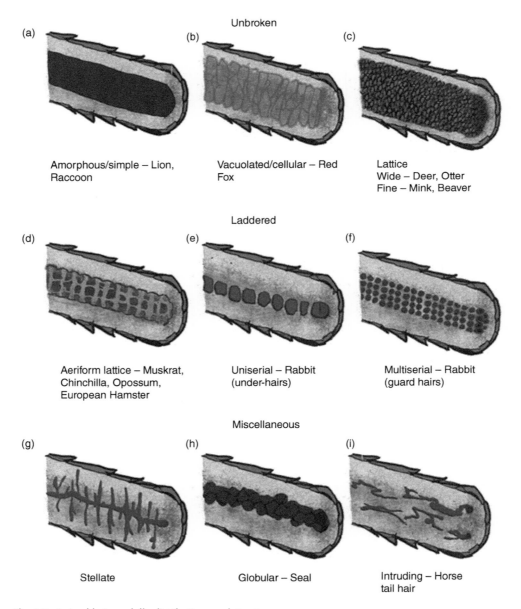

Unbroken

(a) (b) (c)

Amorphous/simple – Lion, Raccoon

Vacuolated/cellular – Red Fox

Lattice
Wide – Deer, Otter
Fine – Mink, Beaver

Laddered

(d) (e) (f)

Aeriform lattice – Muskrat, Chinchilla, Opossum, European Hamster

Uniserial – Rabbit (under-hairs)

Multiserial – Rabbit (guard hairs)

Miscellaneous

(g) (h) (i)

Stellate

Globular – Seal

Intruding – Horse tail hair

Fig. 6.5. Animal hair medulla distributions and structures.

6.7.3   Medullary fraction (MF)
aka medullary index (MI)

The medullary fraction (MF) is the ratio between the width of the hair and width of the medulla. The width of both the shaft of the hair and the medulla are measured in micrometres and can be compared as a quantitative characteristic or used to aid identification; for example, Peabody *et al.* (1983) determined that the medullary fraction could be used to reliably distinguish between dogs and cats.

6.7.4   Colour banding

Pigment distribution in animal hair may not only differ across the width of the hair, but also quite dramatically along its length. The length, order, colour and number of bands can help identify different species. For example, badger hair can be differentiated from dog and fox hair primarily by its distinct white proximal end, black shaft and white tip (Moore, 1988).

6.7.5   Root shape

Further to identifying growth stage, animal hair root bulbs can have particular shapes that are useful in identifying species. Examples of this include deer (wine glass), horse (elongated), cow (elongated but with a medulla present in the root portion), dog (spade) and cat ('paint brush' with the inclusion of fibrils) (Moore, 1988; Linacre, 2009).

6.7.6   Species identification aids

Research into the variation of morphological characteristics in animal hair, comparisons of different species and sub-species, and the development of identification keys, reference collections and interpretation aids are abundant. Examples of specific ID schemes include the following: Stains (1958); Appleyard (1960); Moore (1988); and Petraco (1987). Petraco's (1987) scheme includes 25 genera and was designed to allow quick and effective identification of these genera using only one

complete guard hair. Moore's (1988) scheme mainly focuses upon animal species commonly found in the UK, but also incorporates other species such as camel and llama. A comprehensive atlas of west-European hairs developed by Teerink (1991) provides illustrations and photographs of cross-sections, scale casts, medulla slides and mounted samples of guard and under-hairs from a vast range of animals. Smaller research projects analysing particular species or geographical area either for casework or other environmental or scientific purpose are also very useful to the hair analyst. Examples of these types of study include Williams' (1938) ID of mole and shrew hairs; Hilton and Kutscha's (1978) ID of coyote, dog, red fox and bobcat hairs in Maine; Vineis *et al.*'s (2008) ID of wild goat and domestic goat hair; and Mayer's (1952) examination of Californian mammals. In addition to these works, there are very useful online resources that present photomicrographs of different animal hairs, including Deedrick and Koch (2004).

These guides are very important for forensic analysts who may not have come across certain animal hair types in casework previously. Some of these keys state different characteristics for the same species type but this is to be expected, as different sub-species will have been sampled for the production of the keys and therefore the use of multiple keys, to identify any variation and differences in interpretation, is advised.

The breadth of animal hairs and their microscopical characteristics is huge and it is advisable for a forensic analyst to have reference samples of a large range of animals for comparison (Wildman, 1961). Samples may be obtained from casework, museums, zoos or commercially produced collections, such the Arbidar Animal Hair and Fur Collection.

6.8   Interpretation of Animal Hair in Casework

6.8.1   Conclusions from comparing control and target hairs

The interpretation of the characteristics observed between target hairs and control hairs is different to species identification and must attempt to identify any differences rather than similarities. Differences due to the hairs being from different animals can be difficult to distinguish from differences due to variation seen across hairs from the same animal; therefore care must be taken when interpreting results.

As stated by Deedrick and Koch (2000, 2004) there are three general conclusions that can be reached as a result of microscopic hair analysis: exclusion; no conclusion; or association. Exclusion indicates that the target hair has originated from a different source to the control (exhibiting significant difference in one or more characteristics); association (where the same microscopical characteristics can be seen between the control and the target hairs) indicates that they have a common source; and no conclusion is given when neither of these can be stated with reliability. In order to come to one of these conclusions, the analyst must identify any variation seen in the control hairs and decide whether the target hair falls within this range (Deedrick and Koch, 2004).

When association has been concluded, the certainty placed upon this conclusion will be affected by the number of hair characteristics seen in the target hair that are the same as the control, the condition of the hair and the individuality of the hair: the more characteristics and the less common the characteristics, the greater the confidence that can be placed upon the conclusion.

Where possible, knowledge of the population should be used to provide statistical evaluation of the evidence; for example, knowledge of the commonality of certain characteristics within and across species. This form of information is very difficult to obtain reliably for animal hair and is usually based upon an expert's experience, although the use of statistics to create probabilities for association has been attempted with human hair (Gaudette and Keeping, 1974; Barnett and Ogle, 1982).

Unfortunately, with animal hair, identification of an individual animal without DNA analysis is not normally possible. Studies such as Suzanski (1988), carried out to investigate dog hair from different individuals of the same breed, has indicated that although some individuality can be found in German Shepherds, this does not apply to all individuals, as some hairs show fewer characteristics for comparison.

6.8.2 Transfer and persistence for interpreting animal crimes

Understanding the mechanisms of transfer and persistence of animal hair is very important for establishing the evidential value of any hairs found in animal crimes, and may help to identify time periods within which the hairs were likely to have been deposited upon the object or individual that has been sampled. Animal hair may be transferred in a variety of ways: directly from the animal to an object (for example, to a wooden baton used for dog fighting); from animal to an environment (such as its living quarters); from an animal to a human; and from an animal to another animal. Transfer of hairs can be primary, secondary or even tertiary. Primary transfer is where the hair has been transferred from the donor directly to an object, suspect or victim; for example, from a dog to a weapon used to cause head injuries to the dog. Secondary transfer is where hair is transferred to an intermediary object/person/animal before being transferred to the object/person/animal that it is found upon; for example, a hair being transferred from a person to a chair and then a second person sitting on the chair and the hair being transferred to that individual. Tertiary is the presence of two intermediary objects.

The factors which affect the transfer and persistence of fibred and human hairs is well documented but much less is known for animal hairs, especially in regard to animal crimes (Boehme et al., 2009). Having said that, some factors that affect the number of hairs transferred from an animal to an object will be the same as with human hair or natural fibres, including the following:

1. Length (time) of contact.
2. Surface area in contact.
3. Force of contact.
4. Hair length.
5. Recipient surface, e.g. fur of a different animal, fabric (Boehme et al., 2009).

Specifically for animal hairs, the growth stage of hair (seasonal shedding) will also affect transfer.

Persistence of hairs is the length of time a hair will adhere to an object/person/animal after deposition. Knowledge of how long different hairs persist on different surfaces can help identify time of deposition and therefore help reconstruct a crime scene. To aid with this, reconstruction experiments can be carried out to identify the persistence of particular hairs on particular surfaces.

Factors that could affect the persistence of animal hairs include:

1. The recipient surface.
   a. Another animal as the recipient surface – density and length of fur, cleanliness of fur, position on body.
   b. Other surfaces – smoothness, fibre and weave type (if fabric) (Dachs *et al.*, 2003).
2. Activity since deposition.
3. Washing/cleaning behaviour of the animal.

Research carried out by Boehme *et al.* (2009) on the persistence of animal hairs on different fabrics indicated that hair type is not significant to persistence, although rougher cuticles may affect persistence.

Acknowledgements

Thank you to William Bailey for the production of the diagrams.

References

Appleyard, H.M. (1960) *Guide to the Identification of Animal Fibres*. Wool Industries Research Association, Leeds, UK.

Ayres, L.M. (1985) Misleading color changes in hair that has been heated but not exposed to flame. In: *Proceedings of the International Symposium on Forensic Hair Comparisons*. 25–27 June, FBI Academy, Quantico, Virginia. US Department of Justice, Washington, DC.

Bahuguna, A. and Mukherjee, S.K. (2000) Use of SEM to recognise Tibetan antelope (Chiru) hair and blending in wool products. *Science and Justice* 40(3), 177–182.

Barnett, P.D. and Ogle, R.R. (1982) Probabilities and human hair comparisons. *Journal of Forensic Sciences* 27, 272–278.

Boehme, A., Brooks, E., McNaught, I. and Robertson, J. (2009) The persistence of animal hairs in a forensic context. *Australian Journal of Forensic Sciences* 41(2), 99–112.

Chang, B.S., Hong, W.S., Lee, E., Yeo, S.M., Bang, I.S., Yeo, S.M., Chung, Y.H., Lim, D.S., Mun, G.A., Kim, J., Park, S.O. and Shin, D.H. (2005) Ultramicroscopic observations on morphological changes in hair during 25 Years of weathering. *Forensic Science International* 151, 249–200.

Choudhry, M.Y. (1988) A novel technique for the collection and recovery of foreign fibers in forensic science casework. *Journal of Forensic Sciences* 33(1), 249–253.

Dachs, J., McNaught, I.J., and Robertson, J. (2003) The persistence of human scalp hair on clothing fabrics. *Forensic Science International* 138, 27–36.

Deedrick, D.W. and Koch, S.L. (2000) Microscopy of hair (Part 1): a practical guide and manual for human hairs. *Forensic Science Communications* 2, 3. Available online at: https://www.fbi.gov/about-us/lab/forensic-science-communications/fsc/jan2004/research/2004_01_research01b.htm (accessed 21 September 2015).

Deedrick, D.W. and Koch, S.L. (2004) Microscopy of hair (Part II): a practical guide and manual for animal hairs. *Forensic Science Communications* 6, 3. Available online at: https://www.fbi.gov/about-us/lab/forensic-science-communications/fsc/july2004/research/2004_03_research02.htm (accessed 21 September 2015).

Gaudette, B.D. and Keeping, E.S. (1974) An attempt at determining probabilities in human scalp hair comparison. *Journal of Forensic Sciences* 19, 599–606.

Gratacos-Cubarsi, M., Castellari, M., Valero, A. and Garcia-Regueiro, J.A. (2006) Hair analysis for veterinary drug monitoring in livestock production. *Journal of Chromatography* 834, 14–25.

Hilton, H. and Kutscha, N.P. (1978) Distinguishing characteristics of the hairs of eastern coyote, domestic dog, red fox and bobcat in Maine. *American Midland Naturalist* 100(1), 223–227.

Huffman, J.E. and Wallace, J.R. (2012) *Wildlife Forensics: Methods and Applications*. Wiley, Chichester, UK.

Jackson, A. and Gwinnett, C. (2013) Easylift: a novel tape lifting system. *Interfaces* 73, 22–23.

Lenertz, O. (2001) Retaining physical traces and evidence. *Problems of Forensic Sciences* 46, 68–75.

Linacre, A. (ed.) (2009) *Forensic Science in Wildlife Investigations*. CRC Press, Boca Raton, Florida, USA.

Linch, C.A. and Prahlow, J.A. (2001) Postmortem microscopic changes observed at the human head hair proximal end. *Journal of Forensic Sciences* 46, 15–20.

Locard, E. (1930) The analysis of dust traces. *American Journal of Political Science* 1, 276–298.

Mayer, W.V. (1952) The hair of California mammals with keys to the dorsal guard hairs of California mammals. *American Midland Naturalist* 38, 480–512.

McKenna, F.J. and Sherwin, J.C. (1975) A simple and effective method for collecting contact evidence. *Journal of the Forensic Science Society* 15, 227.

Moore, J.E. (1988) A key for the identification of animal hairs. *Journal of the Forensic Science Society* 28, 335–339.

Ogle, R.R. and Mitosinka, G. (1973) A rapid technique for preparing hair cuticular scale casts. *Journal of Forensic Science* 18(1), 82–83.

Oxford Dictionaries (2016) *Hair*. Available at: http://www.oxforddictionaries.com/definition/english/hair (accessed 16 May 2016).

Pangerl, E. and Igowsky, K. (2007) Changes observed in human head hairs exposed to heat. *Trace Evidence Symposium NFSTC*, Clearwater Florida. Available online at: http://projects.nfstc.org/trace/docs/Trace%20 Presentations%20CD-2/Pangerl.pdf (accessed 21 September 2015).

Partin, K. (2003) A microscopical study of exotic animal hair: Part 1. *Modern Microscopy Journal* (online), The McCrone Group. Available online at https://www.mccrone.com/mm/a-microscopical-study-of-exotic-animal-hair-part-1 (accessed 24 September 2015).

Peabody, A.J., Oxborough, R.J., Cage, P.E. and Evett, J.W. (1983) The discrimination of cat and dog hairs. *Journal of Forensic Science Society* 23, 121–129.

Petraco, N. (1987) A microscopical method to aid in the identification of animal hair. *The Microscope* 35, 83–92.

Robertson, J. (1999) *Forensic Examination of Hair*. Taylor & Francis, London, UK.

Robertson, J. and Roux, C. (2010) Trace evidence: here today, gone tomorrow? *Science and Justice* 50, 18–22.

Rosen, S.I. (1974) Identification of primate hair. *Journal of Forensic Sciences* 19(1), 109–112.

Stains, H.J. (1958) Key to guard hairs of middle Western Furbearers. *Journal of Wildlife Management* 22, 95–97.

Suzanski, T.W. (1988) Dog hair comparison: a preliminary study. *Canadian Society of Forensic Science Journal* 21, 19–28.

Taupin, J.M. (2004) Forensic hair morphology comparison – a dying art or junk science? *Science and Justice* 44(2), 95–100.

Teerink, B.J. (1991) *Hair of West-European Mammals: Atlas and Identification Key*. Cambridge University Press, Cambridge, UK.

Vineis, C., Aluigi, A. and Tonin, C. (2008) Morphological and thermal behaviour of textile fibres from the hair of domestic and wild goat species. *AUTEX Research Journal* 8(3), 68–71.

Wildman, A.B. (1954) *The Microscopy of Animal Textile Fibres*. Wool Industries Research Association, Leeds, UK.

Wildman, A.B. (1961) The identification of animal fibres. *Journal of the Forensic Science Society* 1, 115–119.

Williams, C.S. (1938) Aids to the identification of mole and shrew hairs with general comments on hair structure and hair determination. *Journal of Wildlife Management* 2, 239–249.

7 Firearms and Ballistics

Rachel Bolton-King[1]* and Johan Schulze[2]*

[1]*Department of Forensic and Crime Science, Staffordshire University, Stoke-on-Trent, Staffordshire, UK; [2]Veterinary Forensic and Wildlife Services, Germany and Norway*

---

*Corresponding authors: r.bolton-king@staffs.ac.uk; schulze@vet-for-wild-serv.eu

7.1   Crime Scene Evidence: Firearms and Ballistics

RACHEL BOLTON-KING

7.1.1   Introduction

Crime scenes involving shooting-related incidents can contain a raft of forensic evidence that may be of benefit to the forensic veterinarian and criminal investigating team. The nature of the firearm (Section 7.1.2) and the ammunition (Section 7.1.3) utilized in the shooting have a critical role to play in the resulting injury and trauma exhibited in the body.

The term ballistics is defined as the study of the motion of projectiles. Ballistics is divided into three main categories: internal (Section 7.1.4), external (Section 7.1.6) and terminal (Section 7.1.7); however, there is also a fourth category known as intermediate ballistics (Section 7.1.5). Terminal ballistics (Section 7.1.7) covers both inanimate objects and living organisms; however, the study of projectiles through living organisms is classified as a sub-category of terminal ballistics referred to as wound ballistics (see Section 7.2).

The field of firearms and ballistics is extensive. This chapter, therefore, aims to provide an introductory explanation of the scientific theory underpinning firearms, ammunition and ballistics. The focus will be on the common types of firearm and associated ammunition that are utilized by civilians, which would ultimately be encountered in the majority of cases where veterinarians are involved in forensic investigations. For more in-depth reading into this field, recommended reading includes Farrar and Leeming (1983), Carlucci and Jacobson (2008), Heard (2008), Haag and Haag (2011), Warlow (2011).

7.1.2   Firearms

The legal definition of a firearm differs slightly from the dictionary definition. A firearm is defined by The Firearms (Amendment) Act 1988 (UK Parliament, 1988) as 'a lethal barrelled weapon of any description from which any shot, bullet or other missile can be discharged'; whereas the Oxford English Dictionary (Oxford University Press, 2014) simply identifies a firearm as different types of gun, i.e. 'a rifle, pistol or other portable gun', thus 'gun' is defined as 'a weapon incorporating a metal tube from which bullets, shells, or other missiles are propelled by explosive force, typically making a characteristic loud, sharp noise'. The mechanism of firing the projectile (Section 7.1.2.2) is unspecified; however, the legal definition implies that the weapon must be capable of killing a living target. The dictionary states that an explosive force is required; however, the force may not have to be explosive in order to be lethal. The legislation around firearm ownership, transportation and use will vary extensively depending on the region in which the crime occurred.

7.1.2.1   Types of firearm

The term handgun is commonly used to describe any firearm that is capable of being fired from one hand (AFTE Training and Standardization Committee, 2007). This term includes two types of firearm: revolver (or revolving pistol) and pistol, although the sub-machine gun (SMG) may also be considered in this category. Within the UK, air weapons are currently the most common firearms utilized in gun crime as these are typically legal and unlicensed, but this is closely followed by handguns (Berman, 2012; Smith *et al.*, 2012) due to their small size, making them easy to conceal from other civilians and law enforcement. Air weapons are typically used for recreational use, such as target shooting, whereas handguns are typically utilized for self-defence.

The main difference between a pistol and a revolver is that a revolver has a cylinder containing multiple chambers, each capable of housing a single ammunition cartridge, and the chamber is therefore separated from the barrel. A pistol has a single chamber that houses only one ammunition cartridge and this is integrated into the barrel. A sub-machine gun is a shorter-barrelled, lightweight machine gun, designed to fire pistol-sized cartridges in short or long bursts of fire. Modern handgun barrels are typically rifled with a spiral internal surface profile consisting of alternating spiral lands and grooves to enhance the ballistic properties of the projectile upon muzzle exit. Figure 7.1.1 indicates the key components common to a wide range of firearms.

Rifles also have a single chamber to house one cartridge, but are identified by their longer-rifled barrel and are larger in overall size than handguns. Rifles are designed to be fired by one individual, but using two hands.

A shotgun is differentiated from handguns and rifles due to the smooth-bore barrel

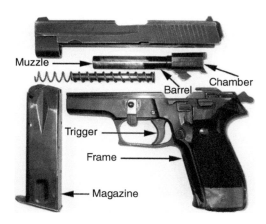

Fig. 7.1.1. Annotated image of a Sig Sauer P226 semi-automatic pistol field stripped into its key component parts listed from top of the image; slide (containing the ejection port), barrel (with integral chamber), recoil guide spring, frame and magazine (housed inside the grip of the frame).

and typically utilizes cartridges measured in gauge rather than calibre. Gauge equates to the number of lead balls with the diameter of the barrel bore, that collectively weigh 1 lb. The calibre is either the internal diameter of the mouth of the cartridge case or the maximum diameter of the projectile (units may be metric or imperial). For example, a 12-gauge shotgun has a barrel diameter of 0.729 in. and 12 lead balls of 0.729 in. weigh 1 lb. Shotguns are usually single- or double-barrelled with the latter having either a side-by-side or up-and-over barrel alignment. Shotgun barrels also may contain a choke at the muzzle end, which can be integral to the barrel or be removable. The choke aims to force the multiple shot together prior to exiting the barrel and there are varying degrees of choke available. To be made more concealable, criminals are known to cut down and shorten the barrel length, which will ultimately reduce the velocity, energy and range of the projectile(s) and increase the spread of lead shot fired from the ammunition due to excessively high pressure (Haag and Haag, 2011) and choke removal.

Tasers and stun guns may also be considered as a firearm in some countries, including Great Britain. Tasers are designed to fire two barbs from a cartridge, which are connected to the weapon by wire reaching up to 10.6 m. When the wired barbs make contact with or penetrate the upper layer of the skin (epidermis) the electrical circuit is complete and current is passed through the target's tissue to incapacitate. Tasers can be used in stun drive mode to cause pain, whereby the cartridge is not used and contact is made directly between the skin and the electrical device.

Other weapons that could be considered relevant within the context of veterinary forensics are bows and crossbows, humane killers such as captive-bolt guns (Warlow, 2011), airsoft weapons and paintball guns. However, by the UK legal definition these are not firearms and therefore not considered within the scope of this chapter.

7.1.2.2   Modern firing mechanisms

Firing mechanisms involve the loading of the projectile/ammunition into the weapon and the functioning of all the firearm's internal components required to propel the projectile out of the barrel. Design and functionality of specific firearms is an extensive topic, ultimately determined by the firearm manufacturer. Forensic veterinarians do not need to know the in-depth details of all firing mechanisms, but need to appreciate the differences in the key firing mechanisms and how these influence the ammunition selected, the properties of the projectiles fired and the potential differences that could be expected for wound examination and interpretation.

Air weapons are relatively low-powered weapons, which use a high-pressure volume of gas, typically atmospheric air or carbon dioxide, to transfer energy to the projectile (pellet) and propel it out of the barrel; these weapons therefore do not require ignition of chemical compounds to generate kinetic energy. Air weapons using atmospheric air typically operate by manually compressing a spring; pulling the trigger releases the spring compressing the air and pushing it behind the pellet. Alternatively, the pellet is fired utilizing a small jet of compressed gas, such as carbon dioxide, released from a small gas canister attached to the weapon when the trigger is pulled. In most of the UK,

the legal limits for an air weapon to be classified as a firearm are higher than 1 ft lb (Home Office, 2014). Criminal use of air weapons was on the rise until 2003/2004 (Berman, 2012), when legislation aimed to reduce this (Squires, 2014). However, injuries to animals caused by air weapons are still more commonly observed by veterinarians. To be legal and unlicensed, air pistols must generate projectile muzzle energy less than 6 ft lbs (8.1 J) and less than 12 ft lbs (16.3 J) for air rifles (Home Office, 2014). However, in Northern Ireland, air weapons firing projectiles with muzzle energy greater than 1 J must be held on a firearms certificate (Northern Ireland Office, 2005).

The ammunition is loaded into the weapon either manually, or automatically from a magazine or belt of ammunition. Automatic loading (self-loading) uses the energy created from discharging a previous cartridge to reload the next live cartridge of ammunition into the chamber ready to be fired again. Heard (2008) and Warlow (2011) discuss the range of firing mechanisms that enable self-loading of ammunition and examples include recoil, blowback and bolt-action. Principally, there are two overarching automatic firing mechanisms: semi-automatic and fully automatic. Semi-automatic means that with one pull of the trigger, one cartridge is fired. With fully automatic, one pull of the trigger causes continual firing and reloading of ammunition until either the trigger is released, or there is no ammunition left to fire from the magazine or belt. There are some firearms designed to fire short bursts of ammunition, whereby continual hold of the trigger will fire a small number of cartridges (usually three to five); to fire further cartridges the trigger will need to be released and pulled again. Modern pistols such as Browning Hi-Power and Beretta 92FS are commonly semi-automatic, whereas SMGs such as MAC-10 and Uzi SMG may also have the capability of fully automatic fire and the AK47 assault rifle may have the additional option of short-burst fire.

For handguns, there are two ways to set the trigger and fire the weapon: single-action and double-action. Single-action requires a manual cocking of the hammer and then a subsequent pull of the trigger to fire. With double-action, a longer and heavier pull of the trigger will first cock the hammer and then release the firing pin/striker on to the cartridge causing it to discharge.

For rifles and shotgun, the firing mechanisms include single-shot, bolt-action (bolt is turned to lock the cartridge into the breech end of the barrel before firing), self-loading (similar to self-loading pistols) and pump-action (breech is linked to the fore-end, which when pulled back, unlocks the breech and ejects the cartridge case; pushing the fore-end forward loads in a live cartridge from the magazine and cocks the weapon).

Other terms used to describe firearms and their firing mechanisms include converted (for example, a blank firing weapon converted to fire ammunition such as Olympic 38 or Baikal), home-made, concealed (firearms made to look like other objects such as pen gun), de-activated (firearms made unable to fire ammunition by machining/removing key components), reactivated (deactivated weapons made to fire again) and imitation (firearms that look real, but do not fire live ammunition).

7.1.3 Ammunition

Like firearms, ammunition has developed over the centuries. However, ammunition is designed first for a specific purpose; the weapon is developed later to fire that ammunition. For example, Georg Luger developed the 9 × 19 mm cartridge in 1902 which was later designed to be fired in the 1908 Luger P08 semi-automatic pistol (Jones and Ness, 2009; Bolton-King, 2012). Thus, a wide range of ammunition with a variety of specifications has been developed for specific purposes (Table 7.1.1); choosing the correct ammunition for a specific weapon can be critical to achieve the intended outcome. To ensure the weapon fires safely and correctly, the dimension(s) of the ammunition (calibre or gauge) must be accurately selected for the firearm in which it is discharged.

7.1.3.1 Composition

Modern ammunition has developed from loading individual components (primer, propellant and projectile) into a self-enclosed cartridge system to create a closed environment for a large amount of gas to be produced and allow the gas pressure to rise exponentially.

The core components of a cartridge are the cartridge case and the projectile. The projectile is positioned at the mouth of the cartridge case and they are crimped together to form the cartridge. The base of the cartridge case houses the primer unit that contains the primer compound. Inside the cartridge case, the propellant is confined between the primer unit and the projectile.

Table 7.1.1. Common examples of modern ammunition calibres and their intended purpose.

Calibre (in.)	Weapon Type (Centre-Fire)	Purpose
0.22 Hornet	Rifle	Small varmint hunting (<200 m)
0.223 Remington	Rifle	Military standard (long range)
0.303 British	Rifle	Military standard (long range)
0.357 Magnum	Revolver	Law enforcement (short range)
0.410	Shotgun	Small varmint/game hunting
0.45 Automatic Colt Pistol (ACP)	Pistol	Close combat, self-defence
0.458 Winchester Magnum	Rifle	Hunting dangerous game
Calibre (mm)		
7.62 NATO	Rifle	Military standard (long range)
9 × 19	Pistol or sub-machine gun	Military standard (short range)
Gauge		
20	Shotgun	Recommended for hunting novices
12	Shotgun	Short range bird hunting

The primer (Section 7.1.4.1) and propellant (Section 7.1.4.2) are both mixtures of chemical compounds designed to ignite, burn and provide oxygen to the combustion process. Priming compounds are typically inorganic compounds that are explosive and more exothermic, whereas propellant flakes are organic in nature, burning slower and slightly cooler.

There are two main classifications of modern cartridge: centre-fire and rim-fire. The difference is due to the location of the explosive primer that ignites the cartridge. As the name implies, the centre-fire cartridge has the primer located in the centre of the base, whereas the primer within the rim-fire cartridge has it located around the rim.

Projectiles are identified for ammunition based on the intended functional purpose of the cartridge and the weapon type the cartridge is designed for. Projectile shape, dimensions and material properties affect the external (Section 7.1.6) and terminal ballistics (Section 7.1.7) following projectile exit from the barrel. Typically the softer the material property of the projectile, the more easily the projectile will deform on impact with a target, increasing surface area and increasing the amount of energy that can be transferred into the target material. For example, a full metal jacketed (FMJ) projectile is harder than a metal jacketed hollow-point (HP) that has an exposed lead cavity at the projectile nose. The HP will deform and mushroom on impact with a target, significantly reducing penetration depth and increasing wounding in comparison to an FMJ. This makes the FMJ more suitable for military use and the HP more suitable to law enforcement and hunting, where only one target needs to be hit.

Air weapons do not utilize a cartridge system, as the compressed air supplies the force to propel a single lead pellet using comparably low gas pressure. More lethal firearms utilizing cartridge-based ammunition create much higher gas pressures during ignition, and therefore have greater muzzle velocity, muzzle energy, range and penetration depth. However, research has shown that even blank firing weapons can be fatal, due to the gas pressures released (Demirci et al., 2011). Projectiles

fired from pistols, revolvers, rifles and machine guns are typically referred to as bullets. Shotgun ammunition, however, commonly contain multiple spherical lead pellets known as shot. However, some shotgun cartridges are designed to fire a single projectile (slug) from a rifled-barrel shotgun, commonly used for beast destruction.

7.1.3.2 Live cartridges

Although fired cartridge cases and fired projectiles (Section 7.1.3.3) are the primary types of forensic firearms evidence recovered from crime scenes, the presence of unfired (live) cartridges is important to forensic firearms examiners. Live cartridges allow an examiner to determine exactly the type of ammunition that was used by the firer and can be used for corroborative intelligence and for test firing to assist in the identification of a specific weapon.

7.1.3.3 Fired cartridge cases and projectiles

Brief examination of fired cartridge cases can provide valuable intelligence to the forensic practitioners investigating the incident. Information can include the manufacturer and calibre of the likely ammunition used, and probable identification of the type of weapon, its manufacturer and model, using class characteristics transferred during the firing process (for example, the shape and dimensions of the firing pin impression). Knowledge of such initial intelligence can aid the forensic veterinarian in their examination of wounds (Section 7.2).

The fired ammunition component that is more commonly encountered by a forensic veterinarian is the fired projectile, which may or may not be located inside the injured species. Ideally, the presence of a forensic firearms examiner or ballistics expert would be very beneficial as they can assist with wound examination and interpretation and recover any firearms-related evidence; however, the overriding purpose of the veterinarian is to preserve life. As a minimum, an X-ray of the wound should be undertaken, as some initial visual analysis of the X-ray images can provide intelligence to the practitioner during their examination. The approximate dimension of the base of the projectile can indicate the calibre of the weapon, and the shape of projectile found may lead to the type of weapon that discharged it. Also, it is possible that the projectile may have fragmented inside the body; this could be due to the design of the ammunition component or because the projectile has struck dense material within the body; for example, bone. Retrieval of fired projectiles will be covered in Section 7.1.8.

Although beyond the scope of this chapter, submission of fired cartridge cases and projectiles to the laboratory for examination by a firearms examiner can further identify the specific weapon that was involved using microscopic examination of the individual characteristics engraved and impressed into the fired ammunition component. Individual characteristics are created by unique toolmarks generated on the surface of the weapon components during the component manufacturing process. The toolmarks are randomly created due to wear of the tool surface used to manufacture the component and these toolmarks are transferred to the component during the firing process. As they are random and unique, the individual characteristics can be used to identify a specific weapon component. Even if a firearm is not recovered, examination of multiple fired cases or projectiles can be used to link shooting incidents together and identify a single weapon used in one or more incidents, known as an inferred weapon.

7.1.4 Internal ballistics

Internal ballistics covers all aspects involving the ammunition and firearm from the moment the firing pin strikes the cartridge to the point at which the projectile exits the muzzle of the firearm. A range of scientific concepts underpin internal ballistics, which include combustion theory, Piobert's law of burning, the ideal gas law, laws of thermodynamics, conservation of energy and linear momentum, and Newton's laws of physics (Carlucci and Jacobson, 2008). This section will not explain these concepts in depth, but will introduce the various stages that comprise the ignition of typical modern cartridge-based ammunition.

7.1.4.1 Primer

When the base of the cartridge is struck by the firing pin, this creates an impression in the metal base known as the firing pin impression. The distortion to the base causes the case to strike a metal anvil positioned directly beneath, within the primer unit, thus creating a spark. The spark detonates the unstable, explosive inorganic primer producing a flame jet of approximately 2000°C (Heard, 2008).

The primer mixture comprises an igniter, an oxidizer and a fuel. The igniter is an explosive chemical compound such as lead styphenate or tetrazine (in lead-free ammunition). Barium nitrate is an oxidizer that aids flame production by providing oxygen during the reaction, and antimony sulphide is an example of the fuel needed to increase the temperature and length of the flame.

The flame is forced through one (boxer primer type) or two (berdan primer type) flash holes in the top of the primer unit, which provides sufficient thermal energy to ignite the propellant flakes housed in the main body of the cartridge case.

7.1.4.2 Propellant

Propellant is compressed grains of organic materials designed to burn at a controlled rate. In modern smokeless propellant (as opposed to black powder), nitrocellulose and/or nitroglycerine is the main component.

The shape and dimensions of the grains (ballistic size) and presence/absence of moderators, stabilizers and/or retardant chemicals within or coated on the grain surface(s) can control the burning rate of the propellant. As the grains combust, they produce a large volume of gas (primarily carbon dioxide and water vapour), which is sealed inside the cartridge case and chamber of the firearm. The temperature and pressure builds inside the cartridge, thereby increasing the burning rate of the propellant and resulting in an exponential rate of combustion. The initial rate of combustion is also determined by the ratio between propellant volume and case volume; a greater volume of unfilled space in the cartridge case will result in a slower combustion rate, as the gas has more space to fill before the pressure can start to rise. When the pressure is high enough in the cartridge it forces the projectile(s) free from the cartridge case; this is known as shot start (Farrar and Leeming, 1983).

7.1.4.3   Projectile

At shot start, the projectile(s) starts to travel down the barrel of the weapon and accelerates due to the work done by the high-pressure gas on the entire surface of the projectile base, which increases energy transferred to the projectile. Due to the increase in space behind the projectile, the pressure is still rising, but the propellant starts to burn at an increasingly slower rate. Peak pressure occurs approximately 0.5 ms after cartridge ignition and can be in excess of 300 MPa (Warlow, 2011).

If the barrel is rifled (see Section 7.1.5.2) then there will be some friction when the projectile engages with the slightly smaller dimension of the barrel bore created by lands of the barrel rifling. Some gas will escape in front of the projectile through the grooves of the rifling as these may be deeper than the maximum diameter of the projectile. If the barrel is smooth bore and multiple projectiles are fired from the cartridge, as with a shotgun, some gas may escape by passing between and around the shot inside the barrel.

At the time of peak pressure, the projectile may have only moved 2 cm. As the projectile accelerates and level of kinetic energy overcomes the initial frictional force, an increasing volume will be left behind the projectile and the rate of burning continues to reduce as the propellant flakes reduce in size and produce less gaseous products. Providing sufficient force is maintained as the propellant burns, the projectile(s) will pass down the barrel to the muzzle exit within 2 ms from the strike of the firing pin (Warlow, 2011).

The precise velocity of the projectile prior to exit will vary to some extent from the ammunition manufacturer's specifications, depending on the specifications of the model of firearm the ammunition is fired from. For example, for a given cartridge, the tighter the fit of the projectile within the barrel bore, the greater the level of friction initially acting against the forward motion of the projectile, and therefore the lower the muzzle velocity. If the barrel is longer, then frictional force may act for longer. There will also be some variability from cartridge to cartridge due to the tolerances during ammunition production and how the cartridge seats in the breech of the weapon.

7.1.4.4   Weapon

The detonation of the primer, combustion of the propellant and friction generated (typically for rifled barrels) between the barrel and the projectile will transfer thermal energy to the metallic firearm components, primarily the chamber and barrel. Lawton (2001) indicates barrel bore temperatures in the region of 1100°C, whereas Warlow (2011) suggests over 2200°C. Contact between firearm components and ammunition, together with these extreme temperatures, even over such a short period of time, will cause surface melting and enhanced wear of the weapon components.

When the propellant combusts, the pressure of the gases does not only act in the direction of the projectile base, but in all directions around the breech of the weapon. As a result, while the projectile remains inside the barrel, the pressure exerted forwards on the projectile is experienced backwards on the weapon, known as recoil. Typically, the greater the recoil velocity, the more uncomfortable the weapon is to fire. The production of high-pressure gas or recoil energy generated can be exploited in the weapon design and be utilized by the firing mechanism to eject fired cartridge cases after discharge and load new cartridges (auto-loading).

As the pressure acts in all directions, the muzzle of the weapon will also lift slightly above its point of aim, especially if the muzzle end of the weapon is unsupported.

Barrel lift will vary depending on the ammunition utilized and will ultimately affect shooting accuracy. This needs to be considered when sighting the weapon and firing in automatic modes.

7.1.4.5   Production of gunshot residue (GSR)

The inorganic primer and organic propellant will not completely burn during ignition of the cartridge. This generates a mixture of unburnt, partially burnt and still burning particles, referred to as gunshot residue (GSR) or firearms discharge residue. GSR will also contain some of the metallic particles produced from the wear of the firearm component surfaces, together with the ammunition materials removed by striated contact with the weapon components, such as the barrel. GSR particles predominantly exit the weapon once the projectile has left the muzzle, but some will escape before the projectile(s) exits and GSR will be carried by the escaping gaseous combustion products in gaps between the projectile(s) and bore surface. GSR will also exit from any opening within the firearm, such as the ejection port (semi-automatic weapon) or cylinder (revolver).

Partially burnt and still burning particles are important with respect to intermediate ballistics (Section 7.1.5), as well as being significant to forensic investigation. In the context of veterinary forensics, presence or absence of GSR can assist with determining firing distance between muzzle and the target, differentiating between initial entry and exit wounds and identification of the type of ammunition used (Heard, 2008; Brożek-Mucha, 2009; Dalby et al., 2010; Haag and Haag, 2011; Warlow, 2011).

7.1.5   Intermediate ballistics

Intermediate ballistics is a transitional area covering the moment the projectile exits the barrel until the projectile is considered to be in free flight. Heard (2008) encompasses intermediate ballistics within the scope of wider external ballistics, whereas more specialized literature (Carlucci and Jacobson, 2008) classifies intermediate ballistics as an area in its own right. The time and distance that intermediate ballistics covers will vary, depending on the type of ammunition used and the ballistic properties of the projectile. This section will briefly discuss how the flow of gaseous combustion products and presence of muzzle attachments influence propellant particles and the motion of the projectile upon muzzle exit.

7.1.5.1   Propellant particles and gaseous combustion products

As previously discussed, high-pressure combustion products escape the muzzle in front of the projectile due to the high pressure release of gas after shot start, together with a column of air that is pushed forwards by the moving projectile. When these high-pressure gases exit the muzzle, a shock wave (precursor blast shock) is created just in front of the muzzle, travelling slightly above 340 m/s (speed of sound) and meets with the 'normal' atmosphere. This shock wave generates a sonic bang and radiates out in a spherical direction away from the muzzle.

Precursor bottle shock and the Mach disk also occurs around the muzzle as the precursor blast shock is trying to travel back inside the barrel, against the flow of gas (Carlucci and Jacobson, 2008). The bottle shock increases as the gas velocity increases; as gas velocity reduces the bottle shock will eventually shrink back inside the barrel.

When the projectile exits the muzzle, the gas seal is broken and a further release of highly pressurized gas is released into the atmosphere. A second high-pressure blast wave is formed, together with further bottle shock and Mach disk. This second blast wave is higher in pressure than the precursor blast wave and is initially non-spherical due to the projectile and flow of combustion gases. This blast wave accelerates the combustion products forwards, creating a turbulent column of gas. The column of gas initially overtakes the projectile, causing a shock wave around the base of the projectile (stern shock), which can accelerate the projectile and produce instability and yawing. The spherical blast shock is travelling faster and has more energy than the precursor blast shock and catches up with it; shock waves lose energy and velocity as they increase in size and the gas molecules dissipate.

Within the gaseous combustion products, still burning propellant particles are also present. These particles exit from the barrel in front of the projectile, but are predominantly built up behind the projectile. As these particles pass through high-pressure shock waves, their temperature and burning rate increases producing visible light (incandescent radiation), known as muzzle flash. Preflash can occur before the projectile exits the muzzle, but primary muzzle flash occurs at the muzzle of the firearm after projectile exit. Intermediate muzzle flash can occur further from the muzzle. As the gases in the bottle shock expand rapidly they cool down and a faint muzzle glow can be seen moving away from the muzzle.

Once all the combustion products have been released from the barrel, there is a void in the barrel bore. As the blast shock radiates out in all directions, the blast wave can then recede down the empty barrel along with some of the combustion products. If a target is in close proximity to the muzzle upon discharge, it is this vacuum effect which sucks the target material back inside the barrel, which can therefore be of forensic significance when interpreting the shooting incident.

7.1.5.2   Projectile

Upon muzzle exit, the projectile is in a turbulent atmosphere and is therefore not fully stabilized. This can have varying degrees of impact on the projectile, depending on its shape. For example, cannonballs and shot are typically spherical and therefore turbulence will affect the object similarly in all directions. With most other types of projectile, however, they are designed to be aerodynamic and stable during free flight and may have characteristic features (such as fins) on the surface to ensure that the projectile arrives at the target nose first.

Turbulence created by the combustion products initially destabilizes these projectiles, causing the projectile to yaw slightly (1.5° for a 0.303-in. rifle bullet (Heard, 2008)), i.e.

the nose to rise or fall above or below the projectile's line of flight base, which increases the surface area presented at the projectile nose. Such increase in surface area increases the air resistance around the projectile, reducing projectile velocity and, without a rotational force about the centre of mass, this would cause the bullet to tumble. Tumbling would ultimately reduce projectile velocity, energy, distance (range), accuracy, precision of fire, but increase damage/wound potential due to an increased surface area upon contact with the target.

To counteract destabilization, the rifling inside the barrel consists of spiral lands and grooves. The higher-profile lands on either side of the grooves in the barrel bore are smaller in diameter compared to the maximum diameter of the projectile and therefore engrave into the surface of the projectile, gripping the projectile and bringing about rotation as the projectile travels down the barrel. Upon muzzle exit, the projectile will be rotating at a pre-defined rate. This rotation helps to re-stabilize the projectile as it travels through the turbulent gas due to gyroscopic nutation and thus, the rate of rifling twist down the barrel is important for optimum stabilization of the projectile.

Depending on the muzzle velocity of the projectile, the projectile will either not reach the blast wave (subsonic projectile), or overtake the blast shock (supersonic projectile) and generate a shock wave and audible sonic bang from the nose of the projectile. With supersonic projectiles, a further shock wave and sonic bang will be created when the base of the projectile subsequently passes through the blast shock.

7.1.5.3   Muzzle attachments

Heard (2008) indicates there are six types of muzzle attachment for pistols, revolvers, rifles and shotguns:

1. Sound suppressors.
2. Recoil reducers (compensators).
3. Flash hiders.
4. Muzzle counter weights (to reduce muzzle lift).
5. Grenade dischargers.
6. Recoil boosters.

Only the first three will be discussed here, as these have a direct influence on intermediate ballistics.

Sound suppressors are predominantly designed to reduce noise generated from an expanding gas pressure wave by 18–32 dB (Heard, 2008). They also act to reduce flash and recoil to some extent. Such attachments lower the energy of the gas by allowing the gases to expand within a closed container, by increasing the volume the gas flows into or by making the gas do mechanical work (moving a rotor, for example), or by reducing the temperature through absorption. Those suppressors that are built into the barrel can also reduce the muzzle velocity of the projectile to less than the speed of sound, thereby preventing the supersonic boom of firing by bleeding off some gas near the muzzle of the weapon.

Recoil reducers (or muzzle brakes) are designed to direct the muzzle gas sideways rather than in a primary forwards motion. Gas deflection is obtained by placing one or more sets of symmetrical ports along the sides of the muzzle attachment for gases to escape.

Modern flash hiders are usually the simplest type of muzzle attachment. These devices are primarily designed to reduce intermediate muzzle flash by dispersing the muzzle gas and breaking up the barrel shock and Mach disk. They are usually cone-shaped, a tube with odd-numbered slots, or a bar style (Farrar and Leeming, 1983; Carlucci and Jacobson, 2008).

7.1.6 External ballistics

External ballistics covers the period of flight from the point at which the projectile is stable and behaving within 'normal' atmospheric conditions until the moment it comes into contact with an object. Like internal ballistics, this aspect is very complex and involves extensive mathematical computation to determine a projectile's flight path. This section considers basic concepts that critically underpin this area of applied physics.

7.1.6.1 Muzzle velocity and kinetic energy

During internal ballistics, approximately 30% of the energy created is actually transferred to the projectile(s) (Warlow, 2011), predominantly in the form of kinetic energy, resulting in acceleration of the projectile(s) to a known velocity. Following muzzle exit and a very short distance past the muzzle, the projectile reaches a maximum velocity, referred to as muzzle velocity. Muzzle velocity is pre-determined by the ammunition manufacturer; however, as previously explained, fired projectiles may not reach the technical specification of muzzle velocity quoted by the ammunition manufacturer.

Kinetic energy and muzzle velocity are two of three linked factors; the third component that affects muzzle velocity and the kinetic energy is the projectile mass. Kinetic energy is calculated by squaring the velocity and then multiplying this by half the mass of the projectile. As the mass of the projectile increases, a greater amount of work, force and energy is required to move the projectile the same amount. Therefore, for two projectiles of different masses to have the same muzzle velocity, more kinetic energy (and therefore a higher gas pressure) is required to fire the heavier projectile. A projectile with higher mass will ultimately enhance its 'carrying power' (Heard, 2008).

When considering terminal ballistics later on, the kinetic energy of the projectile is of greater importance than the velocity of the projectile, as kinetic energy takes into account both projectile mass and velocity. It is also the ability of the projectile design to transfer energy to the other object that impacts on the resulting damage to the object.

As soon as the projectile exits the muzzle, the energy and force acting on the projectile is in the forwards (horizontal) direction away from the muzzle, therefore the velocity vector has a positive value. Initially this will be the dominant direction of force acting on the projectile. However, unless the projectile is fired into a vacuum, there will always be forces acting against the projectile in the opposite direction limiting the forwards progression, reducing the kinetic energy and therefore the velocity of the projectile over time. These opposing forces are from the interaction with molecules within the atmosphere; the phenomenon is known as air resistance (drag). The forward movement of the projectile compresses the air molecules in front of it causing areas of higher pressure which act in all directions around the front of the projectile. Minimizing the cross-sectional area of the projectile and making the projectile less angular will reduce air resistance. The air molecules then flow around the projectile, a small amount of surface (skin) friction is created between the air molecules and the sides of the projectile, further reducing the kinetic energy and velocity of the projectile.

When the air molecules have passed over the sides of the projectile, they have to fill in the space left by the base of the projectile. This again causes high-pressure regions at the back edges of the projectile and leaves a turbulent wake of gas behind the projectile. The shape of the nose and base of the projectile are therefore critical to limiting the effect of air resistance on the kinetic energy and velocity of the projectile. A more aerodynamically shaped projectile will exhibit a slower decline in velocity and kinetic energy due to air resistance. Aerodynamically shaped projectiles will display

a long, sharp and low-angled nose (spitzer) to reduce the cross-sectional surface area initially presented to the air and may even have a slightly angled base (boat-tail) to improve the flow of air particles and reduce turbulence from air molecules behind the projectile. The term ballistic coefficient is used to calculate the decline in projectile velocity due to the air, and takes into account projectile mass and diameter (Carlucci and Jacobson, 2008). Typically, the higher the ballistic coefficient, the better a projectile retains its velocity over time. Using data provided by Forker (2010), Table 7.1.2 and Fig. 7.1.2 illustrate how the projectile energy changes for some common cartridges.

7.1.6.2 Trajectory

Air resistance is not the only force acting on the projectile. Acceleration due to gravitational pull from the Earth is constantly acting downwards in the vertical direction on the unsupported object at 9.81 ms^{-2} (Haag and Haag, 2011). As a result, the natural flight path or trajectory will always ultimately curve downwards towards the ground (bullet drop), unless the trajectory is prematurely interrupted by an object.

Table 7.1.2. Examples of various cartridges.

Firearm Type	Cartridge	Manufacturer	Projectile Type	Bullet Weight (g)	G1 Ballistic Coefficient	Muzzle Velocity (fps)	Muzzle Velocity (m/s)
Revolver	0.357 Magnum	Sellier and Bellot	FMJ	158	0.154	1263	385
Pistol	0.45 ACP	American Eagle (Federal)	FMJ	230	0.178	890	271
	9×19 mm	Sellier and Bellot	FMJ	115	0.102	1280	390
Rifle	0.22 Hornet	Sellier and Bellot	FMJ	45	0.102	2346	715
	0.223 Remington	American Eagle (Federal)	FMJ Boat-tail	55	0.270	3240	988
	0.303 British	Sellier and Bellot	FMJ	180	0.564	2438	743
	0.458 Winchester Magnum	Hornady	DGX	500	0.295	2260	689
	7.62 mm NATO	American Eagle (Federal)	FMJ Boat-tail	150	0.409	2820	860

(a)

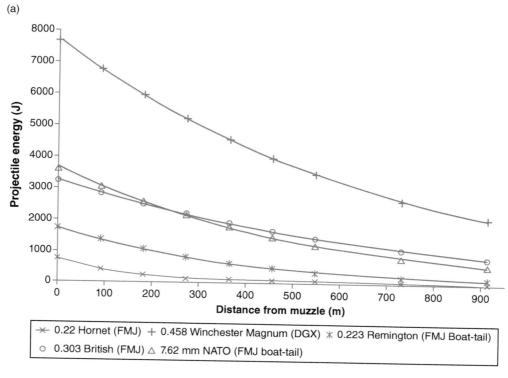

(b)

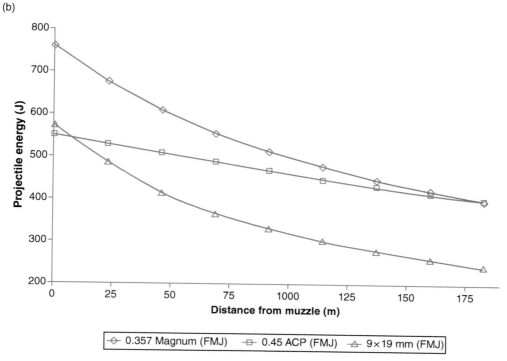

Fig. 7.1.2. Projectile energy changes for some common cartridges.

The initial projectile trajectory will be affected by the muzzle firing angle (angle of inclination). However, it is typical for the projectile not to exit the muzzle aligned with the bore so it will experience vertical and lateral jump (Carlucci and Jacobson, 2008) caused by air resistance. Considering only the effect of vertical gravitation force on a projectile fired in a vacuum at 45°, for example, the trajectory would be a symmetrical parabolic curve about a peak height.

In atmospheric conditions, this parabolic curve is no longer symmetrical due to the effect of air resistance (wave drag, base drag and skin friction). The forces counteracting the forward motion of the projectile will cause the projectile not to reach as high vertical distance or as long horizontal distance (range). The velocity of the projectile will reduce over the time of flight at an exponential rate; therefore, the faster the muzzle velocity of the projectile, the greater the velocity lost per unit of time.

Many firearms are discharged at relatively low-angle (flat) trajectories over relatively short range; however, when the target is positioned at a significant range or the projectile needs to travel over obstacles in the line of sight, higher angles of trajectory are employed, exploiting the curved trajectory.

7.1.6.3   Range

Maximum effective range of real projectile trajectories can be difficult to calculate. Range is affected by the muzzle velocity, the mass, shape and cross-sectional area of the projectile. Other effects include altitude, barometric pressure, crosswind, humidity and temperature. However, to consider the effects of all these variables is outside the scope of this chapter.

As velocity is calculated by dividing distance by time, the greater the velocity of the projectile, the further the projectile will travel in a set period of time. To maximize range, the aerodynamic shape and geometry of the projectile are critical depending on projectile muzzle velocity (subsonic or supersonic). Subsonic projectiles are most influenced by base drag, whereas supersonic

projectiles are most influenced by wave drag, and therefore the nose of supersonic projectiles needs to be designed to minimize drag.

Angle of inclination has a significant role in the maximum potential range of fire for a projectile. For a specific projectile fired in a vacuum on Earth, the time spent in free flight for the same ammunition will be identical, but the maximum range will be obtained when there is as much forwards motion as vertical motion. Maximum theoretical range will therefore occur at 45° inclination due to the trajectory's symmetrical shape; 30° and 60° firing angles will result in identical, but reduced, range of fire compared to 45°.

Considering the impact of firing angle alone in atmospheric conditions, maximum range will typically be generated when fired between 27° and 30° (Carlucci and Jacobson, 2008), although Haag and Haag (2011) indicates 30° to 35° for handgun cartridges. The accent of the projectile to peak height will be slightly lower and of less distance compared to in the vacuum, but the biggest effect to range occurs during projectile descent to ground. Pistol and revolver bullets, when fired at their optimum departure angle can reach a maximum range of 1000–2000 m, whereas rifle bullets can reach between 3000 m and 4000 m (Haag and Haag, 2011).

Shot need to be considered separately. Shot are spherical, symmetrical and do not require stabilization by rotational force. Spheres are less aerodynamic, and these projectiles are not designed to be fired over long distances. Their maximum range in air has been demonstrated to be 1–3% of the range achieved if fired in a vacuum (Chugh, 1982) compared to approximately 20% for bullets. As there are multiple projectiles, shot spread out over range and can be used more effectively for distance determination (Çakir et al., 2003; Haag and Haag, 2011).

7.1.6.4   Accuracy and precision

The accuracy (closeness to the intended point of impact) and precision (spread around the intended point of impact) of the projectile will be affected by the firer, weapon and atmospheric conditions, including wind speed and direction, the extent of which is outside the scope of this chapter; however, some examples are considered.

The weapon type is important to consider. Handguns are typically designed for close combat and therefore less accurate and precise over distance than rifles. Generally, this is due to the shorter barrel and less aerodynamic projectiles. By design, shotguns firing a number of shot are primarily used for hunting and therefore accuracy and precision are less critical as there are multiple shot that spread out as range of fire increases, and therefore the shot are more likely to penetrate and strike the animal.

Firing a brand new weapon from a fixed firing position should provide excellent accuracy and precision. Over time, as weapon components such as the barrel suffer from wear, the tolerance to generate a stable projectile during flight increases and this has a negative effect on accuracy and precision. Incorrect support, handling and aim of the weapon during firing (Goonetilleke *et al.*, 2009) will reduce accuracy and lower precision due to recoil forces, whereas reducing the trigger pull force required to action the trigger mechanism and discharge a round can increase precision and accuracy.

7.1.7   Terminal ballistics

Energy and design of the projectile as well as the density, material properties and surface roughness will affect what happens to the projectile when it hits a target surface. Target materials that are less dense and more malleable than the projectile materials are more likely to deform, be penetrated to some extent and absorb more energy from the projectile, compared to those that are denser and have greater hardness. Yielding surfaces that deform upon impact produce greater angles of projectile ricochet than unyielding surfaces (Haag and Haag, 2011).

The design of the projectile will have an effect on the potential for ricochet. Some projectiles (e.g. soft-point or hollow-point

bullets) are designed to mushroom at the nose to increase surface area and increase the transfer of energy from the projectile to the target. The consequence is a greater damage/wounding potential. FMJ projectiles, however, are not designed to deform on impact and therefore do not transfer as much energy into the target, ultimately reducing the damage/wound potential and increasing the depth of penetration into the target.

The angle at which the projectile hits the target also affects whether the projectile is more likely to penetrate into the target or ricochet, i.e. deflect off the target surface. For every combination of specific projectile design and target surface, there will be a critical angle that determines whether the projectile penetrates or has the potential to ricochet. Generally, the critical angle will be relatively low (oblique) and the projectile typically ricochets off at a comparably lower angle (Haag and Haag, 2011).

The effect of ricochet and tumbling will affect the size and shape of penetrating wounds (Section 7.2). Tumbling or instability in a projectile will cause it to yaw. If the projectile hits an animal in a state of yaw rather than perpendicular and nose first, the surface area where impact occurs is increased and therefore the size of the entry wound may be increased. Such impact angle can also transfer energy into the animal/target more effectively. However, if the projectile is designed to transfer energy effectively (for example, a hollow-point or soft-point) then the energy transfer may be less effective as the nose will not be able to perform as designed.

7.1.8   Retrieval of fired ammunition components

7.1.8.1   Cartridges and fired cartridge cases

If you are called to a crime scene of a suspected shooting, the forensic veterinarian should be aware of the potential for finding live ammunition as well as fired cartridge case evidence. Depending on the nature of the scene and the location of the incident geographically, there will be a variety of policies governing who recovers this physical evidence. The purpose of this section is to remind the practitioner that such evidence has forensic value in inferring the calibre and type of firearm likely to have discharged the cartridge, the number of weapons involved, and has the potential to link crimes utilizing discharge of the same weapon in various cases; and microscopic examination of fired cartridge case evidence can uniquely identify the firearm that discharged it, if a weapon is ultimately recovered.

If unfired ammunition is discovered, the cartridges need to be recovered using good practice to minimize contamination, such as wearing gloves, and should be packaged separately to any weapon recovered to minimize risk and prevent accidental firing. Cartridges should be packaged in paper bags, cardboard boxes or plastic containers (Tilstone et al., 2013) lined with non-abrasive material (not cotton wool) to prevent them rolling around during transportation.

If fired cartridge cases, shotgun wadding (typically made of fibre or plastic) and/ or projectiles are observed in the scene surroundings they should be recovered using *plastic* forceps or tweezers, to prevent damage to the evidence surface (Bruce-Chwatt, 2010). Handling items with metal tweezers of a harder material than the evidence may cause permanent toolmarks on the evidence surface, that could damage or impede forensic examination and interpretation subsequently undertaken by firearms examiners. Fired cartridge cases, like the cartridges themselves, should be packaged as they are recovered from the scene in paper bags, cardboard boxes or plastic containers lined with polythene/non-abrasive material (not cotton wool), with the latter preferably used for fired projectiles and wadding.

7.1.8.2   Fired projectiles and shotgun wadding

Fired projectiles, such as bullets, pellets (air weapons), slugs or shot (shotgun) may be present in the animal. Even legal unlicensed air weapons can penetrate animal skin, but research has shown that the type of animal

(Wightman et al., 2013) and the thickness and material properties of their skin will influence the ability for the pellet to penetrate, together with the energy and shape of the projectile.

As previously stated, any fired projectiles recovered should be handled with plastic tweezers or forceps to prevent damage to the forensic characteristics. Upon recovery of the projectile, this should be washed with sterile water to remove biological hazards (different protocols are required for projectile retrieval from humans) and air-dried before packaging, to prevent any corrosion of the projectile material surface. Packaging for fired projectiles is ideally in polythene and plastic containers, i.e. not containing cotton wool.

Wadding components within shotgun cartridges are ejected from the cartridge along with the single slug or multiple shot. This can travel over 30 m from the muzzle of the weapon (Bonfanti and De Kinder, 2013) and, therefore, finding wadding inside a wound tract or permanent cavity can imply that the weapon has been discharged at close range to the target. Recovery and packaging of shotgun wadding should be as described above for fired projectiles.

7.1.8.3   Gunshot residue (GSR)

GSR can be sampled with commercially available GSR collection kits by swabbing around the area of the wound entry. GSR may be differentiated from other metallic residues (Romolo and Margot, 2001; Dalby et al., 2010; Grima et al., 2012) and can sometimes be uniquely identified to a type of ammunition (Brozek-Mucha and Jankowicz, 2001); for example, if the composition of the primer is very distinctive. GSR can be indicative of close range of fire (Ditrich, 2012), as can the presence of stippling, powder tattooing on the skin and burning of hair from burning propellant flakes and hot gases released from the muzzle of the firearm. However, if an air weapon was utilized, such characteristics will not be present around an entry wound, even at close proximity, as there is no combustion of propellant used to propel the pellet out of the weapon.

7.1.9 Conclusion

This section aimed to introduce some of the key scientific principles underpinning shooting incidents that may influence observed wounding in animals. Variations in the type of firearm and ammunition (internal ballistics) used in the shooting as well as environmental conditions and shooting distances (external ballistics), location of impact, composition of the target material and design of the projectile upon impact (terminal ballistics), for example, may all cause variations in the expected severity of damage and lethality. By understanding how these factors may affect wounding, potential forensic veterinarians may have an increased capacity to interpret the manner in which injuries have been sustained and provide further information to the forensic investigative process.

The essential steps in the forensic examination and investigation of a shot animal were identified, clearly highlighting the requirement for a logical and methodical approach supported by extensive documentation. The approach for animals should be similar to that conducted on humans and all wound ballistics research may be relevant for consideration in application to animal practice. It is vital for external observations to be completed before invasive internal examination commences, and modern noninvasive imaging technologies, including computer tomography (CT) and ultrasound, should be employed at the earliest opportunity. Use of such technologies facilitates the formation of the forensic examination strategy by providing visualization of bullet-wound channels, projectiles or projectile fragments, and the presence of fractures and other damage in the animal prior to invasive action.

Firearms evidence collated from both the crime scene and the injured animal can provide vital information and intelligence to those investigating both domestic animal and wildlife crimes. The form and extent of firearms evidence that may be located at a crime scene will also vary, depending on the firearm, ammunition and ballistic variables. Correct handling and recovery of such evidence is important for any further analysis requested to be probative in the case. Demonstration of the breadth of knowledge required to investigate shooting incidents may highlight the need for forensic veterinarians to get in contact with subject experts to provide support prior to and during forensic examinations and any subsequent investigation. By building a strong prosecution case, including corroborative evidence from firearms examiners, investigators are more likely to be able to link crime series and identify those involved in the crimes, to ultimately increase the probability of prosecution and conviction in forensic cases.

References

AFTE Training and Standardization Committee (ed.) (2007) *Glossary of Association of Firearms and Tool Mark Examiner*, 5th edn. AFTE, Montreal, Canada. Available on CD-ROM.

Berman, G. (2012) *Firearm Crime Statistics*. SN/SG/1940. House of Commons, London, UK.

Bolton-King, R.S. (2012) Classification of barrel rifling transitions for the identification of firearms. PhD thesis. Nottingham Trent University, Nottingham, UK.

Bonfanti, M.S. and De Kinder, J. (2013) Shotgun ammunition on a target. In: Siegel, J.A., Saukko, P.J. and Houck, M.M. (eds) *Encyclopedia of Forensic Sciences*. Academic Press, Waltham, Massachusetts, USA, pp. 48–53.

Brożek-Mucha, Z. (2009) Distribution and properties of gunshot residue originating from a Luger 9 mm ammunition in the vicinity of the shooting gun. *Forensic Science International* 183(1–3), 33–44.

Brozek-Mucha, Z. and Jankowicz, A. (2001) Evaluation of the possibility of differentiation between various types of ammunition by means of GSR examination with SEM–EDX method. *Forensic Science International* 123(1), 39–47.

Bruce-Chwatt, R.M. (2010) Air gun wounding and current UK laws controlling air weapons. *Journal of Forensic and Legal Medicine* 17(3), 123–126.

Çakir, I., Çetin, G., Uner, H.B. and Albek, E. (2003) Shot range estimation based on pellet distribution in shots with a pump-action shotgun. *Forensic Science International* 132(3), 211–215.

Carlucci, D.E. and Jacobson, S.S. (2008) *Ballistics: Theory and Design of Guns and Ammunition*. CRC Press, Boca Raton, Florida, USA.

Chugh, O.P. (1982) Maximum range of pellets fired from a shotgun. *Forensic Science International* 19(3), 223–230.

Dalby, O., Butler, D. and Birkett, J.W. (2010) Analysis of gunshot residue and associated materials – a review. *Journal of Forensic Sciences* 55(4), 924–943.

Demirci, S., Dogan, K.H. and Koc, S. (2011) Fatal injury by an unmodified blank pistol: a case report and review of the literature. *Journal of Forensic and Legal Medicine* 18(6), 237–241.

Ditrich, H. (2012) Distribution of gunshot residues – the influence of weapon type. *Forensic Science International* 220(1–3), 85–90.

Farrar, C.L. and Leeming, D.W. (1983) *Military Ballistics: A Basic Manual*. Brassey's, London, UK.

Forker, R. (2010) *Ammo and Ballistics 4*, 4th edn. Safari Press, Huntington Beach, California, USA.

Goonetilleke, R.S., Hoffmann, E.R. and Lau, W.C. (2009) Pistol shooting accuracy as dependent on experience, eyes being opened and available viewing time. *Applied Ergonomics* 40(3), 500–508.

Grima, M., Butler, M., Hanson, R. and Mohameden, A.O. (2012) Firework displays as sources of particles similar to gunshot residue. *Science and Justice* 52(1), 49–57.

Haag, M.G. and Haag, L.C. (2011) *Shooting Incident Reconstruction*, 2nd edn. Academic Press, San Diego, California, USA.

Heard, B.J. (2008) *Handbook of Firearms and Ballistics: Examining and Interpreting Forensic Evidence*, 2nd edn. John Wiley, Chichester, UK.

Home Office (2014) *Guide on Firearms Licensing Law*. Home Office, London, UK.

Jones, R.D. and Ness, L.S. (eds) (2009) *Jane's Infantry Weapons 2009–2010,* 35th edn. Jane's Information Group, Surrey, UK.

Lawton, B. (2001) Thermo-chemical erosion in gun barrels. *Wear* 251(1–12), 827–838.

Northern Ireland Office (2005) *Guidance on Northern Ireland Firearms Controls*. Northern Ireland Office, Stormont, Belfast, Northern Ireland, UK.

Oxford University Press (2014) *Oxford Dictionaries: British and World*. Available online at: http://www.oxforddictionaries.com (accessed 10 August 2014).

Romolo, F.S. and Margot, P. (2001) Identification of gunshot residue: a critical review. *Forensic Science International* 119(2), 195–211.

Smith, K., Osborne, S., Ivy, L. and Britton, A. (eds) (2012) *Homicides, Firearm Offences and Intimate Violence 2010/11: Supplementary Volume 2 to Crime in England and Wales 2010/11*. Home Office Statistical Bulletin, 02/12 edn. Home Office: London. Available online at: https://www.gov.uk/government/uploads/system/uploads/attachment_data/file/116483/hosb0212.pdf (accessed 28 August 2014).

Squires, P. (2014) *Gun Crime in Global Contexts*. Routledge, Abingdon, Oxfordshire, UK.

Tilstone, W.J., Hastrup, M.L. and Hald, C. (2013) *Fisher's Techniques of Crime Scene Investigation: First International Edition*. CRC Press, Boca Raton, Florida, USA.

UK Parliament (1988) *Firearms (Amendment) Act 1988*. Available online at: http://www.opsi.gov.uk/acts/acts1988/pdf/ukpga_19880045_en.pdf (accessed 10 August 2014).

Warlow, T. (2011) *Firearms, the Law, and Forensic Ballistics* (International Forensic Science and Investigation), 3rd edn. CRC Press, Boca Raton, USA.

Wightman, G., Cochrane, R., Gray, R.A. and Linton, M. (2013) A contribution to the discussion on the safety of air weapons. *Science and Justice* 53(3), 343–349.

7.2   Wound Ballistics

JOHAN SCHULZE

7.2.1   Introduction

A standard rifle projectile like the 308 Winchester travels with a velocity of about 800 m/s (2625 fps). It takes the projectile less than 0.5 ms to penetrate the skin and to create a wound channel approximately 30 cm (1 ft) long (Braathen *et al.*, 2006). The challenge for the medical investigator is to understand the interaction between projectile and body that takes place within this time frame and to estimate how the body responds to this. He then has to relate this knowledge to his investigation, and if possible formulate an opinion appropriate to answer the demands of the legal system. Interpretations of wound patterns which may be appropriate to human cases may not be directly transferable to animal forensic investigation and should be undertaken with caution.

I will first discuss some basic wound ballistics by looking at the interaction between a body and a penetrating projectile. Next, some specifics not discussed in the first part are highlighted. Finally, essential steps in examination of an animal which has been shot will be outlined. Readers with a special interest in wound ballistics are referred to literature including Fackler (1987), Di Maio (1999), Brinkmann and Madea (2004), Munro and Munro (2008) and Kneubuehl *et al.* (2011).

7.2.2   Basics of wound ballistics

When investigating injuries caused by a projectile, the most important topic is the wound channel caused by the passage of the projectile through the body. No two wound channels are alike. Innumerable modifying factors make it impossible to accurately predict the course or form of a particular wound channel. Nevertheless, some important physical mechanisms are well established and knowledge of them is crucial when working with such injuries. The following describes a wound channel caused by a *non-deforming, non-fragmenting rifle bullet*. Other types of projectiles and weapons will cause other effects, and some of these are discussed later in the chapter.

A bullet entering a dense medium, like a body (or ballistic gelatine), transfers energy to the medium into which it penetrates. Wounding mechanisms of stretching, compression and shearing are initiated. Particles directly struck by, or close to, the projectile receive a radial accelerative force causing their temporary displacement perpendicular to the axis along which the projectile travels. The effect of this radial dislocation can be compared with a hard and radiating punch originating from the wound channel. The centrifugal movement of the medium lasts until the transmitted energy is spent or is absorbed by elastic tissues (or gel). At this state, about 2–4 ms after the hit, the moving projectile has not only created a wound channel approximately the diameter of its calibre, but also an additional larger cavity. This cavity, known as the *temporary wound channel*, collapses immediately as the elasticity of the tissue allows the particles to return towards their original position, hereby releasing the stored energy. Depending on the tissue or medium involved, the pulsation away from and towards the permanent wound channel continues until all transferred energy has been translated into friction and thermal energy. Naturally, this forceful radial pulsation causes anatomical and physiological damage in the living tissue.

Anatomical damage is mainly crushing and tearing. Some tissue close to the passing projectile may also be destroyed by the heavy centrifugal acceleration described above. This central core of the wound channel, originated by the destruction of tissue by the projectile, is called the *permanent wound channel*. The permanent wound channel is encircled by the now relocated but previously compressed tissue that had circumscribed the temporary wound channel. In contrast to the debris related to that of the permanent wound channel, this latter tissue zone has (at least for the meanwhile) maintained viability, despite having been through forced radial pulsation.

Though viability may be maintained, it is obvious that tissue close to the permanent wound channel, having been stretched and compressed considerably more forcibly, is likely to show more severe damage than tissue that is more distant. An area surrounding the permanent wound channel, named the *extravasation zone* (Fig. 7.2.1), is characterized by haemorrhage from lacerated capillaries. The haemorrhages are caused more by the stretching of blood vessels, to which they are very vulnerable, than by their being torn (Kneubuehl *et al.*, 2011). Bones are far less elastic. The size of a penetration through a flat bone, like a scapula, can be a very close approximation of the calibre of the projectile (Karger, 2004).

The overall form of the wound channel is far from homogenous. Its shape is a direct result of the amount of energy transferred from the projectile on its path through the tissue. The more energy that is transmitted, the harder is the impact and consequently the greater the dimensions of the permanent and temporary wound channels. The amount of energy transmitted per unit distance (E_{tr}) is proportional to the amount of energy the projectile has stored (E) and inversely proportional to its sectional density (m/A). The sectional density is defined as the ratio of the mass of the bullet (m) to the cross-sectional area of contact between bullet and medium (A).

$$E_{tr} = E/(m/A)$$

A bullet travelling perpendicularly to the plane of contact (*tip-first* position) has a small cross-sectional area. Hence the amount of energy transferred is low compared to the same bullet having rotated and thus presenting a larger cross-sectional area.

In Fig. 7.2.1 below, the longitudinal section in the lower part of the figure covers the total length of the wound channel; the two cross-sections in the upper part illustrate the profile of the wound channel at the levels of the narrow channel (left) and temporary cavity (right).

It is difficult to appreciate a detailed impression of the extent of a wound channel in

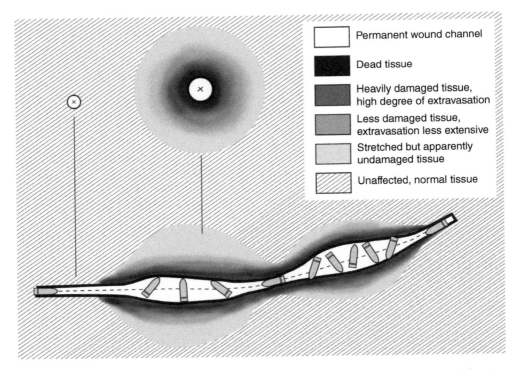

Permanent wound channel

Dead tissue

Heavily damaged tissue, high degree of extravasation

Less damaged tissue, extravasation less extensive

Stretched but apparently undamaged tissue

Unaffected, normal tissue

Fig. 7.2.1. Idealized schematic diagram of a wound channel created by the movement of a non-deforming rifle bullet through tissue (based on Kneubuehl *et al.* (2011) and Karger (2004)).

a body. Fortunately the physical processes involved have been visualized by experiments, mainly through the study of wound channels in simulants for natural bodies such as ballistic gelatine and soap (Nicholas and Welsch, 2004).

Long and slender rifle bullets striking the surface perpendicularly can stabilize themselves in the tip-first position. The exposure of a small cross-sectional area leads to both permanent and temporary wound channels initially being narrow, termed *narrow wound channel*. While slowing down, however, the projectile becomes increasingly unstable and starts to tumble as it proceeds. At this point, the narrow wound channel ends and the second part of the wound channel begins (Fig. 7.2.1). The tumbling motion causes presentation of parts of the bullet's side to the medium. The cross-sectional area of contact increases momentarily while the mass of the projectile, due to the law of inertia, initially ensures the maintenance of its velocity. The dramatic increase of transferred energy is accordingly reflected in the dimensions of the wound channel, which consequently expands, often considerably.

Having lost stability along the longitudinal axis, the projectile rotates around its transversal axis. In general the rotation will first turn the projectile into a position approximately 90° to its direction of movement. Because of inertia, however, the projectile may continue to rotate to 180°, or even up to 270°, out of line. At the same time, the bullet is decelerated far more markedly than in the narrow wound channel.

Clearly, more extensive injuries are to be expected from the tumbling of a long, fast-travelling rifle projectile than from a shorter and slower handgun bullet.

Even in a homogenous medium, the axis of the wound channel is not necessarily straight. When not in tip-first position, the cross-sectional area of the bullet is asymmetric. The sum of the withstanding forces affecting the projectile is not solely directed towards the opposite direction to that of the motion of the bullet. Hence the bullet receives an additional force vectored perpendicularly to its direction of travel. This force can be strong enough to change considerably the previous direction of travel of the projectile. This effect may be increased considerably with passage through heterogeneous tissues.

During the last phase of the bullet's journey, particularly the last part of the wound channel, the projectile stabilizes itself, taking a position with its longitudinal axis perpendicular to its direction of movement. In this phase, the projectile has already transferred much of its embedded energy. The kinetic energy transformed in rotation is more and more matched, and finally zeroed, by the resisting medium. The projectile moves through the medium, oscillating round its centre of mass. If the off-centred positioned tip swings faster forward, it meets a higher resistance than the opposite base, and vice versa. Thus a self-adjusting mechanism stabilizes the projectile until it comes to rest, ending the wound channel.

Projectiles may be found with their tail towards their direction of travel. They may also be found slightly withdrawn from the end of the wound channel. This phenomenon is due to residual negative pressure in the temporary wound channel that pulls the projectile slightly backwards once its forward movement has ceased.

This description of the formation and structure of ballistic wound channels is necessarily simplified, with the discussion focusing on a rifle bullet that does not deform, break up or fragment. There are many modifying variables that can alter this picture, but already certain principles are apparent. Thus, when considering missile wound injuries, we may be able to form conclusions or consider different scenarios.

- *The capacity of a bullet to cause injuries does not primarily depend on its energy or calibre, but on its ability to transmit its energy to the body while travelling through it.* If, for example, no exit hole was found and the bullet came to rest in the body, the conclusion must be that all of the energy with which the projectile was loaded when reaching the target was absorbed by the body. If a long narrow wound channel, in the absence of damage to large bones, was demonstrated, one might suspect a long-distance shot. With knowledge of the ammunition used and the extent of the injuries, such conclusions may be justified.

- *A long narrow wound channel can indicate different things:* it might mean, for instance, that signs of a temporary cavity will be recognized deeper in the body than usual, or that the bullet left the body before becoming unstable or deformed (see Section 7.2.3.1, 'Deformation/fragmentation'). It might be as a result of a short bullet fired by a handgun or the passage of a full-jacketed rifle bullet travelling relatively slowly.
- *A prominent temporary wound chamber does not necessarily equate to extensive injuries* – although this is often the case. It merely indicates that a significant amount of energy has been transferred to the body. If the tissue affected has the potential to cope with stretching and twisting, the consequences might be less severe than might otherwise be expected.

7.2.3   Some specifics of wound ballistics

7.2.3.1   Deformation/fragmentation

The deformation of a projectile travelling through a body is not necessarily merely an incidental result of being exposed to massive decelerating forces. Hunting bullets, for example, are designed to expand directly after skin penetration in order to increase the cross-sectional area and thereby enhance the transfer of energy from projectile to animal. In this case, the onset of the temporary cavity might start very early. Due to the rapid increase of the cross-sectional area of the deforming bullet at the very beginning of the wound channel, the narrow channel can be short or almost absent. The aim of hunting bullets is to guarantee the animal's instant death by maximally injuring vital organs. At the same time it is desirable to create an exit wound. In case of not succeeding in an instant kill, an exit wound bleeding to the outside is almost a prerequisite for retrieving the injured animal. Hence, despite the 'mushrooming' bullet deformation, the aim is to achieve a high penetration depth by maintaining the mass of the projectile, and fragmentation

of the bullet is not necessarily welcome in this scenario. Exceptions to these requirements may be determined by specific needs. Beaver hunters try to avoid large exit wounds to maintain the quality of the fur without making concessions in terms of animal welfare. This is achieved by the use of splinter projectiles designed to fragment after impact (Parker *et al.*, 2006).

Fragmentation, caused either by the bullet's design or by chance, increases the overall cross-sectional area, consequently increasing the volume of the temporary cavity. The mass of the original projectile can be reduced considerably (Fackler *et al.*, 1984). The fragments are dispersed away from the axis of the main wound channel. Typically, the distribution of the fragments is cone-shaped and can be visualized by imaging techniques. On an X-ray image, the configuration of fragments of a high-velocity rifle projectile resembles a snowstorm. The longer penetration depth of larger and heavier fragments can be demonstrated, strengthening the evidential value of imaging techniques regarding the line of departure. However, these findings should be verified; for example, by necropsy. Steady linear embedding of bullet fragments into tissue does not necessarily occur and individual fragments might move from the localization into which they initially settled after the bullet disintegrated. 'Loose' fragments can follow the force of gravity, for instance, and be found at the bottom of body cavities, often embedded in blood clots, or can be moved due to vascular embolization. The secondary translocations of bullet fragments like these must, of course, be differentiated and be recorded as such. Furthermore, one should bear in mind that even slow-travelling projectiles, as shotgun pellets, can disrupt upon collision with, for example, bone (Frank, 1986).

Of course, the penetration depth of fragmented and non-fragmented projectiles cannot be compared.

7.2.3.2   Entrance and exit wound

Every external inspection of the animal will include a close examination of entrance and exit wounds. Though these generally are straightforward to distinguish, the assignment of each wound must be undertaken with care. It is the author's experience that entrance wounds in animals seldom show all the features described in standard literature referring to missile wounds in humans. This may be due to intrinsic differences, such as differing density of hair coat, or to the fact that close-distance shots are generally less frequent in animal cases compared with human shootings. The skin of dogs, pigs, sheep and goats are said to react most similarly to that of man (Schantz, 1979). Notwithstanding these possibilities for variation it remains meaningful to take a generic approach to describing the possible composition of entrance and exit wounds, as the wounding mechanisms are the same, regardless of species.

The entrance wound can be considered the first part of the wound channel. Its importance lies in being the first point of contact between the projectile and the body. The entrance wound potentially conveys valuable information about the angle of impact, characteristics of the bullet and the distance between the animal and the muzzle of the weapon. If shot from very close range, singeing of the fur or feathers may be present, but due to the splashing and oozing of blood in the wound area it can be very difficult to recognize.

The entrance wound may be the object of special interest regarding the occurrence of gunshot residues (GSR). To preserve GSRs, all handling of the wound area must be reduced to a minimum, and absolutely no cleaning of the wound should be undertaken uncritically (Karger, 2004)! Though autolysis, moisture, blood and contamination impede GSR analysis, the safest way of submitting an appropriate sample is to excise a larger skin area around the entrance wound (Di Maio, 1999). The intact wound with its encircling skin can then be stored frozen until processed further. In living animals, or if the entrance wound needs to remain with the body at necropsy, GSR can be sampled using cotton buds. On dry wounds, one can use cotton buds wetted with distilled water, tape-lifts or use a fine-toothed comb in the hair surrounding the wound (MacCrehan *et al.*, 2003). Examination for GSRs may be performed by, for example, scanning electron microscope

(Karger, 2004) or energy dispersive X-ray (Di Maio, 1999).

At the margins of the entry wound, different zones merging into each other may be distinguished. The central penetration is caused by the bullet crushing the skin. A circular wound results when the angle of impact was perpendicular to the surface, while an elliptical wound is formed with a low angle of impact. As a consequence of loss of tissue substance the edges of the wound cannot readily be adapted. Again, tissue fragments from the skin are accelerated radially outwards from the central contact zone by the impact of the bullet. After having been stretched outwards, the elastic skin recoils somewhat, so that the entry wound is smaller than the calibre of the bullet. The edge and an area only a few millimetres wide around the entry wound form a ring of discolouration, due to abrasion and possible deposition of gunshot residues. The surface defect is a consequence of the displacement of debris from crushed tissue, as well as the radial acceleration and stretching of the skin caused by the entering bullet. The margin of distention, an outer reddened ring that merges into the unaffected skin, is characterized by multiple petechial sub-epithelial haemorrhages from lacerated capillaries.

Again, an asymmetric elliptical shape to these changes around the central perforation indicates a low angle of impact, with the larger tail pointing towards the shooter. The extent of the damage (as for the exit wound) does not convey detailed information about the bullet used, but it can indicate the amount of energy transferred at this point in the wound channel. There are many factors that can modify the configuration of the entrance wound from that described above, depending on different underlying physical mechanisms. A large irregular star-shaped wound might, for example, be seen when additional forces transmitted by propellant gases from a close-range shot affect the wounding process.

Skin penetration of an exiting bullet involves different mechanisms to those described for the entrance wound. In the majority of cases, the projectile has lost much of its energy and exposes a larger cross-sectional area when it hits the skin from the inside.

Consequently, the tissue is not crushed but buckled and stretched until the bullet is released by rupture of the skin. As no tissue substance is lost, the edges of the irregular-shaped wound can normally be adapted. If, meanwhile, the localization of the exit wound and the large temporary cavity coincide, loss of substance is obvious.

7.2.3.3   Shotgun

The wound picture created by shotgun pellets is largely determined by the range at which the weapon is fired. However, the design of ammunition used and the barrel characteristics are also important. These three factors determine how densely clustered is the sheaf of pellets just before reaching the point of impact.

A pellet sheaf and its ballistic can be compared with a herd of cattle that is to be driven through a river by cowboys. The cowboys determine how densely and how fast the animals move when the herd reaches the edge of the river. In a widely spread herd, the cows will go separately into the river, thereby slowing down, but still in a group that is heading in the same direction. If the herd stays close together, the first animals entering the water will slow down and, being crowded and pushed by the adjacent animals, will deviate sideways.

The wound channel of a close-range shotgun blast may have a larger diameter than the entrance hole, as the decelerated pellets, like the cattle from the example above, are deviated outwards by pellets clashing from behind. The light spherical pellets lose energy quickly and, consequently, the penetration depth of individual pellets generally declines rapidly with increasing range. Nevertheless, the penetration depth can still be considerable, markedly disrupting internal organs. The tissue damage of shotgun wounds, especially close-range wounds, can be extensive. At longer ranges, larger types of shot (size and weight of pellets) produce more serious injuries (Ordog et al., 1988).

It is important to note that the morphology of the skin wound allows only a rough estimation of the shooting range. From shooting distances of around 3 m, differing characteristics of the barrel of the shotgun

and the ammunition cause variation of the wound pattern. Generally, the shorter the distance, the denser will be the injuries of the entrance wound. If directly after leaving the barrel, the shot sheaf has not spread radially, it creates a single prominent circular wound. With rising distances and wider spreading of the shot sheaf, the edge of the wound starts to become undulating (scalloping) or discrete skin perforations caused by individual pellets are seen immediately peripheral to the central wound. With still wider spread (or larger distance) the larger central wound is not present and instead a wound field composed of many individual pellet perforations is found.

The range estimation is based on the wound pattern as long as a central wound is apparent, but is based on the dispersion pattern of the pellets at longer ranges. Correctly scaled documentation of a representative wound field, showing all points of impact within that field, is necessary to compare the pattern in question to the test-shot pattern fired with the same weapon and ammunition. The resulting range estimation would presuppose that the test field was within the core area of the shot sheaf and that the angle of impact was perpendicular (Karger, 2004).

This may illustrate that detailed statements about shooting distances should only be made with caution, and should include a statement of the underlying preconditions.

Shotgun pellets can be made of many different metal alloys, such as lead, steel, tungsten-bismuth-tin (TBT) and other principal constituents. A first impression of what material the shotgun pellet is made of can be achieved by studying the radiological images (see Section 7.2.4.1, 'Before necropsy'). However, true and detailed information is based on the recovery of the pellets. Besides studying obvious injuries, one should pay attention to possible reactions of the surrounding tissue of each recovered pellet. Kraabel et al. (1996) observed a consistent inflammatory response to steel pellets in mallard muscle tissue, a reaction possibly triggered by corrosion. TBT pellets induced comparatively mild inflammatory responses. Sterile steel shots surgically implanted into dogs corroded and resulted in severe inflammatory responses, sometimes complicated by bacterial contamination and foreign-body reactions (Bartels *et al.*, 1991). Species-specific differences in the responses must be taken into account. Tungsten alloy pellets, for instance, implanted intramuscularly into rats, induced growth of aggressive, rapidly metastasizing high-grade pleomorphic rhabdomyosarcomas in an experimental study (Kalinich *et al.*, 2005).

Sampling of tissue in a state of inflammation or granulation provides an opportunity for approximation of age of the process (Schulz, 1990; Wohlsein and Reifinger, 2011).

7.2.3.4 Airgun

Though air weapons are commonly considered toys, or at least non-lethal weapons, projectiles from air-powered guns cause injuries and fatalities (Smith, 1985; Bond *et al.*, 1996; Campbell-Hewson *et al.*, 1997; Milroy *et al.*, 1998). These weapons have been shown to be dangerous devices for humans and animals, and animals wounded by airguns are relatively frequently presented in veterinary clinics (Cooper and Cooper, 2007; Anon., 2013). Even pellets fired from a comparatively low-powered weapon, such as a ball-bearing gun, can penetrate human skin. Such an injury is reported by Tsui *et al.* (2010). A 15-year-old boy suffered from an infected wound caused by a spherical soft airgun pellet, 0.2 g in weight and 6 mm in diameter, discharged from legal weapons with muzzle energy not greater than 2 Joule. Other authors (Phillips, 1979; Sinclair *et al.*, 2006; Cooper and Cooper, 2007; Merck, 2007; Munro and Munro, 2008; de la Fuente *et al.*, 2013) discuss the ability of airgun pellets, usually .177 calibre (4.5 mm) with a law-regulated maximum muzzle velocity of maximal 7.5 Joule,[1] to penetrate human skin or the cornea of the human eye. Penetration depth in ballistic gel close to 8 cm for 5.5 mm pellets fired from 10 m range has been reported by Ogunc *et al.* (2013). As in anthropocentric forensics (Bond *et al.*, 1996), veterinarians should no longer underestimate the potential for life-threatening injury from these weapons.

As stated above, generalization across species is problematic, as both general anatomical differences and absolute differences can be distinct. The skin of birds is, for instance, generally far thinner than mammal skin (Vollmerhaus *et al.*, 1992), not to mention the vast proportional differences between humans and, for example, a budgerigar with a body weight of 45 g. Wightman *et al.* (2013) mounted fresh skin samples of different animal species on blocks of gelatin to test the effect of the skin on the perforation ability of airgun pellets; chicken skin had no effect, pig skin stopped the pellet and cow skin was perforated by the pellets.

Small calibre and light weight of airgun pellets must not be equated with being innocuous. After discharge, the velocity of the projectiles decreases rapidly and the sectional density of the pellets is comparatively low. There is a need for a high muzzle velocity to counteract these ballistic disadvantages. Therefore, unless the anatomical structures at the point of impact are very delicate, the barrel–target distance must be relatively short to cause serious injuries (Missliwetz, 1987; Kneubuehl *et al.*, 2011). Nevertheless, the transmitted energy can be significant enough to fracture the upper arm bone (Phillips, 1979) or to cause a traumatic cervical spinal cord injury (de la Fuente *et al.*, 2013) in a cat. Indeed, cone-shaped steel pellets are documented to have penetrated 1 mm-thick steel plates (Smith, 1985).

The wound ballistics of air weapon projectiles follows the mechanisms described above. However, bruises and other injuries without penetration of the skin may be considered a blunt trauma, rather than a gunshot wound. The pathoanatomical findings may be delicate and may easily remain undetected, even by the owners of affected animals. In a study of injured urban cats and dogs, as many as 16 out of 19 owners did not suspect a previous shooting incident when veterinary examination discovered their pet to be carrying a small-calibre projectile (Keep, 1970). This may be a consequence of a small-sized entrance wound, a small calibre of the narrow channel and, in many cases, the absence of an exit wound. In this context, radiographic examination is very valuable, especially for the detection of older damage.

The picture of the wound channel at necropsy is dominated by the appearance of crushed tissue and only moderate bleeding. It should be carefully explored along its total length, especially as some types of air-weapon ammunition are embedded in radio-lucent components (sabot) (Smith, 1985). These might be found as a fragment within the wound channel and must be preserved as evidence.

Airgun pellets and remains must, of course, be preserved using standard routines. The secured item can be assigned to the respective type of ammunition. For the foren-sic veterinarian, knowledge of the design of the bullet and composition material are necessary to obtain the best possible picture of the shooting event. In combination with anatomical findings – such as location of the point of impact, penetration depth and type of tissue along the wound path – these ballis-tic specifications can help investigators to form an impression of, for instance, the range of the shot (Missliwetz, 1987). By comparing three different types of airgun pellets, Smith (1985) observed distinct differences in pene-tration depth in ballistic gel, and a more recent British study indicates total penetration depth of gelatin and different animal organs to be around 10–15 cm (Wightman *et al.*, 2013).

The design of the tip and the material from which the pellet is made may not only be of value for the investigation, but will have a great influence on the capability of the projectile to penetrate tissue (Smith, 1985).

7.2.4 Essential steps of investigating a shot animal

7.2.4.1 Before necropsy

The immediate priority in the investigation of a surviving shot animal is to administer appropriate first-aid treatment before pro-cessing potential evidence from the animal or scene. But even in challenging situations, a well-structured approach is obligatory for all forensic work, a *sine qua non* for the forensic veterinary investigator! The evidence with which we are working has a constantly changing dynamic character. Alterations of

potential evidential value in a living animal might be changed by necessary clinical treat-ment, secondary healing, or the animal's behaviour (licking of the wound, etc.). Car-casses change due to autolytic processes. Necropsy, as clinical treatment, is an evidence-destroying investigative method. Even when circumstances suggest a rapid response, one should consider spending time on documen-tation or preservation of evidence. In any case, each step must be carefully considered to ensure correct procedure.

Extensive transfer of information from the crime scene prevents misinterpretation of observations made in the clinic or the nec-ropsy hall. If one does not have the chance to attend the crime scene oneself, one should try to collect as much information as possible by interviewing those involved in the inves-tigation at the scene. Information on who might be the most relevant person(s) to talk to might be found on the chain of custody scheme or from the officer with overall responsibility for the crime scene.

Certain general questions need to be ad-dressed in cases involving the use of weapons: How many shots were fired and from how many weapons? How many victims were there, receiving how many hits each? Did crime scene findings (for example, the blood stain pattern) or the localization of the victims in-dicate a connection to the wound pattern?

Questions specific to each body would be: In what position was the body found? What kind of injuries were there and were there injury-related marks? An example would be the establishment of consistency between the body and surface alterations. If an animal was lying on the ground when it received a *coup de grâce*, one could expect the exiting bullet to cause damage on the underlying sur-face. One should be aware of the possibility of a residual projectile when removing the body. The missile could be embedded in the ground or within the fur, or could even have re-entered the body. The latter event could involve an atypical entrance wound on which the un-informed veterinary forensic examiner may expend unnecessary time and resources at-tempting to form an opinion.

Preliminary first impression conclusions from an adspective on-scene examination of the body might also initiate other types of forensic investigations. For instance, a star-shaped wound in the head indicating a short muzzle-to-target distance would prompt a recommendation to look for backspatter of blood and tissue debris on a suspect's clothing or weapon.

Whenever bullet wounds or other trauma are suspected, the animal should be imaged as soon as possible. Instead of using conventional radiography, one might consider a computer tomographic (CT) examination. In human forensic pathology, imaging techniques such as CT, magnetic resonance imaging (MRI) and 3D surface scanners, resulting in three-dimensional imaging, are increasingly integrated into the investigations, especially within trauma diagnostics. Post-mortem CT has been shown to be superior to autopsy for depicting fractures and locating projectiles or foreign objects (Flach *et al.*, 2014). CT facilities are nowadays widely available and when an animal carcass is sealed in a body bag the requirements of working in an environment governed by human health standards can be observed. For detecting non-opaque items like soft gun pellets, undetectable on X-ray images, ultrasonographic examination is particularly useful (Tsui *et al.*, 2010).

The most outstanding advantage implied using 3D-imaging techniques is the creation of a data set documenting the anatomical proportions within a whole body. This is done time-effectively and without the need to manipulate the evidence by a destructive method (Flach *et al.*, 2014). Structures with deviant density, like a wound channel, can be visualized against a variety of denser structures, such as parenchymal organs and muscles. Bullets or bullet fragments can be identified by their exceptionally high density. The data set can be re-processed and re-assessed at any time, enabling accurate measurements. Presentation of complex changes, that court and jury might otherwise be challenged to understand by verbal description alone, can be facilitated. A bullet wound channel, for example, can be more clearly demonstrated via the clear narrative of CT images (see Box 7.2.1., 'Illegal shooting of wild grey wolf').

The benefits of 3D imaging has enhanced cooperation between radiologists and pathologists (Flach *et al.*, 2014), resulting in the development of the specialism named 'virtopsy', which has shown to be of high value, especially in wound ballistics.

Information from the crime scene and from imaging provide a solid foundation when the forensic veterinarian, whether clinician or pathologist, approaches the investigation of a shot animal. Nevertheless, all these findings need to be recorded by detailed documentation.

7.2.4.2   The practical approach

After having gone through the routine of the external examination, the next step is to focus on the documentation of entrance and exit wounds. For most cases, the line of departure is of special interest. In almost all cases, it provides a strong indication of position of the weapon in relation to the victim. The entrance and exit wounds are the only outer sign of the axis along which the projectile moved. The axis needs to be measured and documented before the invasive part of the necropsy, which will alter the normal relative positioning of the body, proceeds. An estimation of the line of departure based on the position of the entrance and exit wound alone must be considered as preliminary, since the bullet might have changed its direction within the body (see Section 7.2.2, 'Basics of wound ballistics'). Consequently, statements concerning this matter should not be made without verification.

If the animal was hit by several shots, entrance and exit wounds must be aligned. If there is doubt, then all possible permutations must be considered and documented. It is an advantage for the clinicians and pathologist over the radiologist that he can easily manipulate the animal into a variety of different positions to verify a working hypothesis (see Figs 7.2.6 and 7.2.7). Care must be taken, however, not to place the animal in an unnatural body position. This would apply when attempts are made to trace a wound channel on a suspended body in the necropsy room. The body would be stretched and consequently the tracing risks resulting in an exaggeratedly acute angle of shot.

Box 7.2.1. Illegal shooting of wild grey wolf

By combining the documentation achieved by the use of different methods (necropsy and CT-imaging), strong and illustrative evidence could be presented to the court.

In August 2011 the shooting of a grey wolf was reported. A claim of legal self-defence during protection of fenced domestic sheep was made by the defence. Necropsy confirmed that the animal had been shot. The angle of incidence was estimated to be between 0° and 10° from the front-right side. The findings

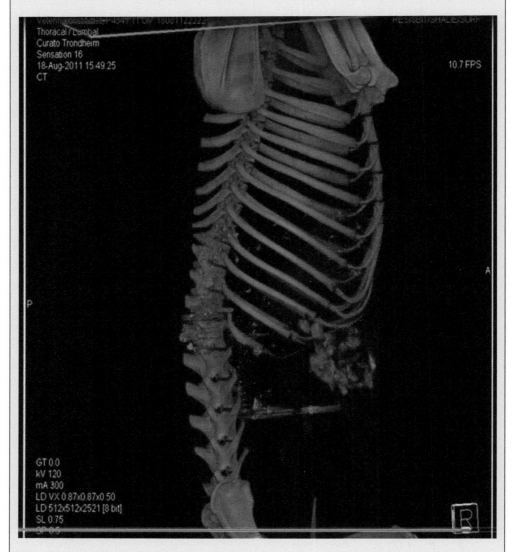

Fig. 7.2.2. Overview picture from lateral aspect of grey wolf (*Lupus lupus*), showing the thorax and luminal skeleton.

Continued

Box 7.2.1. Continued.

were in contradiction to the statement of the shooter. The prosecution appraised the angle of incidence as being crucial to the case. Data from the pre-necropsy whole-body computer tomographic examination was processed with the aim of a best possible demonstration and verification of the wound channel. The narrow channel through the back muscles could be visualized and its angle to the spinal column was measured. The result confirmed previous examinations and added valuable material for the courtroom presentation.

Figures 7.2.2–7.2.5 are from a video presentation made for courtroom demonstration. In Figs 7.2.2 and 7.2.3, there are fractures with loss of bone substance of the caudal four ribs. The wound is funnel-shaped; there are projectile fragments (bright spots) in the wound area. Each fragment on its own renders imprecise estimation of the axis of travel of the projectile before fragmentation. In Fig. 7.2.4, the entrance wound is seen in the upper part of the picture. Before the bullet fractured the 10th rib, it passed three more cranial ribs and their intercostal spaces. This part of the wound channel is not visible. Figure 7.2.5 shows the narrow channel between the entrance wound and fracture of the 10th rib. The perforation of the entrance wound is slightly out of focus and peripheral muscle layers are likely to be located 'out of axis', due to their sliding over the deeper muscles. Thus this outer part of the wound channel is less suitable for the estimation of the angle of incidence and was consequently discounted when the angle between the narrow channel and the spine was measured.

The Norwegian Øvre Romerike tingrett (district court) sentenced the shooter to four months' imprisonment for shooting a grey wolf in claimed self-defence and thereby deliberately violating the right of self-defence.

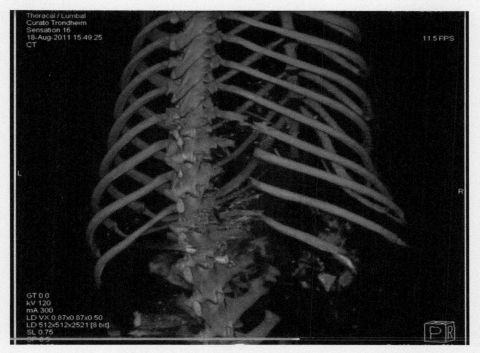

Fig. 7.2.3. Magnification of the image shown in Fig. 7.2.2, now showing caudal thorax and cranial lumbar vertebrae from mainly posterior aspect.

Continued

Box 7.2.1. Continued.

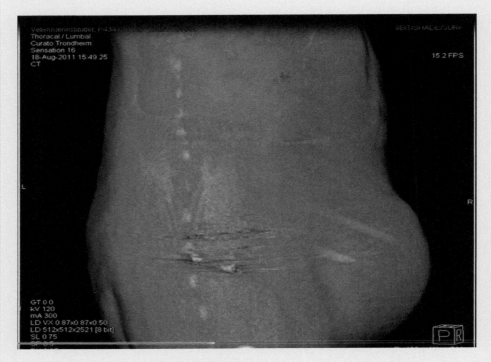

Fig. 7.2.4. Hairless body surface of the same section as in Fig. 7.2.3 and viewed from the same perspective.

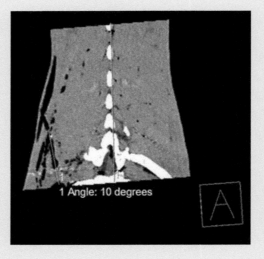

Fig. 7.2.5. Visualization of the narrow channel between the entrance wound and fracture of the 10th rib, viewed from a precise anterior aspect.

Figs 7.2.6 and 7.2.7 show a wounded bear. In Fig. 7.2.7, the probe remains in the same relationship to the wound as that shown in Fig. 7.2.6, but now a possible, near horizontal trajectory of the projectile that caused the injury can be appreciated, and approximations of the angle of shot and line of departure can be achieved.

The first part of the wound channel – the narrow wound channel – potentially yields the most reliable information regarding the angle from which the animal was shot. This portion of the total wound channel may show the best consistency between the axis on which the projectile travelled before and after hitting the target. In order to utilize this information, three conditions must be ensured.

First, the narrow channel must be localized within a part of the body that justifies conclusions regarding the animal's position the moment it was shot. Usually there is a demand to comment on the general position of the animal in relation to the shooter. In this context, the longitudinal axis of the body represented by the spinal column of the trunk is the most appropriate marker for the position of the animal. Parts that have a high degree of freedom such as the tail, the distal extremities and the head and neck region are consequently less reliable than the trunk.

Second, the narrow channel must be long enough that its axis can be estimated with a sufficient degree of certainty. Finally, one must succeed in elucidating and documenting the path of the narrow channel. There are a number of factors which may confound demonstration of the narrow channel. For instance, it may not be possible using modern imaging techniques to demonstrate a collapsed wound channel; the true axis of the channel might not be consistent with the estimated route documented before the body was opened. At necropsy, the carcass may be in a state of advanced autolysis, softening the tissue around the narrow channel. While investigating the wound, extreme care must be taken that the instrument is not inadvertently extended beyond the confines of the narrow channel.

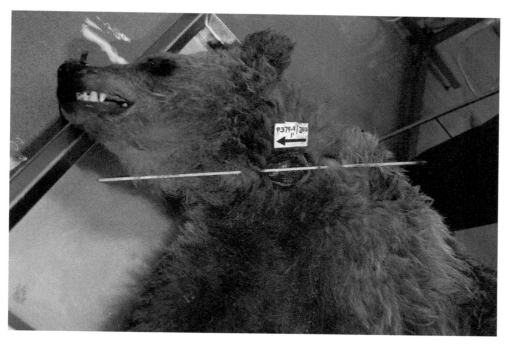

Fig. 7.2.6. A brown bear (*Ursus arctos*) lying in right lateral position enabling a standard left-sided procedure. The probe indicates the longitudinal axis of the wound channel. Entrance wound on the left side of the picture.

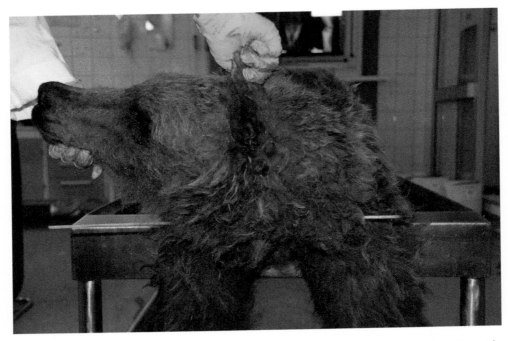

Fig. 7.2.7. The same animal as in Fig. 7.2.6, now mounted in a close to natural, ventrodorsal position with vertical forelegs and head and neck bent to the right.

7.2.4.3   Recovery of bullets

Bullets or relevant fragments recovered from the body must be considered as evidence and must be routinely preserved using standard techniques. They contain valuable information for the case and for the examiner. Submitted to a ballistic lab more information can be revealed from further examination. Determination of the calibre, distinction between rifle and handgun, the linking of the projectile to an individual weapon or type of weapon, and/or establishing contact of the bullets with intermediate target before entering the body, are examples (Brinkmann and Madea, 2004).

Some cast-iron rules must be observed in the process of missile recovery (Wobeser, 1996; Walker and Adrian, 2003; Brinkmann and Madea, 2004).

- Care must be taken not to cut the bullet while dissecting in the proximity of the projectile.
- No tissue must be discarded until the projectile is recovered. If tissue is removed

from the body it should be arranged in a logical manner nearby. If not succeeding in localizing the projectile, one can re-examine piece by piece by palpation or X-ray.

- Bullets must not be handled with metal forceps or other metallic surgical instruments in order to avoid alteration of the fragile markings on the surface of the bullet. Sterile single-use forceps are established tools for this procedure, though Di Maio (1999) recommends removal of bullets with fingers. Preliminary measurements can be taken using a plastic vernier caliper.
- To avoid cross-contamination, clean instruments must be used for each piece of evidence.
- Bullets should be washed to remove tissue and blood. The use of fresh running water will be sufficient in most cases but, if special washing procedures need to be followed, temporary storage at −20°C without washing is preferable.

- The recovered bullet should be briefly described by recording general appearance, deformation/non-deformation, approximate calibre, full- or semi-jacketed, weight, magnetic properties, etc.
- The dried bullets should be placed in wadded packaging (Fig. 7.2.8) and paper envelope for storage or submission.
- It is sufficient to recover a representative sample of pellets from shotgun wounds (Di Maio, 1999). Redundant pellets may be used for preliminary tests, such as testing for magnetism or flame tests.
- Fillers (felt wads, plastic cups, plastic crosspieces, etc.) should be handled in a similar manner to bullets.

Early information about the projectile(s) that are to be recovered is normally based on the assessment of radiographs, pictures or other images. If the recovered projectile matches the imaged structure, that circumstance should be recorded and in due course marked on the picture. It will differ from case to case, whether bullet removal is best performed by

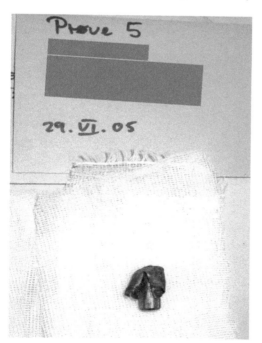

Fig. 7.2.8. The dried bullets should be placed in wadded packaging and paper envelope for storage or submission.

dissecting along the wound track or by more direct approach. At all steps of examination, one should consider the need to take (preliminary) tests, such as flaming, assessing magnetism or swabbing, if a local infectious condition is suspected. Definitive examination of recovered projectile(s) or fragments should be performed at the ballistic lab or at a later phase of the investigation.

It is necessary to know about the further steps of examination regarding each bullet before it is actually removed. Generally, it is a good practice to wash the projectile under fresh running water (Walker and Adrian, 2003). This ensures that the surface of the bullet is cleaned and tissue and blood cannot harden on it. This procedure is contraindicated if the bullet is to be examined for gunshot residues, however, or for all kinds of foreign debris, such as textile fibres, or mineral and biological materials (Walker and Adrian, 2003). To save residues, which may be fragments or soft tissue of intermediate targets, the projectile must undergo special procedures of washing and filtration (Nichols and Sens, 1990). Preservation of traces is possible even with a bullet recovered outside the body after completely traversing the body – a so-called 'through and through' shot. Karger et al. (1996) succeeded in DNA typing cellular debris sampled from hollow point and full-metal-jacket bullets after full penetration of calves, and achieved successful individualization on the basis of STR loci in three human cases (Karger et al., 1997). It is possible also to perform cytological examinations (Nichols and Sens, 1990; Karger, 2004). It can be expected that the amount of gunshot residue obtainable from semi-jacketed and hollow-point bullets is larger than from full-jacket projectiles (Karger et al., 1996).

7.2.5 Conclusion

The appearance of wounds caused by different types of projectiles may range from clear to chaotic. Nevertheless, all modifications are a consequence of the impact of forces falling under the same laws of physics, a consequence of action and reaction. The knowledge about what a bullet does to the body and what the body does to the bullet is crucial for surgeons and pathologists to unscramble – at least parts of – the traumatic modifications they are confronted with when working with animals being fired upon. Hence, being acquainted with the basics of wound ballistics is indispensable to high-quality forensic work.

Case Study 7.2.1. Cat shot by air rifle by David Bailey (images courtesy of Adele Wharton)

Figures 7.2.9a and 7.2.9b show an overview and close-up view of a cat that had been shot by an air-rifle pellet, with an entry wound mid-abdomen. Figs 7.2.9c and 7.2.9d demonstrate massive disruption to the left stifle joint, with the deformed pellet still visible in the radiograph.

It is posited that this animal was lying at rest when it was shot from a cranial direction. The amount of damage done to the stifle joint suggests a close contact discharge.

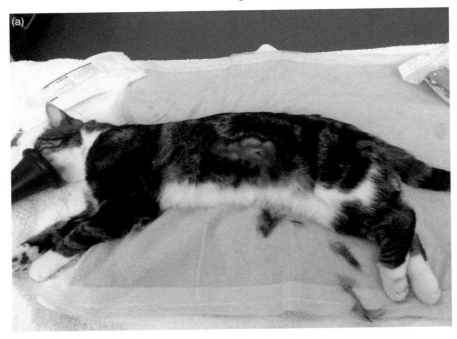

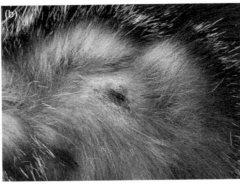

Fig. 7.2.9. The cat shown in (a) to (d) has been shot by an air-rifle pellet.

Continued

Case Study 7.2.1. Continued.

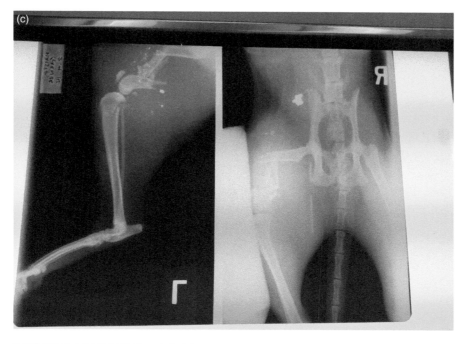

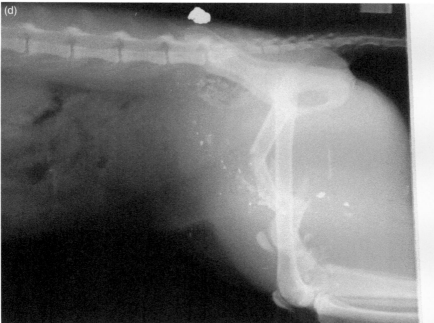

Fig. 7.2.9. Continued.

Note

[1] The specific regulation differs widely between countries. In the UK air weapons are, for the time being, regulated by law to below 12 ft lb (16.3 J) for air rifles and below 6 ft lb (8.1 J) for air pistols (Wightman *et al.*, 2013).

References

Anon. (2013) *Animal Welfare in Scotland*. Available online at: http://www.onekind.org/uploads/publications/animal-welfare-report-2013.pdf (accessed 29 December 2014).

Bartels, K.E., Stair, E.L. and Cohen, R.E. (1991) Corrosion potential of steel bird shot in dogs. *Journal of the American Veterinary Medical Association* 199, 856–863.

Bond, S.J., Schnier, G.C. and Miller, F.B. (1996) Air-powered guns: too much firepower to be a toy. *Journal of Trauma and Acute Care Surgery* 41, 674–678.

Braathen, E., Moen, E. and Lien, J. (2006) *Ladeboken*, 6th edn. HM-Nordic, Oslo, Norway.

Brinkmann, B. and Madea, B. (2004) *Handbuch Gerichtliche Medizin*. Springer, Berlin, Germany.

Campbell-Hewson, G., Egleston, C. and Busuttil, A. (1997) The use of air weapons in attempted suicide. *Injury* 28, 153–158.

Cooper, J.E. and Cooper, M.E. (2007) *Introduction to Veterinary and Comparative Forensic Medicine*. Blackwell, Oxford, UK.

de la Fuente, C., Ródenas, S., Pumarola, M. and Añor, S. (2013) Dural tear and myelomalacia caused by an airgun pellet in a cat. *The Canadian Veterinary Journal* 54, 679–682.

Di Maio, V.J.M. (1999) *Gunshot Wounds: Practical Aspects of Firearms, Ballistics, and Forensic Techniques*, 2nd edn. CRC Press, New York, USA.

Fackler, M.L. (1987) What's wrong with the wound ballistics literature, and why. Available online at: http://www.rkba.org/research/fackler/wrong.html (accessed 27 March 2015).

Fackler, M.L., Surinchak, J.S., Malinowski, J.A. and Bowen, R.E. (1984) Bullet fragmentation: a major cause of tissue disruption. *Journal of Trauma* 24, 35–39.

Flach, P.M., Thali, M.J. and Germerott, T. (2014) Times have changed! Forensic radiology – a new challenge for radiology and forensic pathology. *American Journal of Roentgenology* 202, W325–334.

Frank, A. (1986) Lead fragments in tissues from wild birds: a cause of misleading analytical results. *Science of the Total Environment* 54, 275–281.

Kalinich, J.F., Emond, C.A., Dalton, T.K., Mog, S.R., Coleman, G.D., Kordell, J.E., Miller, A.C. and McClain, D.E. (2005) Embedded weapons-grade tungsten alloy shrapnel rapidly induces metastatic high-grade rhabdomyosarcomas in F344 rats. *Environmental Health Perspectives*, 729–734.

Karger, B. (2004) Schussverletzungen. In: Brinkmann, B. and Madea, B. (eds) *Handbuch gerichtliche Medizin*. Springer Verlag, Berlin, Germany, pp. 593–682.

Karger, B., Meyer, E., Knudsen, P.J.T. and Brinkmann, B. (1996) DNA typing of cellular material on perforating bullets. *International Journal of Legal Medicine* 108, 177–179.

Karger, B., Meyer, E. and DuChesne, A. (1997) STR analysis on perforating FMJ bullets and a new VWA variant allele. *International Journal of Legal Medicine* 110, 101–103.

Keep, J.M. (1970) Gunshot injuries to urban dogs and cats. *Australian Veterinary Journal* 46, 330–334.

Kneubuehl, B.P., Coupland, R.M., Rothschild, M.A. and Thali, M.J. (2011) *Wound Ballistics: Basics and Applications*. Springer, Berlin, Germany.

Kraabel, B.J., Miller, M.W., Getzy, D.M. and Ringelman, J.K. (1996) Effects of embedded tungsten-bismuth-tin shot and steel shot on mallards (Anas platyrhynchos). *Journal of Wildlife Diseases* 32, 1–8.

MacCrehan, W.A., Layman, M.J. and Secl, J.D. (2003) Hair combing to collect organic gunshot residues (OGSR). *Forensic Science International* 135, 167–173.

Merck, M.D. (2007) *Veterinary Forensics*. Blackwell, Oxford, UK.

Milroy, C.M., Clark, J.C., Carter, N., Rutty, G. and Rooney, N. (1998) Air weapon fatalities. *Journal of Clinical Pathology* 51, 525–529.

Missliwetz, J. (1987) Zur Grenzgeschwindigkeit bei der Haut. *Beiträge zur gerichtlichen Medizin* 45, 411–432.

Munro, R. and Munro, H.M.C. (2008) *Animal Abuse and Unlawful Killing*. Saunders Elsevier, Edinburgh, UK.

Nicholas, N. and Welsch, J. (2004) *Ballistic Gelatin*. Available online at: http://www.dtic.mil/cgi-bin/GetTRDoc?AD=ADA446543 (accessed 27 March 2015).

Nichols, C.A. and Sens, M.A. (1990) Recovery and evaluation by cytologic techniques of trace material retained on bullets. *The American Journal of Forensic Medicine and Pathology* 11(1), 17–34.

Ogunc, G.I., Ozer, M.T., Eryilmaz, M., Karakus, O. and Uzar, A.I. (2013) The wounding potential and legal situations of air guns – experimental study. *Australian Journal of Forensic Sciences* 46, 39–52.

Ordog, G.J., Wasserberger, J. and Balasubramaniam, S. (1988) Shotgun Wound Ballistics. *Journal of Trauma and Acute Care Surgery* 28, 624–631.

Parker, H., Rosell, F. and Danielsen, J. (2006) Efficacy of cartridge type and projectile design in the harvest of beaver. *Wildlife Society Bulletin* 34, 127–130.

Phillips, I.R. (1979) A survey of bone fractures in the dog and cat. *Journal of Small Animal Practice* 20, 661–674.

Schantz, B. (1979) Aspects on the choice of experimental animals when reproducing missile trauma. *Acta chirurgica Scandinavica Supplementum* 489, 121–130.

Schulz, L.-C. (1990) *Lehrbuch der Allgemeinen Pathologie*. Enke, Stuttgart, Germany.

Sinclair, L., Merck, M.D. and Lockwood, R. (2006) *Forensic Investigation of Animal Cruelty*, 1. Humane Society Press, Washington, DC, USA.

Smith, W.D. (1985) Air rifle ammunition and its influence on wounding potential. *Archives of Emergency Medicine* 2, 25–29.

Tsui, C., Tsui, K. and Tang, Y. (2010) Ball bearing (BB) gun injuries. *Hong Kong Journal of Emergency Medicine* 17, 488.

Vollmerhaus, B., Sinowatz, I., Frewein, J. and Waibl, H. (1992) *Anatomie der Vögel*, 2. Verlag Paul Parey, Berlin, Germany.

Walker, N.D. and Adrian, W.J. (2003) *Wildlife Forensic Field Manual*, 3. Association of Midwest Fish and Game Law Enforcement Officers, Denver, Colorado, USA.

Wightman, G., Cochrane, R., Gray, R.A. and Linton, M. (2013) A contribution to the discussion on the safety of air weapons. *Science & Justice* 53, 343–349.

Wobeser, G. (1996) Forensic (medico-legal) necropsy of wildlife. *Journal of Wildlife Diseases* 32, 240–249.

Wohlsein, P. and Reifinger, M. (2011) Todeszeichen und Wundalterbestimmung. In: Baumgärtner, W. and Gruber, A.D. (eds) *Allgemeine Pathologie für die Tiermedizin*. Enke Verlag, Stuttgart, Germany, pp. 342–358.

8 Blood and Blood Pattern Analysis

David Bailey*

Department of Forensic and Crime Science, Staffordshire University, Stoke-on-Trent, Staffordshire, UK

*Corresponding author: daysbays@yahoo.co.uk

8.1 Introduction – Analysis versus Observation

The Locard principle is used by forensic scientists to explain the transfer of evidence. It is not possible, according to Locard's principle, to enter an environment and not change it in some manner by either leaving something behind or taking something with you. *Every contact leaves a trace* and with blood there is an initial non-specialist observation that blood spilled at a crime scene is just too messy and adheres to everything.

'Why?' asks the lay observer 'do you need Locard to explain a bloodstained crime scene?'

Crime scene blood pattern analysis is an observational tool. You can take a blood sample from an animal or a crime scene, but you cannot take a blood *pattern* from either. You must first record a blood pattern in order for it to be analysed and interpreted.

Blood pattern analysis is a highly specialized form of forensic science and consists of three independent and linked components.

1. Analysis.
2. Photography (and documentation).
3. Interpretation.

8.2 Definition

Blood pattern analysis means to examine, inspect and record the shape, location and distribution patterns of bloodstains.

The underlying premise upon which all bloodstain analysis depends is that all patterns, shape, location and distribution of bloodstains are characteristic of the forces that created them.

And in this simple descriptor we have the physicists and mathematicians taking the guesswork out of a biological sample investigation. Blood samples will always vary in appearance, but the forces that create them are always the same.

8.3 Blood

Blood is an imprecise medium to examine forensically. No two circulating red blood cells will behave in the same manner or have the same colour, appearance, weight, hue or oxygen saturation. Some red blood cells have nuclear (DNA) material, while others (most) don't. With large variations in size, shape and chromaticity, blood is too difficult to be described in a forensic sense.

Forensic scientists who are experienced at blood pattern analysis, then, don't describe blood that has been found deposited outside the body at a crime scene, but instead they attempt to describe the patterns that blood forms which are *characteristic of the forces* that have created them.

All blood cells are slightly but sufficiently different between species – we know that one can't give a dog a blood transfusion from a cat. There are differences between the blood from individuals of the same species (blood type) and even blood from within the one animal (blood maturity): all red blood cells are similar, but they are not the same.

Regardless of this variation, there are some facets that blood can share with other blood. All blood cells, regardless of inter- and intra-species variation, will obey the rules and laws of physics, fluid dynamics and motion. It is these forces that forensic scientists utilize to describe the creation of blood patterns. This chapter is, by necessity, a bloody lesson in physics and motion. And while there is variation between one red blood cell and its immediate neighbour, there is no variation in the *type* of forces that will act on any number of red blood cells to produce a bloodstain pattern. The shape which the blood pattern will take when blood is deposited on a receptor surface is due to the forces of motion, fluid dynamics, friction, surface tension, viscosity, adhesion, cohesion and gravity.

The blood leaves a telltale pattern of the forces that created it and this is captured by a camera, a sketch or a video recording.

This is what bloodstain pattern analysis is: a *force pattern analysis*, captured by photography and documentation. This step in the process is relatively simple; it is the next, the same issue that affects all aspects of forensic analysis, which is complicated – the interpretation.

8.4   Analysis versus Interpretation

When presenting bloodstain patterns in court, it isn't (usually) the analysis that will be argued against. In that case, you would be (foolishly) arguing against Isaac Newton, Robert Brown, Archimedes and their colleagues, and, in a legal dispute, the barristers find it easier to argue with you, not them, over *your interpretation* of *their laws* of physics and motion applied to the blood pattern analysis.

Beginners in this area should focus on the analysis at the crime scene through accurate documentation and, in particular, the taking of methodical photos. You can then hand over the photos to a more qualified, competent or confident expert to interpret in a laboratory or office setting.

And here we can be discussing blood spatter, hair microscopy or soil samples, as one of the fundamentals of forensic science is entwined with the skill of blood pattern *analysis* and the subsequent procedure and art of *interpretation* of the patterns formed by the forces acting on the blood to create that pattern. While many vets and animal workers are familiar with the taking, analysis and subsequent interpreting of a blood sample from a sick animal to arrive at a clinical decision (based on haematology and biochemistry) for that animal, they are also aware that two vets will arrive at different interpretations of the same clinical blood result. Bloodstain analysis is no different. Two independent blood pattern experts can interpret one blood pattern in two different ways, and this is the basis for the competitive nature of science and an adversarial philosophy of legal disputes.

Most readers will be able to take photos of a blood pattern. This is part of the analysis; however, many need to understand the separation of the analysis step from the interpretation step in forensic science. While very few responders will (willingly) be able to interpret the blood pattern left at a crime scene correctly, most of them can take accurate images and process the scene accurately enough for another expert to assist later in the investigation. You are in this field first as an analyst in the form of a photographer and documenter, and second as an interpreter of the patterns you record. This is where there are differences between crime scenes involving animals and humans; wherein the latter will always attract a skilled blood pattern analyst, and perhaps a proficient forensic photographer, while the former will attract whoever happens to be available and has a good camera.

Blood shed outside an animal's body becomes clotted due to the clotting factors within and the external temperature of the environment it has been deposited in. Deposited blood sticks to hair, clothing, furniture and buildings, and is a persistent witness to a crime. Blood yields a lot of information, clinically, temporally and forensically.

Another chant repeated throughout this book is the discrete independent effect. Blood patterns or any piece of evidence should not be taken in isolation. There should always be at least two independent sources of evidence gathered from any crime scene. For example, a photograph from a bite wound and a salivary swab for DNA analysis taken from the bite wound. Another example is an eyewitness statement and an image produced from a CCTV camera. As long as there is more than one source of evidence and one source is independent from the other. One hundred photographs are 100 different types of the same singular source of evidence. Blood is ideal in that it comes with its own built-in secondary evidence source – DNA. This is useful if DNA is what you need. If you recover blood from a scene for later DNA or toxicological analysis, always photograph it first as a pattern, drop, stain, smudge, spurt, misting, drip, satellite pattern, low-, medium- or high-velocity deposit, back spatter, wipe or cast-off stain, because the pattern created cannot be reproduced after you have sampled it for a secondary source of evidence.

Blood provides many clues as to the temporal sequence of events that have occurred, as well as distance from an animal to determine whether, for example, a shooting incident was accidental or deliberate. Blood also provides information as to the behaviour of the animal. The correct analysis of blood patterns can provide a great deal of information for both prosecution and defence experts to interpret.

Photography of blood and the patterns and stains it can make can be described as evidence collection and analysis, but already an interpretation has been made. This dull red pattern that has collected under this dead animal – is it blood?

How do you know?

8.5   Presumptive Screening of Blood

When we see a red, thick and clotted stain that is expanding slowly under a dead animal, it is likely to be blood. We transcend the boundary between veterinarian (it is blood) to forensic scientist (it is likely to be blood). But even before we approach this question we need to run through the PREGS protocol (see Chapter 5, this volume) at our scene to make sure it is a safe place. We then inspect (look) or examine (look and touch) the animal to determine life-extinct status. Once we have satisfied ourselves the scene is safe and the animal is no longer alive, we then protect the scene and start to gather and document available evidence. In this case, photos, sketches and video.

To ensure we can answer the question in court, 'How do you know it was blood?', we test it.

Presumptive testing of blood can be done in a variety of ways, but the most common manner that many vets and animal workers will be familiar with is the simple Hemastix – see Fig. 8.1.

Most blood presumptive tests rely on the catalytic properties of blood and the presence within a red blood cell of the haemoglobin protein. So a presumptive test for animal blood will be the same, regardless of the species tested for. And armed with the knowledge that very few things in nature contain haemoglobin, we can satisfy ourselves after testing that the bright red thick material is blood. We have analysed the blood from two sources. The first is our prior knowledge, experience and expectation of dealing with what blood is and what blood looks like, and the second, independent source is the presumptive test for blood – these two independent sources provide two separate analyses and one interpretation: *we have blood.*

While the Hemastix presumptive test suggested has been used by veterinarians in clinical practice (there are rules for the admissibility and reliability of any evidence you introduce to a court), for simplicity, the evidence must satisfy two criteria. It should be accepted by your peers *and* it needs to be verifiable. While the lack of a presumptive test for blood prior to subsequent scene processing and analysis should not affect the admissibility of the evidence (photograph and documentation) to a court, it may affect the weight which the court attributes to that evidence.

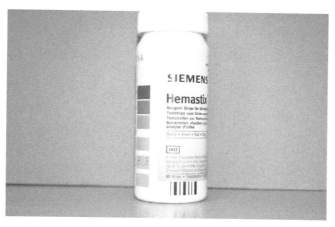

Fig. 8.1. Hemastix test for blood.

8.6   What Is Blood?

Blood consists of red and white blood cells, nutrients, dissolved gases and blood platelets carried around in plasma. Erythrocytes (the red blood cells) have the role of transporting oxygen to the cells of the body. These body cells have an obligate demand for oxygen molecules (O_2) in their respiration cycle and willingly donate a carbon dioxide molecule (CO_2) to the plasma after this exchange, allowing the erythrocyte to spend the second part of its journey oxygen and carbon dioxide free and as a willing servant awaiting the next oxygen molecule to bind with in the lungs, air sacs or gills of its host.

It is the liquid plasma component of blood that acts as the main carrier of CO_2 back to the lungs. This can be visualised when comparing bright red arterial oxygenated blood with that of the venous dull hue of de-oxygenated blood. It is this colour differential that has allowed the application of pulse oximetry in determining the oxygen saturation of a patient's blood in veterinary and human *clinical* medicine. This is our first forensic observation – what colour is the blood?

Colour of blood is determined by the amount of oxygen present in the blood at the time of recording the blood pattern, as well as the time that has elapsed since blood has been deposited on the surface.

Anhydrous blood should not be confused with clotting stage. This is not a clinical examination of blood, and the ability of the blood to dry out depends on volume and shape of the stain as well as environmental conditions such as humidity, temperature and wind exposure.

It is also the colouration of red blood cells and subsequent discolouration due to breakdown of this haemoglobin/iron molecular complex that can cause considerable difficulties in the ageing and interpreting of the appearance of a bruise in *forensic* medicine. Haemoglobin and iron molecule complexes exist within an erythrocyte to transiently capture and transport a molecule of oxygen around the body, allowing it to diffuse through the erythrocyte cell membrane

to the target cell. In order for a red blood cell to get close enough to a target body cell, it needs to be able to squeeze through a capillary. Red blood cells are approximately 25% larger than the diameter of their capillaries (Snyder and Sheafor, 1999). There is (naturally) variation between species as to this exact figure; however, the overriding principle remains that the erythrocyte must be bigger than the capillary it enters. This counter-intuitive set-up prevents carbon dioxide-rich plasma from interfering with the transfer of oxygen between the erythrocyte cell membrane and the target cell, a process that requires uninterrupted membrane-to-membrane contact between the erythrocyte and target cell.

This process of transient cell-to-cell contact requires a red blood cell to retain a rigid cell membrane while maintaining surface flexibility. Like skin cells, all mature mammalian red blood cells have no nuclear material. Most, but not all, mammalian erythrocytes are shaped like biconcave discs; when squeezed through a small capillary this shape and integral membrane rigidity allows the blood cell to assume a cigar shape, thus allowing maximum surface area for oxygen transfer from the red blood cell to the target cell – a passive diffusion process that must not be interfered with by the presence of a surrounding layer of carbon dioxide-rich plasma. This design also allows the erythrocyte to act in many ways like a bullet travelling through a gun barrel. Bullets are (also counter-intuitively) larger than the barrel they travel in and this ensures that the gas build-up behind them pushes them out of the barrel.

Different mammalian and non-mammalian species have distinctive shaped and nucleated erythrocytes, and this allows them different properties with respect to blood flow (laminar or turbulent), blood viscosity, oxygen transfer and cell membrane flexibility.

8.7   Blood Spatter – Overview

Bloodstain pattern analysis is the evaluation of the size, shape and distribution of patterns that are identified in blood. The purpose is to possibly identify the activities that took place to deposit the blood, and to identify the location of the individual animal victim(s) during the bloodshed. The first step involved is identifying basic patterns. By identifying patterns an analyst can then draw conclusions as far as what type of activity took place to create those patterns. Those are recognizable patterns and they are reproducible patterns.[1]

Although in-depth interpretation of blood spatter and bloodstains requires some training and experience, an investigator should be able to look at blood patterns, make some basic deductions, and document these. A simplified introduction would ask the reader to recognize and describe the basic blood pattern and focus on the forces that caused the patterns. The use and application of trigonometry and an understanding of physics, applied to biological material (blood) is what the forensic scientist needs and the courts prefer. While a biological component will always exist to blood and blood patterns, and these biological properties are of use in a clinical sense, the forensic examination of blood compels us to preferentially observe the forces used to create the blood pattern and not biological components.

Correct interpretation of blood spatter can reveal the position and location of the animal victim at the time of death. A dead animal found in a pool of blood may have died in that pool of blood and an animal that is found on a clean floor may have been killed somewhere else and placed at the scene.

Blood spatter patterns and an understanding of the forces that created them can determine the injuries suffered; location of the victim with respect to other physical evidence; which events occurred and, importantly, which did not; and the temporal sequence of events that other forms of static evidence can't provide.

Temporality of events is perhaps not surprising given the abundance of equations in the physical science that require forces, speeds and distance to be measured over a period or function of time.

When analysing a blood pattern, the absence of blood or blood spatter may be just as important as the presence of blood spatter.

Blood spatter requires full documentation primarily by photographs and sketching and should be considered as part of the analysis of the whole scene.

Specialist lighting and chemical enhancement are particularly important in photographing bloodstain patterns.

8.8 Record: Mnemonic – CAPSS

a. *C*olour of the stain
A trained examiner (e.g. a veterinarian) can determine whether a bloodstain is venous or arterial blood by the brightness of the red hue, which is caused by the amount of oxygenated haemoglobin present. It should be noted that the oxygen/haemoglobin bond is, by necessity, a weak bond, so that arterial blood deposited on a surface for a significant period prior to examination may not retain its characteristic bright red hue.
b. *A*nhydrate
Wet, dry, drying (avoid use of the term 'clotting', as we are making a transition from clinical veterinary science into forensic veterinary science).
c. *P*osition of a stain
Wall, floor, ceiling, under animal.
d. *S*ize of the stain, as well as the border characteristics of the stain
Diffuse, discrete.
e. *S*hape of the stain
Amorphous, round, pooled.

Once we have our PREGS protocols (see Chapter 5, this volume) and subsequent CAPSS analysis completed, we can analyse and interpret the recorded evidence with an accumulated forensic knowledge of physics and fluid dynamics, and then combine this with our clinical knowledge of animal behaviour, clinical and gross pathology, clinical disease, and prior crime scene processing and clinical experience to describe *what events occurred* to create those patterns. We have transferred from being an analyst to interpreting the signs, and again we need to ask for an independent (second source of evidence) person to assist with their view of the analysis.

8.9   Forces Acting in Blood

8.9.1   Cohesion

Cohesion is a force that acts within a drop of blood (or any liquid) that gives the liquid certain properties such as surface tension. It allows molecules within the blood drop to resist separation and causes a blood drop to form a distinctive tear shape characteristic of this force (see Fig. 8.2).

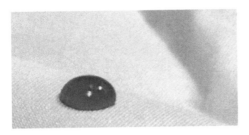

Fig. 8.2. Cohesive forces acting on a blood drop.

8.9.2   Surface tension

Surface tension is a result of cohesion forces, the elastic-like property of blood or any liquid that makes it tend to contract, caused by the cohesive forces of attraction between the molecules *within* the liquid. The molecules on the liquid surface have a net force on them that pulls them toward the centre of the liquid. All other molecules in that liquid will have equal forces of attraction to them as they are surrounded by other molecules. However, the surface molecules are incompletely surrounded by other molecules. This results in a net attraction toward the underlying molecules and away from the surface, causing a 'skin' to be formed on the liquid surface (see Fig. 8.3).

8.9.3   Viscosity

Viscosity of a liquid is a measure of that liquid's resistance to changing shape. *Thicker fluids are more viscous fluids. Thinner*

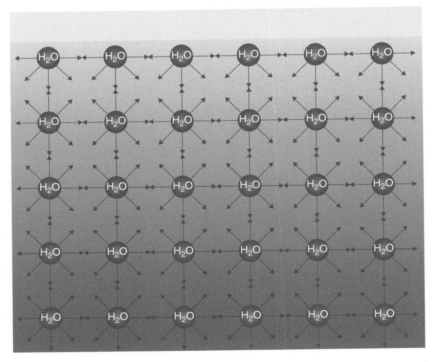

Fig. 8.3. Surface tension: the top layer of molecules (only) is pulled downward; every other layer of molecules is pulled equally in all directions.

fluids are less viscous fluids. Blood is (literally) thicker than water and four times more viscous.

When a liquid such as water is squeezed and projected out through a water pistol, the harder you pull on the trigger, the faster the water comes out of the pistol. This is called a constant viscosity – the harder you squeeze the water, the more resistance the water exerts back against the trigger, and the faster it exits the water pistol.

Blood is slightly different to water in that it doesn't act with a constant viscosity; while blood is four times more viscous than water, when there is a force applied to blood it becomes less viscous (and *thinner*). So when squeezed through a syringe (or small capillary) it becomes easier to squeeze out the harder you press. This property of blood allows it to flow easily through small blood vessels.

8.9.4 Adhesion

When blood strikes a recipient object, it sticks to that object through adhesive forces. Adhesion forces differ from cohesive forces, and for blood to stick to an object the forces of adhesion must exceed those of surface tension cohesion.

8.10 Forces Acting on Blood

1. Force of ejection – arterial spurt or external force (usually a trauma).
2. Gravity.
3. Elasticity of the surface it is in contact with.

Blood will usually leave the body through some form of trauma or externally applied force. It is then immediately affected by gravity and the 'bounce' or the elasticity of the recipient surface.

All three external forces combine to impart a pattern that can be seen in the blood drop or stain.

A blood drop striking a surface with little or no distortion will appear 'perfect' (see Fig. 8.4).

Fig. 8.4. Blood striking a glass surface with little or no distortion to its edge.

8.10.1 Biological forces acting in blood serum

Clotting factors: when we describe clotted blood as forensic scientists we use terms such as dry, drying or wet to assist in the transition from clinical veterinary science (clotted appearance).

8.11 Photography and Analysis

Photography is the key tool for the documentation of bloodstain patterns. When used correctly, a skilful photographer can not only document the scene, but also assist in the post-scene analysis through the correct use of perspective in the taking of photographs. In an animal crime scene that does not involve humans, it is unlikely that a trained blood pattern analyst will attend; however, if required, a trained human blood pattern analyst can look at photos that have been taken at the scene and can assist with or provide an interpretation post-scene.

A blood pattern examiner can provide an interpretation of a scene through careful evaluation of accurate and precise photography. A requirement for a small amount of knowledge in photography is needed beyond 'point and shoot' capabilities; however, the extra photographic skills required are not outside the aptitude of most people and modern digital cameras.

All evidence at scenes, including blood pattern-containing scenes, usually require three starting shots. Overview, approach and close-up – usually with the same numbered indicator in the photo that corresponds to a photographic log to assist with evidence identification and continuity.

Figures 8.5–8.7 show an overview (Fig. 8.5), approach (Fig. 8.6) and close-up (Fig. 8.7) of a bloodstain in a trailer. No photographic markers have been used in these images and no scale has been used in the close-up. It would be difficult to understand the sequence of events if only Fig. 8.7 was adduced as evidence.

8.11.1   Close-up of bloodstains

Have the camera at a perpendicular angle to the surface that is being photographed. This is important as, with the addition of a measuring scale and basic computer programming, the measurements can be made of blood drop size and the spacings between them (see Fig. 8.8).

In the example in Fig. 8.8, I have taken a photo of blood on a horizontal surface with my camera perpendicular to the surface, and included a scale. I have uploaded the image to my computer, opened a software program and cut-and-pasted the scale to overlay the blood drop. So I know that the diameter of the blood drop of interest is 5.5 mm (see Fig. 8.9).

Similarly, I can calculate the distance between drops in the photo after the scene has been processed, not necessarily at the scene.

The only requirements for this to be accurate are:

1. Camera perpendicular to the object being photographed.
2. Inclusion of an accurate scale.
3. Access to a PC or Mac that can perform cut-and-paste tasks – Microsoft Paint is a good one for non-Mac users.

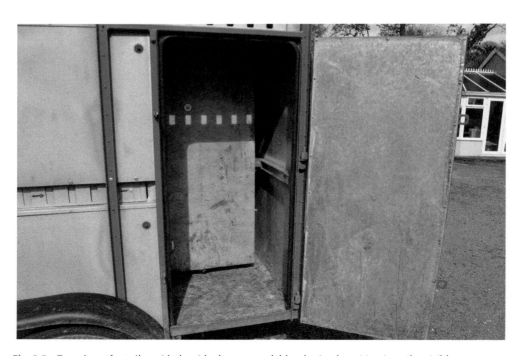

Fig. 8.5. Overview of a trailer with the side door opened: bloodstained partition in trailer visible.

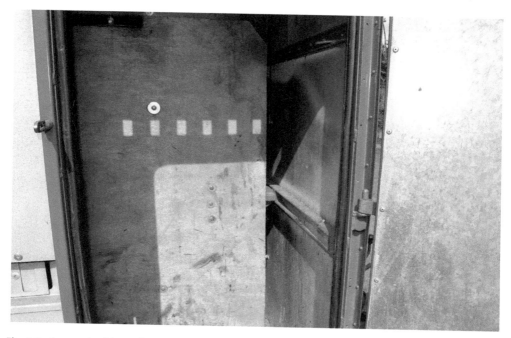

Fig. 8.6. Approach of the trailer door with the partition as the area of interest.

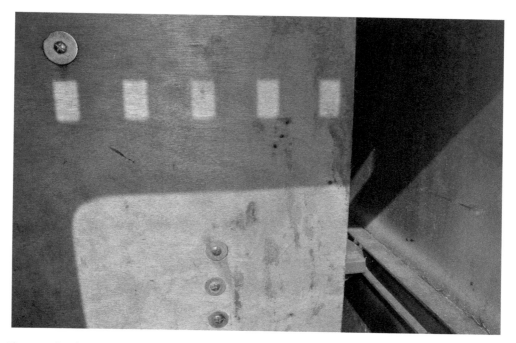

Fig. 8.7. Bloodstained partition visible and overall position in trailer clear with the prior overview and approach shots.

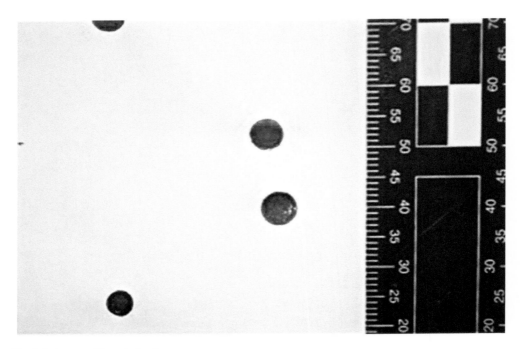

Fig. 8.8. Image with scale in place.

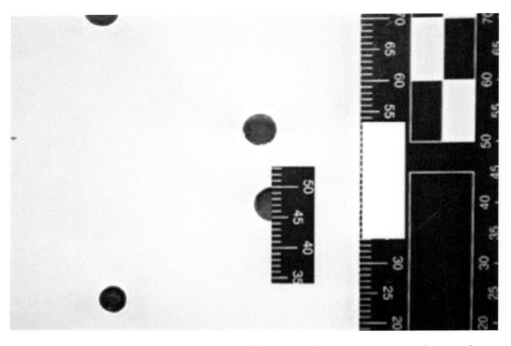

Fig. 8.9. Image with scale and measurement made of blood drop of interest on computer after scene has been processed.

8.12 Blood Patterns

8.12.1 Categories of bloodstains

There are three general categories of blood-stains; each one is defined and described in terms of the force required to form the pattern that is observed.

1. Passive.
2. Transfer.
3. Projected.

Again, we must describe the forces acting on bloodstains and not the bloodstains themselves. Therefore, passive bloodstains are bloodstains formed by gravity as the only *external* force acting on the bloodstain. In reality, all passive stains are a combination of gravity and adhesion with the resulting bloodstain formed by the blood adhering to the contact surface.

Passive bloodstains include drops, drips, clots and pools.

Transfer bloodstains are created when the principle acting force to cause the stain is adhesion only. If an object encounters something bloody, blood will pass between the two objects through the process of adhesion. Transfer stains differ from passive stains by having no gravity component to their formation.

Transfer stains can be further subdivided into contact bleeding, swipes, smears, wipes or smudges.

Projected stains are caused when a force greater than gravity acts to create the bloodstain. Projected stains can be further divided into spurts, cast-off stains, impact stains or spatters.

8.12.2 Directionality of bloodstains

Blood falling in a direction perpendicular to a surface will leave a rounded bloodstain. It will be circular (see Fig. 8.10).

For a bloodstain caused by blood falling from the end of a needle onto the paper, the external forces acting are gravity and adhesion. There will also be a level of distortion to the drop, depending on the type of surface the blood lands upon. The material

Fig. 8.10. Bloodstain falling from a short height onto a paper surface with little or no edge distortion.

of this surface and the elasticity of this surface will affect the final shape of the visible bloodstain.

Directionality of a bloodstain can be indicated by the bloodstain pattern observed that has adhered to a surface.

The 'pointed' end of the bloodstain assists in determining from what direction the blood travelled. The telltale finger-like projection at the end of the bloodstain points in the same direction of travel and away from the point of origin.

8.12.3 Point of convergence

Once the directionality of a bloodstain has been determined, it is then possible to determine the directionality of a group of bloodstains. By drawing a line through the long axis of a group of bloodstains, the point of convergence can be determined.

8.12.4 Number of bloodstains required to make an observation?

The number of bloodstains required to interpret or form a conclusion upon is as many as the expert feels is relevant or appropriate. There is no minimum number of bloodstains required to make an interpretation.

Case Study 8.1 Regina versus XY

The defendant was charged with the offence of stag-carting. It was alleged that the defendant transported two stags to a location for the purpose of releasing and hunting them on horseback. The deer were born and raised in enclosed premises and transported and released for the purpose of hunting them.

At the point of this dispute was the domestic nature of these animals. Wild animals are not covered by the animal welfare act in Northern Ireland; however, this act extends to domesticated and captive animals.

The animals were loaded onto a trailer and transported and released for hunting. The hunting involved the pursuit of these animals on horseback by members of an organized hunt. Hounds followed and often the deer involved would escape into the environment.

A trailer was seized, and evidence collected from it included deer hair, deer antler and blood.

The defendant claimed that the trailer had not been used for this purpose before and the trailer was cleaned prior to each use.

A number of bloodstains were identified in the trailer. These stains were interpreted by the prosecution expert as an indication of bleeding during transit. A number of stains indicated cuts that occurred in transit and demonstrated that the transported deer may have fallen over during transit.

Bloodstains that were overlaid by mud stains demonstrated a temporal sequence to the bleeding.

The bloodstains in the trailer indicated to the prosecution expert that the deer had bled in transit and therefore had suffered during transit. The suffering was not at issue, but the necessity of the suffering was argued. The deer *had to* be transported to be released to be hunted. It was argued that this suffering as evidenced by the bloodstains in the trailer was unnecessary.

8.13   Bruises

Bruise – superficial discoloration due to hemorrhage into the tissue from ruptured blood vessels beneath the surface of the skin without the skin itself being broken.
(Blood and Studdert, 1999, p. 163)

Assigning any forensic significance to bruises in animals can be problematic, due to the lack of visibility of animal bruises. There are very few studies focusing on bruising in animals and the problems inherent to biological systems of variability of presenting signs describing a bruise in a living or dead animal.

These problems are exacerbated by hair covering the skin, thick skin in some species (cattle) preventing visibility of any bruising, as well as deeply pigmented skin in many animals, which further reduces the visibility of bruises.

The mechanism of bruising is the same in animals as in humans – bleeding under the skin into the tissue without the skin being broken. The colour changes seen in bruises are due to the breakdown of the red blood cells and their functional component –

haemoglobin. Blood in new bruises is a red colour. As the haemoglobin breaks down and loses its ability to retain its shape, it becomes converted to biliverdin, which is green in colour. This breakdown progresses to bilirubin, which is yellow in colour. And this in general follows the breakdown process and subsequent age process of a bruise in the skin of a non-pigmented animal.

Langlois and Gresham (1991) examined 369 photographs of 89 human subjects (age range 10–100 years, grouped into <65 years and >65 years) presenting to a casualty department (in addition to staff and in-patients) with bruises, the age and cause of which was known. A standard colour chart was included, and in some, but not all cases, repeat photographs were taken.

The key finding of this study was that yellow was not seen in bruises less than 18 h old, but that not all bruises developed this colour before resolving, and so a bruise without yellow colouring could not be said to be less than 18 h old.

They also indicated that the colours in bruises were dynamic, and could 'reappear' days later, and that separate bruises on the same person, inflicted at the same time, did not necessarily exhibit the same colours, nor undergo equivalent changes in colours over time.

Skin colouration affected the evaluation of bruising, and the study findings were therefore limited to white-skinned human individuals.

Following this study, Munang *et al.* (2002) looked at bruises in children, and observers were asked to describe the predominant colour *in vivo*, and then again later from a colour photograph. Inter-observer variation was also assessed. They found that in only 31% of cases was there complete agreement of colour description by the same observer, between the *in vivo* examination and assessing the photograph. Agreement between observers for a bruise examined *in vivo* was seen in 27% and between photographs of the same bruise in only 24%.

In only one in ten bruises examined at the same time and in the same place did three individuals completely agree as to the predominant colour seen.

Reliance on the colour yellow was thus beginning to be questioned, and Hughes *et al.* (2004) showed subjects a series of photographs of bruises in which the yellow 'saturation' was digitally altered, in order to evaluate differences in yellow perception. They found that there was a variability in yellow perception and that an individual's ability to perceive yellow declines with age. All subjects used in this study had normal colour vision, as assessed using Ishihara plates (the standard tool used to assess colour blindness in children).

8.14   Qualifications to Give Testimony on Blood Spatter and Blood Pattern Analysis

While qualifications vary, courts are willing to hear evidence from experts on seemingly minimum bases (James *et al.*, 2005).

Evidence may be admitted to the court; however, the weight the evidence will be afforded will be determined by the experience, skill, knowledge and training of the expert.

8.15   Ante-mortem versus Post-mortem Injury

Existing forensic techniques are limited in their capability to deliver an accurate assessment of when a wound was inflicted. Wounds can be delivered to a body after death as well as prior to death. This can be due to the action of scavenging animals or, in some cases, the wounds can be deliberately or accidentally inflicted. A dead animal that has autolysis of the external cells can have its hair and skin slough off quite easily from handling while picking it up, and this will need to be differentiated from an ante-mortem wound. Bodies that are buried in a shallow or partial grave can be punctured with a search rod used to find them.

Oehmichen *et al.* (2009) at University Hospital of Schleswig-Holstein in Kiel, Germany, found that counting the number of mast cells at a wound margin can assist in determining whether a wound has been inflicted pre- or post-mortem.

In a living body, if tissue is damaged then many white blood cells, including mast cells, are preferentially diverted to the area through the inflammatory process. The mast cells assist in wound healing by release of granules to assist in new tissue growth and dead tissue destruction. After release of this enzyme, the mast cells lose the ability to make an enzyme called chloracetate esterase, so they will no longer show up when examined microscopically with a dye.

Consequently, a gradient of mast cells is seen microscopically, with the wound margins having less or no visible mast cells and the undamaged areas of the wound with a greater number of mast cells. Any wounds inflicted post-mortem would have no mast cell enzyme release and so, under the dye the researchers used, there would be a uniform distribution of mast cells from wound edge to wound body, indicating a post-mortem-inflicted wound.

Case Study 8.2 Bruising in Animals

Bruising can age a wound clinically, but not forensically. Bruises change colour after death. Here is an example of how bruising can change in a dead animal and how incorrect storage of the animal can lead to bruising colour changes.

In this example, the dog was euthanized after sustaining a dog bite. The animal was photographed immediately after euthanasia (see Fig. 8.11).

The dog was autopsied some time later and the visible colour changes in the external appearance of the skin and bruises were attributed to ante-mortem wounds in the animal (see Fig. 8.12).

The message from this example is that bruising in non-pigmented animals can be used as a clinical indicator (only) and should not be used as a post-mortem finding to interpret wound age.

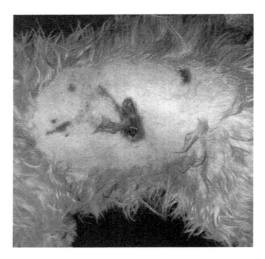

Fig. 8.11. Note the colours of the bruising that ranges from red and blue to areas of yellow discolouration.

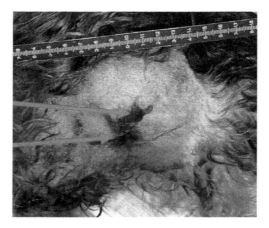

Fig. 8.12. In this image of the same animal, the post-mortem alteration of the skin should not be attributed to any ante-mortem condition in the animal.

Note

1 *State vs Ordway* (1997) 261 Kan. 776. 934 P.2d 94, at 809.

References

Blood, D.C. and Studdert, V.P. (1999) *Saunders Comprehensive Veterinary Dictionary*. Harcourt Publishers Ltd, London, UK.

Hughes, V.K., Ellis, P.S., Burt, T. and Langlois, N.E. (2004) The practical application of reflectance spectrophotometry for the demonstration of haemoglobin and its degradation in bruises. *Journal of Clinical Pathology* 57, 355–359. Available online at: http://doi.org/10.1136/jcp.2003.011445 (accessed 22 September 2015).

James, S.H., Kish, P.E. and Sutton, P. (2005) *Principles of Bloodstain Pattern Analysis*. CRC Press, Boca Raton, Florida, USA.

Langlois, N.E. and Gresham, G.A. (1991) The ageing of bruises: a review and study of the colour changes with time. *Forensic Science International* 50(2), 227–238.

Munang, L.A., Leonard, P.A. and Mok, J.Y.Q. (2002) Lack of agreement on colour description between clinicians examining childhood bruising. *Journal of Clinical Forensic Medicine* 9, 171–174.

Oehmichen, M., Gronki, T., Meissner, C., Anlauf, M. and Schwark, T. (2009) Mast cell reactivity at the margin of human skin wounds: an early cell marker of wound survival? *Forensic Science International* 191(1–3), 1–5. Available online at: http://doi.org/10.1016/j.forsciint.2009.05.020 (accessed 22 September 2015).

Snyder, G.K. and Sheafor, B.A. (1999) Red blood cells: centerpiece in the evolution of the vertebrate circulatory system. *Integrative and Comparative Biology* 39(2), 189. Available online at: http://doi.org/10.1093/icb/39.2.189 (accessed 22 September 2015).

9 Understanding the Nature of Document Evidence

Nikolaos Kalantzis*

Chartoularios Laboratory of Questioned Document Studies, Piraeus, Greece and Department of Forensic and Crime Science, Staffordshire University, Stoke-on-Trent, Staffordshire, UK

9.1 Introduction

The title of this chapter is very descriptive of both the positive and negative aspects of documents when treated as evidence. The term 'document' in a forensic aspect includes all aspects of a document, i.e. handwriting, signature, printing, the ink and the paper itself. As such we all have personal experience of some or all of these aspects. That personal experience, varying from one person to another, can provide useful insight, but can also limit one's view or perception of the evidence.

The basic question posed to document examination is the authenticity of handwriting; therefore, the comparison always takes place between the questioned writing (i.e. the writing of unknown or contested origin) and the specimen material (i.e. writing of known and confirmed origin). The same stands for documents (e.g. passports, banknotes, etc.).

In this chapter the principles of the holistic examination of documents is presented, giving an initial comprehension of the forensic approach.

*Corresponding author: nkalantzis@chartoularios.gr

9.2 Handwriting Evidence

The most common but also most important piece of evidence located on a document is handwriting, in any form. The process of handwriting and signing is essentially the same, and therefore are treated as different aspects of the same behaviour throughout this chapter following the same rules and principles of analysis and examination.

9.2.1 Handwriting as evidence

The essential features of handwriting that allow it to be treated as forensically valuable evidence are uniqueness and repeatability. When these two criteria are not met, forensic handwriting examination cannot take place within scientific boundaries. The problem of proof for the uniqueness of handwriting and signatures appeared intensely during the 1990s as an application of the Daubert Rulings (Berger, 2005) on handwriting evidence (Zlotnick and Lin, 2001), forcing the forensic community to research and prove the scientific validity of their methodology.

On a theoretical level, the function of the neurons in the brain and their synapses provide a very complex network through which hand movement produces handwriting (Hecker, 1993; Caligiuri and Mohammed, 2012). Not only that, but through years of practice the process of writing moves from the conscious competence to the unconscious competence, and the muscles are trained and grown to accommodate pen movement. This leads to the formation of a unique combination of individual characteristics, allowing them to be studied, examined and compared by the trained examiner.

On a practical level, a series of blind tests and proficiency trials carried out mainly from La Trobe University (Found et al., 1999; Sita et al., 2002) proved both the validity of handwritten evidence (meeting the two aforementioned criteria) and the ability of trained document examiners to determine authenticity through specific methodological examination, meeting the Daubert standard.

9.2.2 Feature examination

The methodology followed by the trained document examiner, using first the naked eye and then appropriate magnifying equipment (loupe, stereomicroscope, etc.), requires the analysis and then the comparison of specific features. Comparison always takes place among similar writing features, i.e. capital letters of the questioned writing are compared with capital letters of the specimen material. The main styles of handwriting are block capitals, disconnected lower case, connected lower case and mixed writing forms.

The general characteristics that are most commonly identified, analysed and compared include the following.

- Style and legibility, describing the general appearance of the writing.
- Size and proportions, referring both to the individual letter within a word and to segments of the letter.
- Spacing of words within a sentence and of letters within a word.
- Slant and slope.
- Fluency and pressure of handwriting, which is also evidence of the skilfulness of the writer.
- Additional features might be also discussed, depending on each case (e.g. punctuation, layout, etc.).

Detailed examination then takes place of the more individual characteristics of handwriting, including the following.

- The individual character shape, referring both to the execution parameters (smoothness of curves) and to the structural form.
- Individual character proportions and construction, analysing the direction and speed traced by the writing instrument, the number of strokes used.
- Character combination and connections, both in usual joins (e.g. 'th') and in unique combinations that can possibly be found in the analysed writing.

The next step of the analysis requires the comparison of the analysed features between the questioned writing and the specimen material.

An important factor to be considered during the comparison phase of the examination is natural variation. Writing is a dynamic aspect of human behaviour, and as such it undergoes continuous but not always discerning differentiation, due to numerous influences and various degrees of natural change. A person can produce writings that present subtle differences of no importance as a whole, that shape a concrete pattern. This set of resembling writings in their total is unique for each person and cannot be simulated or copied.

Equally to be considered is the quality (referring to the type of writing in relation to the questioned material, and the timeframe in relation to the assumed date of writing of the questioned document) and quantity (to establish the range of natural variation) of the specimen material. As time progresses, writing also progresses and changes. This aspect of handwriting needs to be taken into account, and be well documented in the specimen material, otherwise gaps of information appear and specific forms of variation might be erroneously misinterpreted as dissimilarities rather than variations of authentic writing. For example, if the authenticity of a last will and testament that was assumed to be written in 2007 is examined, and the specimen material dates from 1974 to 1984, that material is limited, not necessarily exhibiting the full range of the handwriting features of the testator (author of the will) at the assumed time of writing. Comparison with only that material might lead to erroneous conclusions. For such a case, in order to come to a safe conclusion, additional specimen documents may be required, dating as close to the year of the testament writing as possible.

Finally, other special factors can be introduced in the analysis, depending on the specific case details and the assumed author's background history. Outside factors like drug or medication use, alcohol consumption, mental illness or even injury (e.g. a broken arm that is recovering), may affect the writing procedure. In addition, environmental conditions might come into play (e.g. completing a form while standing up, in haste or under duress) and may need to be taken into account.

From a forensic point of view, the comparison of characteristics is not a simple addition and subtraction of similarities and dissimilarities. Even if only one unexplained dissimilarity persists (and cannot be interpreted as accidental), then, regardless of number of similarities, the examined writing should not be considered authentic.

9.2.3   Forgery

When unexplainable dissimilarities persist in the questioned material, a conclusion of forgery is very likely to be formed. Forgery can take place in several forms, including the following.

- Simulation, when the forger attempts to imitate the victim's natural handwriting or signature.
- Freehand forgery, when the forger either is unfamiliar with the victim's specimen or puts no effort into copying it.
- Tracing, when the forger uses an authentic writing or signature as a guide, tracing it to the forged document.
- Transfer, when the forger scans and prints an authentic handwriting or signature through mechanical means.
- Disguise, when the writer attempts to mask his characteristics in order to deny authorship.

When simulation occurs, the forger has access to documents containing the authentic material of the victim, and faces the following challenge: he has to replicate the process of years of training (of both the brain and the muscles of the arm) of his victim, in order to produce (for example) a signature with accuracy of form (drawing the exact same features) and dynamics (exhibiting the same speed and pressure characteristics). This task is unfeasible, and the forger usually balances between two extremes, either successful execution of the structure of the signature by slowly building it (producing slow and carefully plotted lines, with heavy unnatural pressure in order to control the movement of the writing instrument), or pre-forms a speedy and fluent formation that lacks the unnatural characteristics of the slow execution, but also lacks the accuracy of the signature formation (as the forger is not trained in natural execution of the victim's signature).

In freehand forgery, the forger will execute a fast and fluent formation (as there is no effort to 'copy' an original form). The resulting forgery will probably have no resemblance to the specimen material (and may even contain spelling mistakes). Most importantly, as freehand forgeries are quickly executed, they may include parts of the authentic signatures of the forger, that survive and are included in the fraudulent formation by accident (as it is part of the unconscious competence). For example, a forger signing a cheque as 'Mr Philip Morton', in an effort to add natural characteristics and fluency to the freehand forgery, adds a double underline in the same manner as he does with his own true signature.

This does not always happen, but when it does, it gives the document examiner the opportunity to investigate the authorship of the forgery (provided that the surviving unconsciously executed part contains enough information to provide a link to the forger's authentic signatures).

When the forger has access to original material, and has the luxury of time, tracing can be attempted, using that material as a guide. Several approaches of tracing can be followed, all of which leave evidence on the resulting forgery. Main characteristics of tracing include unnatural execution of curves, inclusion of pen stops and pen lifts, unnatural pressure and slow speed of execution. Also, depending on the method used, signs of the trace can be found on the document (e.g. a pencil or indentation used to form the trace of the signature).

Similar to tracing conditions, a forger with basic skills in computers and access to specimen material may use everyday computer equipment to scan, manipulate and print 'authentic' writing and signatures on fraudulent documents. These forgeries are very dangerous, as, without proper caution on the examiner's part, they can be misinterpreted as genuine. If examined in their original form, the microscopic examination will straightforwardly reveal the writing to be a product of printing (or other method of reproduction) and not normal writing (via a writing instrument). If these forgeries are photocopied and then examined (without access to the 'original'), the document examiner will not be in a position to determine whether the writing represented in the document was originally written there or printed.

Disguise is the most difficult forgery type to be encountered. The author already knows his writing features and can easily attempt to hide them from the examiner. Depending on the penmanship of that person and the knowledge of the principles of handwriting examination, it is possible to produce a signature or handwriting that cannot be scientifically linked to the original writer. Again, as with the double underline feature in the freehand forgery example, there is the possibility that the resulting disguised handwriting product contains formation too complex and unique to belong to anyone other than the original writer, allowing the examiner to state that even though the disguised writing is not 'authentic' (i.e. it is not similar to *all* of its features to the specimen material), it is too similar to belong to anyone else and therefore is still linked to the author; but this is the exception rather than the rule.

9.2.4 Further comments

One common misconception regarding handwriting evidence is the assumed link between the writing product and the psychological state of the writer, the study of which is called graphology. It is undeniable that heavy emotional burden or duress (e.g. signing a contract at gunpoint) will affect some handwriting features (most likely causing tremor). However, these features cannot be tracked to one unique cause (for instance, exhaustion from quickly climbing four flights of stairs will also introduce tremor in handwriting) and therefore do not meet the aforementioned criteria or reproducibility. When forensic handwriting examination was first introduced, it was believed that such a link existed, but academic and field research (especially in the post-Daubert era) found no supporting evidence for graphology (Jennings *et al.*, 1982; Furnham and Gunter, 1987).

Another aspect of handwriting that needs to be taken into account is class characteristics. Specific cultural or regional groups may contain in their handwriting features that are uncommon to persons outside these groups, e.g. people who use English as a second language and have a non-Latin alphabet in their mother tongue may exhibit uncommon characteristics. If such peculiarities are not familiar to and taken into account by the examiner, they may be inaccurately evaluated, leading to an erroneous conclusion. The most well-known example of such misinterpretation is the identification of German handwriting class characteristics as individual handwriting characteristics in the Lindbergh kidnapping case (Saferstein, 2007).

Graffiti is also a form of handwriting. The physics and the position of arm and body are different to those encountered in everyday handwriting, but the mental process is the same. Therefore, in principle, graffiti is also subject to the methodology of forensic handwriting examination. Studies have established repeatability and uniqueness in forms of graffiti-like 'tags' (a way of graffiti signing), allowing the examiners to form conclusions on authorship (Hussong, 2001; Sadorf, 2001).

Finally, serial skilful forgers with in-depth knowledge of the principles of handwriting examination can produce forgeries that can be difficult to detect. Such forgeries lack the spontaneity and the natural variation of the authentic signatures and, therefore, if more than one forgery exists they are bound to be too similar (i.e. without variation) allowing the examiner to properly identify them as forgeries.

9.3 Document Evidence

The document itself can provide a lot of useful information for a forensic examination, depending on the case and the mandate (i.e. the request for examination).

9.3.1 Ink/writing instruments (sequence)

Apart from the handwriting features pertaining to the writer, every writing instrument introduces its own category of characteristics to the examined writing. These features derive from both the ink that is deposited on the writing surface and the method of delivery of that ink to the paper surface. The examination of these features can provide helpful information (and proof) regarding alterations on a document, i.e. additions to the originally written document. For example, a cheque bearing the amount of €18,000 is contested, and the person issuing the cheque claims that the original amount was €3000.

The type of ink affects the image of the ink line, as more viscous inks (e.g. fountain pen) will soak the paper surface much more than paste-based inks (e.g. biro). The delivery mechanism also leaves a pattern on the paper surface, distinctive of its class (i.e. unique to fountain pens or ballpoint pens, etc.). With the cheque example, the forger might have used a different type of pen (i.e. a different class of writing instrument) to transform €3000 into €18,000. For example, the revolving ball of rollerball fluid ink pens will 'push' the ink to the sides, leaving a distinctive pattern on the written line, which is very different from the fibre tip pen, which only deposits the ink on the paper (with no revolving parts).

Apart from distinguishing the class of the writing instrument used, which on its own can provide helpful information, the colour properties of the ink used are also examined. Ink is a mixture of different chemical components, some of which provide the colour perceived by the human eye (i.e. in the 390–700 nm part of the electromagnetic spectrum), while others have to do with the kinetic and storing properties of the mixture. Different inks have different compositions and therefore can be distinguished chemically.

Chemical examinations for ink analysis involve chromatography: usually Thin Layer Chromatography (TLC), High Performance Liquid Chromatography (HPLC), Raman spectroscopy, or other chemical procedures destructive to the document (Brunelle and Crawford, 2003).

Apart from the destructive analytical approach, there are visual and spectroscopic methodologies that can provide ink differentiation. Every object reflects light in a specific set of wavelengths, depending both on the source wavelength(s) and the chemical properties of the object. As a result, the human eye perceives colours, i.e. a specific combination of wavelengths reflected by the object. Our eyes are limited to the visible spectrum as they cannot perceive anything above or below, but objects are not limited to it and can reflect in other areas of the electromagnetic spectrum. Therefore two inks that look identical in colour to the naked eye (i.e. reflect light in the same way in the visible spectrum) may behave differently in other parts of the electromagnetic spectrum, and specifically the infrared and ultraviolet areas of the spectrum.

To investigate this behaviour, special instruments are required with infrared sensitive cameras, and controlled light conditions. The instruments (usually called Video Spectral Comparators) control the source light and filter the reflected light appropriately into the recording camera, achieving infrared reflectance, infrared absorption or infrared luminescence of inks.

Other potentially useful information that can be deduced by ink analysis involves line crossings and sequence. For example, a printed document is presented, bearing a signature that overlaps with the last printed line of text, the owner of the signature claims that when he signed the document the last line was absent. In such a case, the sequence of the overlapping lines (i.e. the line of the signature and the line of the printing of the last sentence) will be examined. If the sequence can be determined, then the claim of the owner of the signature can be proved or disproved.

The deduction of sequence is very difficult and there is no uniform method that applies in all ink or printing combinations. The type of inks or printing involved in the crossing defines the possibility to determine the line sequence. Methodological approaches to this problem involve study under the stereomicroscope with perpendicular light, examination with an ElectroStatic Detection Apparatus (ESDA™), or even Scanning Electron Microscopy (SEM). Research is still being carried out to create a definitive methodology to determine sequence by analysing the depth of the strokes, and there is potential for 3D Raman Spectroscopy as the tool for this purpose.

9.3.2 Printed media

Following the same principles as for writing instruments, printed documents bear the class and individual characteristics of the ink or toner used and the method with which it was delivered to the paper surface. There are several different types of printing devices, depending on their mechanism. Typewriters and dot matrix printers once were commonplace in the work environment, but now the most common types encountered in the workplace and at home are inkjet printers and laser printers. The main difference between these two devices is the substance used to print (i.e. form the desired image or text on the paper surface). Inkjet printers use formulations of fluid ink, while laser printers use toner.

Furthermore, the delivery mechanism is different as inkjet printers mainly spray the ink on the paper surface, while laser printers transfer the toner particles through the use of charged drums within the rolling mechanism of the printer. What is important is the difference in features of the resulting printing each type of printer leaves on the document.

Inkjet printers spray the ink while reproducing the original image or text, resulting in printing of only medium detail, if examined under the microscope. On the other hand, laser printing allows for more accurate printing, with sharper detail.

Accurate identification and differentiation of these two printing methods can be detected using a microscope. Additionally, other characteristics that provide printer class identification include ink or toner spatter patterns. When the inkjet printing head delivers the desired ink quantity on the paper, additional small ink droplets will randomly fall, creating a spatter pattern around the printed text. That pattern, even though it is not unique, is located around the printed areas of the document. Laser printers also exhibit a toner spatter pattern, but this is due to a different phenomenon, pertaining to the different printing mechanism. The drum of the laser printer is charged appropriately to guide the toner particles to the specific areas required on the paper surface to reproduce the image or text desired. Due to electrostatics, there will be random flaws in the charging of the drum that result in a random pattern of small toner particles. The main difference from the inkjet spatter pattern is that because the entire page passes through the charged drum, the entire page is exposed to the random flaws of the electrostatic field, and therefore the toner spatter will appear throughout the printed page.

Apart from class identification, unique printer identification may be achieved, provided that the printer used produces identification marks on the paper surface. Such marks can be caused unintentionally by wear of the paper-loading mechanism or by flaws in the printing system.

A device-specific feature that provides complete identification of the printer that is unique to certain laser printers is the yellow dots pattern (Li and Leung, 1998). Many colour laser printers have been manufactured to include a faint pattern of yellow dots in every print they produce. That pattern can be decoded through a program available to government agencies; this may provide the maker, the type, the model and the serial number of the printer used, and sometimes it will include the date and time of the printing. Regardless of the information encoded on the yellow dots, consistency throughout each print job is of value to the examiner. For example, if a ten-page document is printed on a cloud laser printer, then each of those ten pages will have the same yellow dot pattern. If a page is substituted, that page will have a different pattern. Furthermore, if a page is reprinted (adding a sentence or paragraph to the originally printed text) then there will be twice as many dots, indicating that the same page was processed/printed twice.

9.3.3 Paper

Chemical analysis of the paper will not provide a lot of interesting information, as continuous recycling has led to the use of the same pulp over and over again. Still, the paper type in a multi-page document can offer a way of alteration detection. For example, an eight-page contract that bears signatures only on the last page is contested, and one party claims page 6 has been altered. The colour of the paper (even the different tint of white), the weave of the paper surface, or even additional staple holes may hint at the substitution of an original page.

Furthermore, depending on the severity and the use of each document, additional security features may be used. The most common examples of paper documents full of security features are bank notes, bank cheques and passports.

A traditional way of embedding security features on documents going as far back as the 13th century is watermarking, which creates an image within the paper itself. The image is observable with the use of light transmitted through the paper itself. This feature is still used on all bank notes – such as exhibiting the head of the queen in UK notes.

Another feature commonly used in all aforementioned documents is ultraviolet ink. The bank logo with intrigue patterns is usually found printed with UV ink on bank cheques, information regarding currency is printed with UV ink on bank notes, and nearly all the information visible on a passport is also 'hidden' with the use of UV ink in other areas of that passport (including the cover).

UV ink is invisible under normal light, but when hit with UV light (electromagnetic radiation above the visible spectrum; specific wavelengths commonly used are 365 nm, 313 nm and 254 nm) it will absorb and re-emit that radiation near the visible spectrum and be observed. The use of UV ink is a helpful feature as it poses two problems to forgers: first, they have to know of its existence and be able to observe it; second, they have to be able to reproduce it.

A very good security measure that is encountered in highly important documents is microprinting, which consists of very small print of text that without magnification appears as a thick line. It is very difficult to detect unless one knows where to look, and can be found on the lines of bank cheques (usually one of the lines under the signature) and on lines on banknotes. Furthermore, microprinting is nearly impossible to copy with commercially available computer peripherals. The detail is too fine for a common computer scanner to detect, and even if that information was somehow fed into a computer, commercial printers cannot produce such microscopic printing in detail.

Other security features that are used include holograms, security metallic strips embedded in the paper (either visible, semi-visible or completely invisible) and UV fibres inside the paper itself.

Finally, the paper surface can provide an amazing amount of information if carefully examined. Writing by hand on a stack of papers creates indentations on the underlying pages of paper. The indentation is caused by the pressure of the tip of the writing instrument used, and passes by contact from the front page (the one that is written on) to those underneath. Indentations can be very subtle and invisible to the naked eye. A first approach to detect possible indentation involves the use of side light (i.e. a strong light source shining from the side of the document), but this method will reveal only the strongest indentations and does not go further than the first or second page.

A device known to document examiners for more than three decades that detects indentations is the ElectroStatic Detection Apparatus (ESDA™). The ESDA™ essentially involves a vacuum pump fixed in a metallic box, and a metallic plate (with holes) on top. The document is placed on the plate, a Mylar® film is set on top of it, and the configuration is held together by the suction from the vacuum pump. The surface of the Mylar® film is then electrically charged and the charges sit differently on the surface depending on whether there are indentations or a substance on the surface (existence of

ink or printing). After that, toner particles are deposited on the surface and are held by the electrostatic field to those features that attracted the electric charges.

With this methodology, the ESDA™ can clearly reproduce indentations as deep as four or five pages, where they would no longer be visible to the naked eye. Such examinations can provide insight into case specifics and provide solutions to problems that cannot be solved with handwriting comparison alone. For example, an anonymous poison letter is brought in for examination. No specimen material is available because the author (or possible author) of the letter is not known. If the letter was written on a notepad, then the letter will carry the indentations from the writing on the previous pages of that notepad, possibly including information that leads to the author.

Additionally, line-crossing sequence, writing and indentation sequence or even fingerprint deposition and printing sequence can be investigated with the use of the ESDA™, as the subsequent writing or substance deposition sequence might be accurately depicted in the indentations left on the surface, and then picked up by the ESDA™ examination (Mohammed, 1998; Kalantzis, 2007; Fieldhouse et al., 2009). Therefore the examiner can offer insight into whether all the writing was completed in one session, whether the indentations on a document were created before or after the writing on that same document, and whether the fingerprints detected on the document were deposited before or after printing.

9.4 Additional Issues Regarding the Evidential Value of Documents

Having covered the basics of the evidential value of documents, some issues have to be discussed.

9.4.1 Photocopies as evidence

Photocopies or computer-generated (and printed) reproductions of original documents are essential to our everyday life and as such they are routinely encountered in the course of normal casework of a document examiner. Photocopies, reproducing all the visible information of the source document, can substitute for the original and, depending on the legal environment, in some countries they are treated as originals. Still, from the document examiner's point of view, the reproduced handwriting or signatures lack so many characteristics of the original that it increases the difficulty of the analysis and the forensic examination.

As mentioned earlier, handwriting and signatures are described by their pictorial and dynamic characteristics. The dynamic characteristics (i.e. pressure, speed, etc.) are lost in the reproduction process. The fluency of a written line, the accumulation of ink inside loops, feathering and other delicate features of the written line are not recorded by the photocopier and cannot be reproduced. Pen stops, corrections, retouching or small gaps in the written line may be reproduced as one solid (black) line depending on the model of the photocopier used, and therefore the reproduced signature (or handwriting) can be misleading in features of continuity, creating the danger of an erroneous conclusion if these flaws are neglected.

Still, the forensic examiner does not choose his cases nor his evidence, thus photocopies are often the only document evidence available.

The document examiner should be aware and should state in his report the aforementioned dangers of the examination of photocopies or reproductions. Then the examination should be based on the pictorial characteristics that survive the reproduction process. Photocopies are not stripped of any evidential value. For example, if a photocopied document bears a signature assumed to belong to Mr X, but which has no resemblance to the original signatures, then a conclusion of forgery (i.e. the questioned signature is not an original signature of Mr X) can be safely reached, *under the assumption that the examined photocopy is a faithful representation of the originally signed and photocopied document.*

When pictorial differences are spotted, it can be easy to reach a conclusion, as such differences are not expected to be overturned from the examination of the source document. On the other hand, if only similarities are spotted, then the document examiner is on dangerous ground. The fact that no differences are apparent from the photocopies does not mean that none exist – as mentioned earlier, pen pressure, pen stops, pen lifts, retouching, etc. is not reproduced in the photocopy, so all such information (if it exists) is lost. This situation makes it difficult to detect traced forgeries, but the real danger hides with altered documents.

Imagine the forger has access to a genuine signature. With modern equipment, he is able with relative ease to scan, crop and print the genuine signature, discarding the rest of the document it was signed on, and then reintroducing that genuine signature onto a new document. This can also be done (in a more crude manner) with scissors and sticky tape. As long as the product of this forgery is photocopied, the transfer of the genuine signature to a new document cannot be detected (unless the process was done without care and the forger left hints of his forgery, such as shadow lines from the cropping, etc.).

If the original product of such forgery is examined, it is very easy to determine the method used with a microscopic examination (that would reveal the signature was printed and not signed on the document). However, if only a photocopy remains, then all the surviving features point towards authenticity – as expected, since the reproduced signature has indeed originated from a genuine signature.

One common mistake encountered in such forgeries, which enables the examiner to identify it as such, is the use of the same signature again and again in the same or multiple documents. As mentioned earlier, each signature is unique, and no two signatures are 100% identical. This detail is unknown to most forgers who choose their source based on how 'genuine' they look. If the image of several signatures is identical then the only explanation is forgery.

9.4.2 Age and dating of documents

A very interesting and important aspect of document examination revolves around attempts to date documents and writing. Historical documents have many direct or indirect methodologies of being dated: based on the chemical examinations of paper and inks used; the composition of inks (much like similar examinations for authenticity of paintings, i.e. by analysing the components of the dyes and correlating that information with the assumed date of creation to determine whether these components were actually used during that time or not); with radiocarbon dating; or even stylistically, by examining the font system's compatibility with the assumed era of creation.

With modern documents, as briefly discussed earlier, the information deduced by such methodologies is inconclusive, due to the extensive use of recycling. For example, a last will and testament surfaces, dated 1 July 2007. The testator died in 2008 and no specimen material can be located. One party challenges the authenticity of this will, claiming that the other party forged it after a controversy over estates in 2013. The time difference in such a case would be only six years.

Depending on the inks used to create the questioned document, ink-dating methodologies can be used. As mentioned before, ink is a mixture of substances, some of which are volatile (able to evaporate). As ink is deposited from the ink cartridge to the paper surface, it starts drying. That drying process differs from ink type to ink type, but the most common methodologies apply to ballpoint pen ink, which dries out completely in about four to five years.

With chromatographic techniques (usually High Performance Thin Layer Chromatography, HPTLC) the different components of the ink mixture are identified, and their relative proportions are measured. The components are then referenced to curves of known aged inks and by comparison with the proper database, an estimate of the ink age can be achieved. There are two problems with such techniques: the time limit, meaning an ink cannot be indefinitely aged, as from some point on it is completely dry;

and the ability to artificially age a document through heating, causing the more volatile components to evaporate more quickly.

9.4.3 Stipulation of conclusions

An important aspect of document examination and the introduction of documents as evidence in any procedure is the stipulation of conclusions. As the methodology used in handwriting and signature comparison is not a quantitative one, but qualitative, the wording used has to correspond to a context understandable and accessible by all. For example, a signature is questioned as a forgery, and the examination exhibits a majority of similarities, but includes some differentiations from the specimen material, which can be explained and are not significant enough to challenge the authenticity of the signature. In such a case the examiner will not reach a conclusion with the highest certainty, but will express his conclusion regarding the authenticity of the signature with the use of words such as 'possible', 'very high probability', etc. These words, even though familiar to the layperson from everyday activities, do not correspond to a comprehensive scale of conclusions.

Efforts have been made by several countries and government agencies to create and adopt a standard form of conclusion reporting, and what they all have in common is that an explanation of the context descriptive to the specific case needs to follow the phrasing of the conclusion, regardless of the phrasing itself. For example, the currently used German scale (Köller *et al.*, 2004) uses the following wording and context steps.

- Probability bordering on certainty: The entire configuration of findings compiled, discussed and assessed as having high evidential value is in complete conformity with the hypothesis in all respects.
- Very high probability: The entire configuration of findings compiled, discussed and assessed as having high evidential value is in complete conformity with

the hypothesis in all respects. Findings which are not completely concordant and in no way relevant can be explained on the basis of method.

- High probability: The entire configuration of findings compiled, discussed and assessed as having sufficient evidential value is largely consistent with the hypothesis. Minor findings-related, irrelevant restrictions and/or inadequacies attributable to material are insubstantial and can be explained and justified on the basis of method.
- Predominant probability: The entire configuration of findings compiled, discussed and assessed as having sufficient evidential value is in agreement with the hypothesis in many respects. Findings-related, irrelevant restrictions and/or inadequacies attributable to material are insubstantial and can be explained and justified on the basis of method.
- Slightly predominant probability: The entire configuration of findings compiled, discussed and assessed as having meaningful evidence value conforms with the hypothesis but not entirely without inconsistency. Findings-related, restrictions and/or inadequacies attributable to material are significant and cannot be explained entirely on the basis of method.
- Indifferent probability – *non liquet*: The entire configuration of findings compiled and discussed is contradictory and does not support the identification of a tendency with respect to conformity with the hypothesis. Findings-related, restrictions and/or inadequacies attributable to material are significant and cannot be explained sufficiently on the basis of method.

In 2013, the European Network of Forensic Handwriting Examiners (ENFHEX), part of the European Network of Forensic Science (ENFSI) began to establish a uniform system of reporting conclusions for use of member laboratories (government and private) throughout Europe. The consequences of this effort could lead to consistency in reported results from European laboratories and examiners.

References

Berger, M.A. (2005) What has a decade of *Daubert* wrought? *American Journal of Public Health* 95(S1), S59–65.

Brunelle, R.L. and Crawford, K.R. (2003) *Advances in the Forensic Analysis and Dating of Writing Ink*. Charles C. Thomas, Springfield, Illinois, USA.

Caligiuri, M.P. and Mohammed, L.A. (2012) *The Neuroscience of Handwriting*. CRC Press, Boca Raton, Florida, USA.

Fieldhouse, S., Kalantzis, N. and Platt, A.W. (2009) Determination of the sequence of latent fingermarks and writing or printing on white office paper. *Forensic Science International* 206(1–3), 155–160.

Found, B., Sita, J. and Rogers, D. (1999) The development of a program for characterizing forensic handwriting examiners' expertise: signature examination pilot study. *Journal of Forensic Document Examination* 01(12), 69–80.

Furnham, A. and Gunter, B. (1987) Graphology and personality: another failure to validate graphological analysis. *Personality and Individual Differences* 8(3), 433–435.

Hecker, M.R. (1993) *Forensische Handschriftenuntersuchung: Eine systematische Darstellung von Forschung, Begutachtung und Beweiswert*. Kriminalistik Verlag, Heidelberg, Germany.

Hussong, J. (2001) Case study: graffiti. Paper delivered at the 5th International Congress of the Gesellschaft für Forensische Schriftuntersuchung (GFS) e.V., Bingen am Rhine, Germany (not published).

Jennings, D.L., Amabile, T.M. and Ross, L. (1982) Informal covariation assessment: data-based versus theory-based judgments. In: Kahneman, D., Slovic, P. and Tversky, A. (eds) *Judgment under Uncertainty: Heuristics and Biases*. Cambridge University Press, Cambridge, UK, pp. 211–238.

Kalantzis, N. (2007) The use of the Electrostatic Detection Device (ESDA) in the forensic examination of documents. *Penal Justice/Ποινική Δικαιοσύνη* 12(December), 1449–1454 (in Greek).

Köller, N., Nissen, K., Reiβ, M. and Sadorf, E. (2004) *Probabilistische Schlussfolgerungen in Schriftgutachten*. Luchterhand, Munich, Germany.

Li, C.K. and Leung, S.C. (1998) Identification of colour photocopiers: a case study. *Journal of the American Society of Questioned Document Examiners* 1(1), 8–11.

Mohammed, L.A. (1998) Sequencing writing impressions and laser printing or inkjet printing using the ESDA. *Journal of the American Society of Questioned Document Examiners* 1(1), 40–42.

Sadorf, E. (2001) Difficulties with reproducing graffiti handwriting, a case study. Paper delivered at the 5th International Congress of the Gesellschaft für Forensische Schriftuntersuchung (GFS) e.V., Bingen am Rhine, Germany (not published).

Saferstein, R. (2007) *Criminalistics: An Introduction to Forensic Science*, 9th edn. Pearson, Upper Saddle River, New Jersey, USA.

Sita, J., Found, B. and Rogers, D.K. (2002) Forensic handwriting examiners' expertise for signature comparison. *Journal of Forensic Sciences* 47(5), 1117–1124.

Zlotnick, J. and Lin, J.R. (2001) Handwriting evidence in federal courts – from Frye to Kumho. *Forensic Science Review* 13, 87–99.

10 Forensic Toxicology

Ernest Rogers*

*American Board of Forensic Medicine, American College of Forensic
Examiners Institute, Springfield, Missouri, USA*

10.1 Introduction

The practice of forensic toxicology differs from that of clinical toxicology. The difference resides in the fact that suspicion and confirmation of intoxication must be supported by analytical assessment and not necessarily the response to treatment. The analytical investigation starts and ends with:

1. The heightened suspicion of intoxication based on clinical or post-mortem signs.
2. The appropriate identification of the toxin or class of the intoxicating agent.
3. The collection and handling of the appropriate samples to ensure accurate poison or toxin identification.
4. The selection of an appropriately certified forensic laboratory.

5. The documentation, chain of custody, of samples collected and submitted.

Toxicological diagnosis must also include the timeline associated with the biological steps of absorption, distribution, metabolism and, if known, excretion of the intoxicant.

Safety during the investigation of a possible intoxication must take priority for the investigator and their staff. Toxins may be viable at the crime scene and during the ante-mortem and post-mortem examination.

Finally, the forensic report should be inclusive of all findings, the reasonable suspicion (signs or symptoms) for the initiation of an investigation and the conclusions based on toxicokinetics, chemical analysis and the biological evidence.

---

*Corresponding author: forensicinvestigations@comcast.net

10.2 Forensic Toxicology Scope of Practice

Current criminal and civil investigations often rely on many specialized experts. Among these scientific experts is the Forensic Veterinarian. In particular, the veterinary forensic toxicologist provides an integral function in the exploration of illegal activity involving the death of animals. Forensic toxicology is the art and science of the identification of drugs (medically significant), poisons (chemical origin) or toxins (natural origin) that are of medico-legal interest. The goal set forth for the forensic toxicologist is to develop a narrative and timeline related to the events in question using their advanced education in investigative techniques coupled with an understanding of internal medicine, toxicology, pharmacology, biochemistry, chemistry, anatomical pathology, clinical pathology, physiology and anatomy.

The incidence of malicious poisonings is thought to be in the order of 1% of animal cruelty cases investigated in New York City (Wismer, 2014). This low incidence is likely to be due to a number of factors: failure to recognize the possibility of a poisoning event; failure to complete a thorough crime scene investigation; failure of veterinarians, law enforcement and animal control officers to report suspected poisonings; and the possibility that owners find their pet dead and dismiss the possible cause, disposing of the remains without investigation. The recognition of a toxic or poisoning event requires both observation and investigatory skill.

Suspicion of a poisoning event should be heightened by the following features: an otherwise healthy animal that dies acutely; residue or odour of a chemical nature on the coat, mouth, stomach or intestinal contents. Staining of the tongue, lips or peri-oral areas are also signs that should raise the level of suspicion of a toxicological event (see Table 10.1; Gwaltney-Brant, 2007).

The investigating veterinarian or agent must take precautions during the investigation. The ante-mortem signs of intoxication vary with the poison. The post-mortem examination of the remains must be carried out with extreme caution, as some toxins (e.g. zinc phosphide) have been known to affect the individuals in contact with the remains (Guidechem, 2006; Papenfuss, 2012). Many dangerous chemicals have been restricted in their availability to the general public; however, some quantities of restricted or prohibited poisons and pesticides may be available from stored stockpiles and be accessed by ranchers, farmers and agriculturalists. The forensic veterinarian is well advised to perform all necropsies in well-ventilated areas with the appropriate protective equipment to avoid self-contamination, injury or even death.

The forensic toxicologist should always be aware of possible confounding evidence that could be misinterpreted as a malicious poisoning (e.g. carbon monoxide death after a fire event, sudden livestock deaths after exposure to local toxic plant). In each of these cases a complete crime scene investigation and necropsy should assist in the differentiation of malicious and accidental intoxications (Smith, 1996).

Forensic veterinarians differ in their application of toxicological principles from the veterinary clinical toxicologist. The forensic practitioner uses documentation to record significant events during the investigation. The permanent written record of the collection, maintenance and storage of evidence is also termed the chain of custody. The chain of custody includes all findings related to the initial scene of activity, the patient or cadaver and every aspect of the samples of evidentiary value collected (e.g. the time, location, the person collecting the samples or tissues, methods of storage or transport and the identity of all individuals handling the samples). In the ante-mortem patient, the condition of the patient (signs and symptoms), the timing of treatments and the collection of forensic samples (e.g. blood, urine or biopsy tissue) must also be noted. This documentation is maintained for all samples and events from the crime scene through the final judicial process.

10.3 Sample Collection

Obtaining appropriate samples involves an understanding of: the nature of the investigation (e.g. questions being asked by lead investigators); the crime scene; the species

Table 10.1. Examples of common poisons of forensic concern (Gwaltney-Brant, 2007; Wismer, 2014).

Poison	Exposure	Chemical State	Mode of Action	Ante-mortem Signs	Post-mortem Signs	Toxic Dose (LD50)
Ethylene Glycol	Oral	Liquid	Oxalic acid crystal and renal tubule blockage	Vomiting, ataxia, anorexia hypocalcaemia	Birefringent crystals in kidney	Cat 2–4 mg/kg Dog 4–5 mg/kg
Rodenticide -Strychnine	Oral	Powder or pellet	Block neuro-inhibitory transmission	Stiffness, tense abdomen Tetanic seizures started by startle	Rapid rigor Cyanosis Petechial/ecchymotic haemorrhage	Bovine 0.5 mg/kg Equine 0.5 mg/kg Canine 0.75 mg/kg Feline 2.0 mg/kg
Rodenticide -Anticoagulant -Warfarin -Dicumerol -Diphacinone, etc.	Oral	Pellet	Block Vitamin K-dependent coagulation	Skin haemorrhage: -ecchymotic -petechial weakness Anaemia Bloody froth mouth and nose	Haemorrhages: -pulmonary -intraocular -subdural -cerebral, etc. Free blood in body cavities Heart flaccid	Dog 50 mg/kg Cat 25–50 mg/kg
Rodenticide -Metal-Phosphine -Zinc phosphide, etc.	Oral	Powder or pellet	Phosphine gas blocks mitochondrial respiration, protein and enzyme synthesis	Convulsions Vomiting Dyspnoea Weakness Sudden death	Congestion -lungs -kidney (tubular degeneration) Liver (yellow mottling)	Dog 300 mg/kg Very toxic to human investigators[a]
Rodenticide -Bromethalin, etc.	Oral	Pale crystalline powder	Uncouple cellular oxidative phosphorylation	Ataxia Extensor rigidity Clonic seizures Respiratory arrest Muscle Fasciculation Hyperexcitability	CNS Spongy demyelination Cerebral oedema Inflammation of: -liver -kidney -Bowman's capsule	Cat 1.8 mg/kg Dog 4.2 mg/kg
Rodenticide -Calciferol, etc.	Oral	Powder	Increase circulating calcium	Cardiac arrhythmia Depression Inappetance Polyuria Polydipsia Increase blood pressure	Mineralization -blood vessels -kidney -stomach -lungs	Cat - low toxicity Dog 4.7 mg/ml
Dipyridyl herbicide -Paraquat	Oral Skin	Liquid Pellets	Pulmonary free radicals	Vomiting Depression Acute dyspnea Cyanosis	Alveolar fibrosis Atelectisis Hemorrhagic -intra alveolar	Dog 25–30 mg/kg Cat 40 mg/kg

of animal involved; ante-mortem signs and symptoms; and a review of the investigation documentation (police reports, witness reports, crime scene photography) (Young and Ortmeier, 2011). Further, the forensic practitioner should anticipate the questions that could reasonably be asked in the future, including in the court and depositions.

In ante-mortem toxicology, the practitioner should conduct a physical examination (including laboratory evaluation) of all live animals before continuing to the post-mortem patient(s). In the case of the ante-mortem examination (hair, fur, blood and urine) samples should be collected before medical treatment is initiated. Similarly, in the investigation for performance-enhancing drugs, samples should be obtained as soon as the animal athlete is finished with the competition. Any delay after the completion of the competition may taint results or break the chain of custody (Gwaltney-Brant, 2007).

Questions that surround a post-mortem examination may involve the effects of a chemical substance either found at the scene or in the possession of a person of interest. Due to the labile nature of many toxins, drugs or poisons, the accuracy of an analysis depends on a number of factors: time since ingestion or administration; the nature of the substance of interest; ambient weather conditions; amount of decomposition and location of the remains (buried above ground versus below ground versus in water). Investigation of the primary crime scene may reveal evidence of vomitus, salivation, lacrimation, significant toxic flora, chemical staining, unusual odours or residue on tissues or infestation by insects (Gwaltney-Brant, 2007; Rao, 2012). In post-mortem cases, without ante-mortem signs the diagnosis of the toxicological cause of death can be very challenging and solely dependent on the necropsy and the analytical evaluation of entomological samples (AFMES, 2012). Sufficient samples should be obtained and stored in order to ensure access to testing by other appropriate parties (defence attorney, governmental agencies, etc.) and to repeat and confirm initial results (see Table 10.2).

When possible, the direct collection of evidence from the crime scene (fur, faeces, vomitus, suspected debris, chemical residue, and used or discarded containers) is optimal.

In the case of a post-mortem investigation, samples include all body tissues and fluid samples that are available.

Hair and fur should be shaved down to allow examination of the skin for signs of parenteral drug or toxin administration. All body orifices must be examined for evidence of drug or toxin placement. Radiographs may reveal unusual substances, foreign bodies or other evidence in the gastrointestinal tract or body cavity. Though not well established in animal forensic investigations, the fur/hair sample may be used as circumstantial evidence to establish identity between an unknown fur source and an exemplar of fur from a suspect animal. Some initial research has been completed in hair or fur analysis for cortisol levels over time (Bryan et al., 2013). Human hair analysis for illicit drugs has been a forensic investigatory technique to establish and monitor illegal drug use (Ledgerwood et al., 2008). The future of these techniques to analyse and match drug concentrations in animal hair may be another method of comparison and identification of a known and unknown sample.

The submission of specimens should be accompanied by suggestions of the suspected class of poison, toxin or drug. The chemical class may be suspected from: ante-mortem signs and symptoms (from clinical examination, review of witness reports, etc.); necropsy findings; crime scene evidence; and in some cases following a court warranted search of suspect premises. Without guidance as to the nature of the toxin/poison, many laboratories may be unable to complete a forensic analysis of the samples submitted.

False positives and false negatives may be obtained due to unexpected chemicals, poor evidence collection or contamination. To ensure accurate and appropriate test results, the forensic scientist and the forensic analyst must be aware of test limitations and the possible existence of interfering agents. Many of the issues of contamination are addressed by maintaining strict chain of custody protocol and paperwork from the crime scene to the laboratory. Not all analytical laboratories can maintain the chain of custody. Samples are best submitted either by commercial courier or other traceable delivery system. Transport by a member of the

Table 10.2. Appropriate toxicological samples collected during ante-mortem and post-mortem examinations (Cooper and Cooper, 2007; AFMES, 2012).

Ante-mortem Samples	Collection Transport	Post-mortem Samples (fluid)	Collection Transport	Post-mortem Samples (tissue)	Collection Transport
Urine	Fresh sample Glass/plastic vial	Vitreous humour	All, 2%Na fluoride	Liver (right lobe deep)	50–100 g unfixed, plastic or glass
Venous blood[a]	15 ml Na fluoride tube 10 ml K EDTA tube Extra aliquots (50 ml)	Stomach contents	Fresh, unfixed plastic or glass	Brain	100–200 g, fresh, fixed in plastic or glass
Hair/fur	100–200 mg Envelope or aluminium foil[b]	Blood[a] -cardiac (rt. atrium) -inferior vena cava	30 ml Na fluoride 30 ml K oxalate Extra aliquot (50 ml)	Subcutaneous fat	100–200 g, glass or plastic
Vomitus	All collected Glass vial	Urine	Fresh sample	Kidney	25–50 g, glass or plastic
Faeces	All collected Glass vial	Bile	All, fresh sample	Skeletal muscle Psoas, deep thigh, spinal muscle	100 g, fresh in glass or plastic
		Cerebral spinal fluid	All, glass or plastic	Lung	Apex tissue 25–50 g, glass or plastic
				Hair/fur	100–200 mg Envelope or aluminium foil[b]

[a]Avoid serum separation tubes as the gel may absorb drugs or toxins.
[b]May use glassine or paper.

forensic team or police force directly to the laboratory is also acceptable. When submitting toxin, drug or poison samples for chemical evaluation, the practitioner must be aware of the receiving laboratory limitations and strengths. In many cases, failing to follow the specific sample submission protocols may result in compromising both the chain of custody and the overall criminal or civil investigation.

Often, the biological remains are infested by insects after death. Entomology measures the assessment of the time since death and is well-established science based on the presence and growth of various insect species, including assessment of the stages of the Green Bottle fly (order Diptera) (Amendt et al., 2007; Cooper and Cooper, 2007). Where degradation is advanced, the collection of arthropod samples for entomotoxicology is an alternative to direct tissue/body fluid analysis. Entomotoxicology is the established science of assessing the effects of common drugs on the growth rate and activity of arthropod species in decomposing animals. This technique allows the investigator another tool to assess the presence of drugs in the remains, weeks or months after death (Beyer et al., 1980; Gagliano-Candela and Avetaggiato, 2001). In human forensic sciences, controversy exists among analysts who disagree over the usefulness of the analysis of maggots, since there appears to be little correlation between chemical analysis of arthropods and the quantification of drug in the cadaver (Tracqui et al., 2004). However, unlike our forensic physician counterparts, the establishment of any quantity of illegal drug in an animal cadaver is cause for suspicion of abuse. To appropriately submit samples for entomotoxicology, the forensic veterinarian should visit the crime scene and confirm the presence of arthropods on the remains: in particular the larva of Diptera and the beetles (order Cole-optera), which feed directly on the larva (Gagliano-Candela and Avetaggiato, 2001). Collected arthropods should be sampled while on, or in, the body as opposed to those found in the environment surrounding the remains.

10.4   Animal Athletes and Performance-enhancing Drugs

The forensic veterinarian may be called to ascertain whether an animal athlete is using performance-altering drugs. This type of investigation follows the human concerns of athlete doping and chemical enhancement of performance. The World Anti-Doping Agency (WADA) concerns itself with the evaluation of the human athlete performance by monitoring the use and abuse of drugs altering human physiology.

The animal athlete may also be chemically altered to enhance performance, reduce signs of over-exertion and mask injury. The use of performance-enhancing drugs in horse racing and dog racing has resulted in tragic injury following the catastrophic failure of the animal in full race mode, resulting in both animal and human injury (Huntington, 2011; Animal House, 2013; Richardson, 2013).

Monitoring of performance drugs is limited to animal sports regulatory agencies, animal cruelty monitoring agencies (e.g. People for the Ethical Treatment of Animals), and overseeing bodies for the horse and dog racing industries. The veterinarians used to monitor and collect appropriate samples from those animals in the top tiers of a race, are often under the control and regulations of the state or federal governmental agricultural or gaming agencies. Though not a direct responsibility of law enforcement, the forensic veterinarian may still have need to investigate the illicit or illegal use of performance-enhancing drugs in animals.

There are efforts under way in the USA to ban illegal drugs in the horse racing industry so as to reduce the risk of death and injury to animal and jockey. Currently in the USA there are no national testing systems in place (Butler, 2010). Further, some state legislatures have proposed that an organization similar to WADA be established. In the north-east USA there is a governmental bill to establish an enforcement organization for the regulation of the prohibition of animal doping (e.g. Horseracing Integrity and Safety Act of 2013). This trend of calling for increased oversight and enforcement of animal doping is likely to expand across North America (Racing Medication and Testing Consortium, Kentucky, USA), and Europe (Fédération Equestre Internationale, Lausanne, Switzerland).

In many cases, where the forensic veterinarian is alerted and activated to investigate a case of animal doping, there are criminal or civil issues beyond the importance of the successful completion of an athletic event. Many insurance claims, wrongful death litigation and events with consequential human injury may be tied to animal performance drugs. The forensic veterinary toxicologist should have some familiarity with the illegal use of performance drugs in animal sports (Table 10.3).

In some cases the forensic toxicologist may be asked to evaluate performance-enhancing drugs related to reproduction, growth or bio-production (e.g. milk). Forensic investigations may also require the investigation of the use of antibiotics in food animals (European Union) or restricted antibiotics (North America and Asia). In many cases, the use of restricted pharmaceuticals in food-producing animals is monitored by the department of agriculture for the country or region involved. The forensic toxicologist when activated to investigate these occurrences should use the appropriate agricultural or food animal testing laboratory to ensure accurate results.

10.5   Selection of a Forensic Laboratory

The selection of an appropriate laboratory for toxicological analysis is intimately tied to the legal acceptance of the expert analysis and the testimony of a forensic veterinary toxicologist, and establishes the nature of the challenges from the opposing attorney or their expert witnesses.

Historically, in the USA, the accreditation of laboratories is required to ensure the highest standards of analytical science and toxicology. Two court decisions in the USA resulted in

Table 10.3. Performance-enhancing drugs in animal athletes (Butler, 2010; Huntington, 2011; Richardson, 2013).

Drug	Species	Use	Bio-samples	Detection Method	Comments
Sildenafil (Viagra)	Equine	Vasodilatation Increase lung perfusion	Plasma, serum, whole blood	Chromatography Mass spectrometry	
Anabolic Steroids (Stanozolol, etc.)	Equine, Canine	Increase muscle mass and endurance	Urine	ELISA	
Corticosteroids	Equine, Canine	Decrease inflammation Analgesia	Urine	ELISA	
Sodium bicarbonate (Milk Shake)	Equine	Decrease lactic acidosis Decrease fatigue	Blood	Plasma total carbon dioxide (TCO2)	Confound: commercial forage/grain
Arsenic	Equine	Low dose stimulant Higher dose decrease performance	Blood, hair, urine, soft tissue	Multiple tests: Marsh Test Atomic absorption Neutron activation	
Dimethyl sulfoxide (DMSO)	Equine	Analgesia Decrease inflammation	Urine	Chromatography Mass spectrometry	Confound lucerne grass
Methyl xanthenes (caffeine)	Equine	Stimulant Bronchodilator Vasodilator	Urine	ELISA	

setting the quality standards and expectations for use of science in the court system. The Frye Standard[i] and the Daubert Standard[ii] were the basis for challenging 'junk science' testimony in the court. Combined with other rulings, these decisions resulted in the establishment of the US Federal Rules of Evidence guiding the use of science techniques and testimony in a medico-legal forum. Science must be based on well-founded research when used to establish or refute criminal guilt, innocence or responsibility, in a civil hearing. The Federal Rules of evidence set forth four standards for the acceptance of good science in the court:

1. The scientific technique or method must be tested and considered valid by the educated scientific community.

2. The error rate for any technique (e.g. false positives versus false negatives) must be known and within acceptable scientific limits.
3. The techniques used must have been reviewed and be acceptable in peer-reviewed journals for their accuracy, specificity, selectivity and repeatability.
4. The testing and the equipment used must be generally accepted by the scientific community as appropriate for the test completed.[1]

Though these rules are only binding on the acceptance of scientific evidence and expert testimony presented before the US Supreme Court, many other courts have accepted this guidance for the evaluation of the quality and validity of scientific evidence. To this goal, forensic laboratories in general, and forensic toxicology laboratories in particular, should meet all regulatory standards for techniques, equipment, staff, training and facilities. Only those laboratories compliant with the regional standards, with appropriate certifications and qualified staff, should be engaged by the veterinary forensic toxicologist to ensure acceptance of the expert scientific and toxicological conclusions presented in the legal forum.

[i] Frye vs United States (1923) 293 F.1013, D.C. Circuit Court. Available online at: http://www.law.ufl.edu/_pdf/faculty/little/topic8.pdf (accessed 25 August 2014).
[ii] Daubert vs Merrill Dow Pharmaceuticals Inc. (1993) 509 US Supreme Court 579. Available online at: https://www.law.cornell.edu/supct/html/92-102.ZS.html (accessed 25 August 2014).

Specifics of the laboratory-accreditation procedures and processes vary among the multiple regulatory organizations and countries. In general, laboratory accreditation indicates that there is regular external oversight and monitoring of forensic laboratory procedures, techniques, calibration of equipment, and continuing education standards for technical and supervisory staff. Quality control programmes must be in place to ensure accurate results. There is proficiency testing of technical staff using unknown samples interspersed with regular forensic samples.

Internationally, the establishment of forensic and crime laboratory standards involves several nations in North America, Europe and Asia. The International Organization for Standardization (ISO) has set laboratory accreditation standards, ISO 17025. These are standards for performing tests and equipment calibration. In the European Union (EU), the forensic laboratory accrediting body is the International Laboratory Accreditation Cooperation (ILAC). The European Network of Forensic Science Institutes (ENFSI) also oversees laboratories in more than 20 EU nations. The combination of oversight and regulatory standards issued by ISO, ILAC and ENFSI support forensic laboratory accreditation for the majority of the crime laboratories outside the US and Canada. ISO standards are recognized by forensic laboratories in North America (What-when-how.com, 2010).

In North America forensic laboratories follow several standards to be qualified for forensic investigation analytical work. The College of American Pathologists (CAP) issues written standards for evaluation of the proficiency of laboratory testing. CAP has several areas of laboratory accreditation for human testing. The accreditations that are ensuring accuracy for forensic testing include:

1. Laboratory Accreditation Program.
2. Forensic Urine Drug Testing.
3. Athletic Drug Testing Program.

The American Society of Crime Laboratory Directors (ASCLD) offers a laboratory certification programme. Finally the American Board of Forensic Toxicology Inc. (ABFT) is another certification accepted by the court as

ensuring quality testing and standards (What-when-how.com, 2010). To date, the laboratory certification programs are acknowledged to monitor primarily human-testing laboratories. The excellent standards set by these certifications allows confidence in the toxicological results for animal samples, and acceptability by the court and legal system.

10.6   Methods of Toxicological Analyses

In the selection of an analytical testing laboratory, several criteria should be considered. The nature and robustness of any forensic testing procedure depends on its accuracy, precision, specificity, selectivity and sensitivity. Technical analytical procedures depend on a number of factors:

1. Type and quality of the samples submitted (fluid versus tissue).
2. Availability of analytical techniques and equipment.
3. Expertise of the laboratory and analytical toxicologist.
4. Nature of the suspected toxin (drug or poison).
5. Complexity of the specimen preparation for analysis (the more complex the procedure the more likely the defence will dispute the results).
6. The legal and scientific acceptability of the method to be used.

The molecular nature of toxicants suspected will determine the requirements for the upper and lower limits of detection (LOD). The selection of the signal must be significantly greater than the background noise to ensure an acceptable signal to noise ratio (S/N) and therefore acceptance in method validation and hence in a court of law (Peters and Maurer, 2002). Often the presence of a poison in a body is sufficient to confirm criminal activity (e.g. strychnine, cyanine). Quantification of a drug, toxin or poison may be necessary in the case where there is interference from metabolic products or feeds. Decisions made for the analysis of forensic evidence should be completed with the assistance of an experienced laboratory toxicologist.

There are both screening tests and confirmatory tests. Screening tests can be used to differentiate a presumptive positive test for a drug from a negative. There should always be sufficient biological samples so that screening tests may be followed by a confirmatory test. The confirmatory test is used to definitively identify the toxin, poison or drug and to avoid false positives or false negatives (Dolinak, 2005; What-when-how.com, 2010; Caplan and Kwong, 2012).

Screening tests may be used either at the crime scene or in the clinical setting. This is a common method of analysis for the drugs of abuse or performance-enhancing drugs (Caplan and Kwong, 2012). Obtaining immediate samples of urine and blood may allow the use of field drug tests to identify the drug(s) in the system. Tests are available through law enforcement and forensic suppliers. Many types of urine/drug analysis kits are available as over-the-counter products at local pharmacies. This information must not be relied upon to the exclusion of other possible toxins or poisons. Often a confirmatory test is supportive to the diagnosis.

Confirmatory tests are performed in a laboratory setting. These tests occur in two stages, beginning with the separation of the suspected chemical analyte from the biomaterial submitted, and then the detection of the chemically unique characteristics of the analyte for identification. Separation methods include enzyme-linked immunoassay (ELISA), chromatography and capillary electrophoresis (CE). Once separated, the chemical analyte is detected based on a unique molecular or chemical characteristic for a definitive identification. Selection of the method of separation and detection may be limited either by standards against which the unknown is compared or due to a limited library of detector results available to identify the unknown (Caplan and Kwong, 2012).

ELISA is often used for the identification of drugs (performance-enhancing, abuse) or known chemical substances of abuse. The method involves using the unknown sample antigen (analyte) attached to the surface of a non-mobile phase or well. The known detection antibody is intimately linked to an enzyme and allowed to interact with the antigen. Multiple liquid agents are then added to the analyte. The analyte is washed and eventually leads to a colour change, concluding with the identification of the sample (Gomolka, 2012). The ELISA tests are limited by the availability of known standard detection antibodies. Although many enzyme-linked antibodies are available, the development of additional testing antibodies is often an expensive and time-consuming task. Another separation method, and one that is more widely used as a laboratory method, is that of chromatography coupled with a mass spectrometer.

Chromatography separates an unknown chemical entity for analysis from biological material. Chromatography methods vary, based on their use of either a liquid or a gas mobile phase for separation. These techniques include liquid chromatography (LC), gas chromatography (GC) and high-performance/pressure liquid chromatography (HPLC). Once separated, the components pass through a detector that is continuous with the chromatography unit. The unique properties of the analyte are then detected and changed to an identifiable signal (e.g. electrical or photometric). The detector output is translated to a data format stored either in a computer interface or as a printed paper record. The selection of a separation method and detector used is critical to the medico-legal validity and conclusions drawn by the forensic scientist.

The most commonly used detector is the mass spectrometer (MS). The MS identifies and quantifies drug of abuse and illicit pharmaceuticals based on their unique chemical characteristics (Cody, 2003). For the MS there are known libraries identifying specific known compounds. The standards contained in the known library are compared to the unknown chemical analyte. This results in the identification and confirmation of the unknown sample. Several detectors are modifications of a basic MS detector. These include quadrupole MS (QMS), ion trap MS (ITMS), time of flight MS (TOFMS), and Fourier transform ion cyclotron resonance MS (FTMS) (Stafford *et al.*, 1984; Ojanpera *et al.*, 2005). The various

MS techniques differ in cost and ease of operation, LOD and availability of known standards. Choice will be dictated by the nature of the sample analyte presented or suspected. Currently the gold standard for forensic analysis is HPLC-MS. The use of the HPLC-MS (FTMS) is considered of superior forensic value because of its greater sensitivity, specificity and accuracy compared to other chromatographic mass-spectrometer techniques (Valaskovic et al., 1996). Currently, HPLC-MS (FTMS) is of limited use in forensics due to the extreme high cost of the equipment and ultra-low vacuum requirements for use (Smith et al., 2007).

Capillary electrophoresis (CE) is of increasing use in forensic toxicology laboratories due to its relatively low cost, and its ease of set-up and use. This separation method uses either a liquid or solid medium phase for separating chemical components based on electrophorectic direction and mobility (differentiation based on molecular positive and negative electrical charges). Detectors available for use with CE include ultraviolet light, visible light, florescence spectrophotometers, mass spectrometers and pulsed electrochemical detectors (Smith et al., 2007).

10.7   Principles of Toxicokinetics

Toxicokinetics and toxicodynamics refer to the nature of the distribution of toxins, poisons or drugs through the body from absorption to excretion. In many cases, the method of absorption can determine the toxicity of a chemical. The method of exposure to an agent may be determined by a close external and internal examination of the victim for oral, rectal or parenteral administrations (both ante-mortem and post-mortem). The rate of absorption is critical, as some toxins, if absorbed slowly, may be significantly less toxic than when rapidly absorbed. The chemical nature of the toxin, poison or drug may allow for the establishment of a timeline prior to death. The rate and method of absorption, target organs, mode of action, mode of metabolism and excretion all play critical roles in determining the motivation of an

intoxication. This is a significant medico-legal issue in the consideration of criminal or civil culpability (Dolinak and Matshes, 2005).

Exposure to a lethal substance often results in variations in the toxic and lethal response of individuals to the same dose and toxin. The toxin in a group of animals results in some percentage of morbidity versus mortality. The toxic effect of a chemical is described as the lethal dose resulting in death of 50% of animals exposed (LD50). Variability of the lethal effects of a toxin, poison or drug is based on multiple factors. Toxicity of a chemical is described by its concentrations in target organ(s) (Rao, 2012).

The forensic toxicologist must be cognizant of all of the factors that may affect the lethality of a chemical entity. This describes the risk assessment for the exposed animals. Biological variability of individuals and among species is based on differences in genetics, physiology and biochemical metabolism. Other factors that act to enhance variability include type of exposure (acute versus chronic, route), and age, health and reproductive status of the animals exposed. Finally the environmental conditions may have a synergistic or antagonistic action on the chemical lethality. Considering the physiological and genetic factors of the organism, and the influence of the molecular chemistry of the toxicant on tissue concentrations (and therefore its lethality) may be defined as toxicokinetics. It is the science of toxicokinetics that determines the rationale for tissue and fluid sampling of the previous sections (Poklis, 1996).

Toxins may enter the body either through dermal, inhalation, ingestion or injection routes. The absorption characteristics of each of these methods of exposure are very different and contribute to the eventual mortality of the animal. Bioavailability is also dependent on the chemical phase and molecular structure of the toxicant. Tissue levels will rise very rapidly with inhalation, ingestion or injection, while dermal exposures are often more slowly absorbed. The rapid rise in toxin concentrations at the target organs for the toxin or poison may be the difference in an acute versus a chronic lethal event (Dolinak and Matshes, 2005).

Once absorbed, the poison will be distributed via the vascular or lymphatic systems, diffusion or active transport, facilitated passive transport or pinocytosis. Distribution is not the same to all organs and tissues due to different blood perfusion percentages, varying lipid content, tissue pH and cellular activity or metabolism. The distribution of a toxicant in the body is described as the volume of distribution (Vd, reported as milligrams of toxicant/millilitres of blood volume). Rarely is the dose of a toxicant known at the time of the investigation; however, the identification of the toxin or poison and knowledge of the volume of distribution for a given chemical entity will help the forensic toxicologist understand the concentrations of the drug in the individual tissues sampled and analysed (Rozman and Klassen, 1996; Rao, 2012).

The metabolism of a toxin or poison may either decrease toxicity or enhance toxicity, dependent on the nature of the metabolites formed. Metabolism can involve the liver, lungs or kidney. In many cases, the original chemical entity will be metabolized to increase its ability to be excreted from the body. The rate of metabolism varies between individuals. Once formed, the metabolites will be excreted by the kidney in the urine, by the liver in the bile or by the lungs as exhaled gas (Rozman and Klassen, 1996; Rao, 2012).

Excretion of the metabolic products results in decreasing toxicity as they are removed from the body. In some cases the decreasing toxicity may result in morbidity without mortality. In cases where the metabolites have a higher toxicity than the parent compound, mortality may be delayed as the metabolites concentrate in the body system. The distribution and metabolism of a toxicant must be considered when examining the antemortem patient (Dolinak, 2005).

10.8   Conclusions

Veterinary forensic toxicology involves the scientific assessment of animal intoxications by various chemical, pharmaceutical or toxic agents. The role of the investigator is to gather all the pertinent data relating to the suspected crime from the crime scene.

This evidence must then be catalogued, recorded and secured. The conclusions drawn from the necropsy, along with reviewed police reports, medical records and witness reports, allows the veterinarian to establish a level of suspicion as to the possibility of a toxic event. There may even be sufficient evidence to give an indication as to the class of poison/toxin or a specific poison. The forensic investigator may then submit the body tissue and fluid samples to an analytical laboratory. The forensic investigator is responsible for selecting an appropriately qualified laboratory for the toxicological analysis. Once received, the investigator must assess the laboratory analytical report for validity and accuracy based on all the evidence gathered.

The veterinary forensic investigator plays a pivotal role in establishing the narrative of the sequence of events leading to the suspected crime. The narrative should encompass the biological, pathological and toxicological evidence that has allowed an informed opinion to be reached regarding the possible nature of death of the animal. A reconstruction of the timeline of events immediately preceding the death is the ultimate goal of these investigations.

The diversity of veterinary patients requires that toxicological conclusions be supported by the most current and accepted scientific and medical documentation. Therefore, veterinarians involved in the investigations of crimes against, or involving, animals should be cautious of assigning blame. Forensic scientists are not concerned with justice or injustice, guilt or innocence; they are only interested in the use of the best medical science and investigatory procedures to establish, support or disprove other evidence collected. In an effort to continually improve its art and science, veterinary forensic toxicology is currently utilizing the most modern scientific and investigative techniques.

This chapter has reviewed the salient factors that may be considered during a forensic investigation involving toxins or poisons. As crimes become more sophisticated, so must our observations, and levels of suspicion must become more acute. Technological equipment and chemical analysis allows the toxicologist the ability to detect smaller quantities of toxins or poison that can result in morbidity or mortality. For each forensic investigator, working within the criminal legal system, there must be considerations of the cost/benefit of each test requested. Multiple testing without cause or scientific direction is to be avoided.

In conclusion, the critical link in the process of a toxicological investigation is the ability of the investigator. The astute perception and understanding of the elements of intoxication is the key to a successful conviction. The forensic toxicologist is responsible for the appropriate documentation and presentation of the evidence and conclusions.

Note

[1] Committee on the Judiciary, 112th Congress (2012) Federal Rules of Evidence 2013, in Federal Evidence Review. Available online at: http://federalevidence.com/downloads/rules.of.evidence.pdf (accessed 1 August 2014).

References

AFMES (2012) Guidelines for the collection and shipment of specimens for toxicological analysis. Armed Forces Medical Examiner System, Division of Forensic Toxicology, Dover Air Force Base, Delaware, USA, pp. 1–3. Available online at: http://www.afmes.mil/assets/docs/toxguidelines.pdf (accessed 23 September 2015).

Amendt, J., Campobasso, C.P., Gaudry, E., Reiter, C., LeBlanc, H.N. and Hall, M.J.R (2007) Best practice in forensic entomology-standards and guidelines. *International Journal of Legal Medicine* 121, 90–104.

Animal House (2013) Dying for an edge: performance-enhancing drugs in the animal world. Available online at: http://wamuanimalhouse.org/shows/2013-08-10/dying-edge-performance-enhancing-drugs-animal-world (accessed 23 September 2015).

Beyer, J.C., Enos, W.F. and Stajic, M. (1980) Drug identification through analysis of maggots. *Journal of Forensic Sciences* 25, 411–412.

Bryan, H.M., Adams, A.G., Invik, R.M., Edwards, K.E.W. and Smits, J.E.G. (2013) Hair as a measure of baseline cortisol levels over time in dogs. *Journal of the American Association of Laboratory Animal Science* 52, 189–196.

Butler, L. (2010) 3 most common performance enhancing drugs & steroids in horse racing. Available online at: http://www.testcountry.org/3-most-common-performance-enhancing-drugs-steroids-in-horse-racing.htm (accessed 25 August 2014).

Caplan, Y.H. and Kwong, T.C. (2012) Evaluation of toxicology test results – characterization and confirmation of analytical methods. Available online at: http://www.cap.org/apps/docs/committees/toxicology/toxeval.pdf (accessed 25 August 2014).

Cody, J. (2003) Mass spectrometry. In: Levine, B. (ed.) *Principles of Forensic Toxicology*. AACC Press, Washington, District of Columbia, USA, pp. 139–153.

Cooper, J.E. and Cooper, M.E. (2007) Clinical work. In: Cooper, J.E. and Cooper, M.E. (eds) *Introduction to Veterinary and Comparative Forensic Medicine*. Blackwell Publishing, Ames Iowa, USA, pp. 145–147.

Dolinak, D. (2005) Toxicology. In: Dolinak, D., Matshes, E. and Lew E. (eds) *Forensic Pathology: Principles and Practice*. Elsevier Academic Press, Burlington, Maine, USA, p. 490.

Dolinak, D. and Matshes, E. (2005) The forensic autopsy. In: Dolinak, D., Matshes, E. and Lew E. (eds) *Forensic Pathology: Principles and Practice*. Elsevier Academic Press, Burlington, Maine, USA, pp. 65–70.

Gagliano-Candela, R. and Avetaggiato, L. (2001) The detection of toxic substances in entomological specimens. *International Journal of Legal Medicine* 114, 197–203.

Gomolka, E. (2012) Immunoassay in toxicology diagnosis. In: Abuelzein, E. (ed.) *Trends in Immunolabelled and Related Techniques*. In: TechOpen.com, pp. 67–82. Available online at: http://library.umac.mo/ebooks/b2805037x.pdf (accessed 25 August 2014).

Guidechem (2006) Material Safety Data Sheet, Zinc Phosphide (CAS 1314-84-7). Available online at: http://www.guidechem.com/msds/1314-84-7.html (accessed 28 September 2014).

Gwaltney-Brant, S.M. (2007) Patterns of non-accidental injury: poisoning. In: Merck, M.D. (ed.), *Veterinary Forensics: Animal Cruelty Investigations*. Blackwell Publishing, Oxford, UK, pp. 169–183. doi: 10.1002/9780470344583.

Huntington, P. (2011) Prohibited substances, feed and the performance horse. Equinews, 22 June. Available online at: http://www.equinews.com/article/prohibited-substances-feed-and-the-performance-horse (accessed 25 August 2014).

Ledgerwood, D.M., Goldberger, B.A., Risk, N.K., Lewis, C.E. and Price, R.K. (2008) Comparison between self report and hair analysis of illicit drug use in a community. *Addictive Behaviour* 32(9), 1131–1139.

Ojanpera, I., Pelander, A., Laks, S., Gergov, M., Vuori, E. and Witt, M. (2005) Application of accurate mass measurements to urine drug testing. *Journal of Toxicology* 29(1), 34–40.

Papenfuss, M. (2012) Dog dies, people sickened in Edwards after chemical exposure. Available online at: http://www.vaildaily.com/article/20121208/NEWS/121209845 (accessed 23 September 2015).

Peters, F. and Maurer, H., (2002) Bioanalytical method validation and its implications for forensic and clinical toxicology: a review. *Accreditation and Quality Assurance Journal* 7, 441–449.

Poklis, A. (1996) Analytic/forensic toxicology. In: Klassen, C.D. (ed.) *Casarett and Doull's Toxicology: The Basic Science of Poisons*. McGraw-Hill, New York, USA, pp. 951–967.

Rao, D. (2012) General toxicology. Available online at: http://www.forensicpathologyonline.com/e-book/poisons/general-toxicology (accessed 23 September 2015).

Richardson, J. (2013) Vets test Yukon Quest dogs for performance-enhancing drugs. Available online at: http://www.newsminer.com/sports/yukon_quest/vets-test-yukon-quest-dogs-for-performance-enhancing-drugs/article_6e39465a-703b-11e2-9b35-0019bb30f31a.html (accessed 25 August 2014).

Rozman, K.K. and Klassen, C.D. (1996) Absorption, distribution and excretion of toxicants. In: Klassen, C.D. (ed.) *Casarett and Doull's Toxicology: The Basic Science of Poisons*. McGraw-Hill, New York, USA, pp. 97–99.

Smith, M.L., Vorce, S.P., Holler, J.M., Shimomura, E., Magluilo, J., Jacobs, A.J. and Huestis, M.A. (2007) Modern instrumental methods in forensic toxicology. *Journal of Analytical Toxicology* 31(5), 237–253, 8A–9A.

Smith, R.P. (1996) Toxic responses of the blood. In: Klassen, C.D. (ed.) *Casarett and Doull's Toxicology: The Basic Science of Poisons*. McGraw-Hill, New York, USA, pp. 343–344.

Stafford, G.C. Jr., Kelly, P.E., Syka, J.E.P., Reynolds, W.E. and Todd, J.F.J. (1984) Recent improvements in and analytical applications of advanced ion trapping. *International Journal of Mass Spectrometry and Ion Processes* 60, 85–99.

Tracqui, A., Tracqui, C.K., Kintz, P. and Ludes, B. (2004) Entomotoxicology for the forensic toxicologist: much ado about nothing? *International Journal of Legal Medicine* 118, 194–196.

Valaskovic, G.A., Kelleher, N.L. and McLafferty, F.W. (1996) Attamole protein characterization by capillary electrophoresis-mass spectrometry. *Science* 223, 1199–1202.

What-when-how.com (2010) Accreditation of forensic science laboratories. Available online at: http://what-when-how.com/forensic-sciences/accreditation-of-forensic-science-laboratories (accessed 23 September 2015).

Wismer, T. (2014) Personal communication from Director. American Society for the Prevention of Cruelty to Animals, New York City, USA.

Young, T. and Ortmeier, P.J. (2011) Physical evidence collection and analysis. In: Young, T.J. and Ortmeier, P.J., *Crime Scene Investigation: The Forensic Technician's Field Manual*. Prentice-Hall, Upper Saddle River, New Jersey, USA, pp. 7–78.

11 Bitemark Analysis

David Bailey,[1] Jennifer Hamilton-Ible,[2]* Lucy Leicester,[3]
Louise MacLeod[4] and Adele Wharton[5]

[1]Department of Forensic and Crime Science, Staffordshire University, Stroke-on-Trent,
Staffordshire, UK; [2]Highcroft Veterinary Group, Bristol, UK; [3]School of Veterinary
Medicine and Science, University of Nottingham, Nottinghamshire, UK; [4]Hills
Veterinary Surgery, London, UK; [5]Saphinia Veterinary Forensics, Bottesford,
Nottinghamshire, UK

11.1 Introduction: Dog Bitemarks – Pathology and Outcomes

Dogs are often referred to as 'man's best friend', but conflicts between the two species are common with potentially catastrophic consequences for both parties.

Serious injury, disfigurement or even death of the victim can occur, and an incident will frequently lead to euthanasia or abandonment of the animal involved. The effects on the victim also may not be purely physical. Peters *et al.* (2004) examined 22 children who had been victims of dog attacks and, of these, 12 were found to have symptoms of post-traumatic stress disorder 2 to 9 months after the incident. In adult victims, there may also be financial consequences due to loss of income, as well as the psychological consequences of disfiguring injuries. There may be legal consequences for the owner of an attacking dog, if a link between it and the victim can be demonstrated.

Fatalities occur uncommonly, and incidents of fatality followed by predation of the victim have been reported, usually involving more than one dog (Avis, 1999). The most visible injuries resulting from dog bites will tend to be penetrating injuries, usually from the canine teeth. Canine dentition is designed to crush and tear prey, meaning that there is often significant blunt trauma. This can lead to circulatory or neurological compromise, which may not be immediately apparent (Calkins *et al.*, 2001). Depending on breed, an adult dog can exert 200–400 pounds per square inch (psi) of pressure with its jaws.

In non-fatal incidents, infection of the wounds following the attack is also a major

---

*Corresponding author: jhamiltonible@gmail.com

concern. These are usually infections caused by a mixed population of pathogens. In any case involving a dog bite, both the dog and victim should be tested for rabies (Kullberg *et al.*, 1991; Talan *et al.*, 1999).

The features of an injury considered to be pathognomonic for dog bites include puncture wounds (caused by the canine teeth), lacerations and avulsions leading to irregular wound edges, and associated claw marks (De Munnynck and Van de Voorde, 2002). However, depending on the severity and duration of the attack, some of these features may not be present. For example, there may not always be avulsion of tissue resulting in a three-dimensional wound (although where dog bites are concerned, this is frequently the case). Many variables may affect what is actually seen as a result of a bite, including the anatomical region bitten, positioning, and age of the victim, with the result that a bite may not be initially recognized as such.

In this chapter we will examine the risk factors and epidemiology of dog bites, prevention strategies, as well as providing an overview of the forensic approach to a suspected bitemark, case studies and a review of the current literature.

11.2   Risks and Relative Incidence

It is estimated that 30%–40% of households in the UK, Belgium, the USA and Australia own dogs (Wise and Yang, 1994; Collier, 2006; De Keuster *et al.*, 2006; Murmann *et al.*, 2006). The incidence of dog bites in people across all age groups is approximately 1.5% annually; or between 8 and 18 per 1000 subjects (Sacks *et al.*, 1996; Weiss *et al.*, 1998; Overall and Love, 2001; Kahn *et al.*, 2003; De Keuster *et al.*, 2006; Gilchrist *et al.*, 2008; Cornelissen and Hopster, 2010). It is hypothesized that most dog bites are not reported to the authorities (Overall and Love, 2001; Kahn *et al.*, 2003; Cornelissen and Hopster, 2010), and so the incidence is likely to be higher than these figures suggests. Fatalities due to dog bites are fortunately rare, with the incidence estimated at 1 fatal attack per 5 million dogs per year (Overall and Love, 2001).

Approximately 70% of dog bite-related fatalities occur in children under 11 years old, and 10.2% in adults over 69 years old (Sachs *et al.*, 1989; Sacks *et al.*, 2000; Overall and Love, 2001).

Children are more at risk of dog bites than adults, and studies have shown that children are two to five times more likely to experience dog bites than adults (Sacks *et al.*, 1996; Overall and Love, 2001; Kahn *et al.*, 2003). De Keuster *et al.* (2006) suggested that 'dog bites represent a significant and under reported part of accidents in children'. Children are more likely than adults to receive medical attention for dog bites (Weiss *et al.*, 1998; Sacks *et al.*, 2000; Gilchrist *et al.*, 2008) and severe dog bites most frequently occur in children under 9 years old (Brogan *et al.*, 1995; Weiss *et al.*, 1998). This may be partly related to the area of the body that children tend to get bitten on. Children are more likely to be bitten on the head and neck (Chin *et al.*, 1982; Brogan *et al.*, 1995; Weiss *et al.*, 1998; Avis, 1999; Kahn *et al.*, 2003), whereas adults are more likely to be bitten on the extremities (Weiss *et al.*, 1998; Overall and Love, 2001). This is in part due to their small physical size, but also due to the way children interact with dogs. It has been shown that young children explore novel objects, especially those that are mobile, such as dogs, with their face (Meints *et al.*, 2010). Young children are often poor at reading dog body language, and can misinterpret a dog snarling for one that is smiling (Meints *et al.*, 2010). Young children also tend to look into the face of a dog to make a decision about the dog's behaviour (Lakestani *et al.*, 2005). Males are more likely to get bitten by a dog (Brogan *et al.*, 1995; Weiss *et al.*, 1998; Overall and Love, 2001) and account for a higher number of dog bite-related fatalities (Overall and Love, 2001). The highest incidence of dog bite-related injuries is for boys aged between 5 and 9 years old; approximately 3.6% of emergency department visits in the US by male children between 5 and 9 years old are dog bite-related (Weiss *et al.*, 1998; Overall and Love, 2001). Unsurprisingly, children are more likely to get bitten if they are left alone with a dog (Kahn *et al.*, 2003; De Keuster *et al.*, 2006; Náhlík *et al.*, 2010).

Náhlík *et al.* (2010) interviewed 92 children in the Czech Republic about their experiences of being bitten by a dog. A proportion reported having provoked the animal by teasing or deliberately inflicting pain, and the authors highlight the concern about behavioural changes seen in children as a result of exposure to age-inappropriate content via media and computer games.

Most dogs involved in dog bite-related injuries and most dogs inflicting fatal bites are normally reported to be large breeds (Overall and Love, 2001). There have been many studies looking at breed-related incidence of dog bites in people, with variable conclusions. Overall and Love (2001) found German Shepherds, Rottweilers, Pit Bull-type dogs and Siberian Huskies to be over-represented in cases of dog bite-related injuries (Overall and Love, 2001). Another study also found German Shepherds and Rottweilers to be over-represented, but surprisingly identified the Labrador, a breed that is not normally categorized as a 'dangerous' dog, to be over-represented in cases of dog bite-related injuries (Kahn *et al.*, 2003). However, Duffy *et al.* (2008) found the Labrador to be among the least aggressive group of breeds, and found that the breeds most likely to exhibit serious aggression towards people included Dachshunds, Chihuahuas and Jack Russell Terriers, all small breeds of dog. Numerous studies have identified Pit Bull-type dogs to be over-represented in breeds of dogs causing fatal bites and severe trauma; they were reported to be involved in 42% of dog bite-related deaths between 1979 and 1988, and in 40% of incidents where an infant was pulled from a crib (Sachs *et al.*, 1989; Overall and Love, 2001). In another study, looking at dog bite-related fatalities in the US between 1979 and 1998, Rottweilers were the most commonly reported breed involved in fatal attacks, followed by Pit Bull-type dogs. Together, these two breeds have been reported to be responsible for approximately 60% of human deaths (Sacks *et al.*, 2000). German Shepherds have also been identified as a breed over-represented in studies of fatal dog bite incidents (Overall and Love, 2001).

Much of this research has been used to create breed-specific legislation, such as the Dangerous Dogs Act (1991) in the UK, which controls ownership of the Pit Bull Terrier, Japanese Tosa, Dogo Argentino and Fila Brasileiro (http://www.legislation.gov.uk/ukpga/1991/65/contents). The authors urge care in interpreting breed-specific data relating to dog bite-related injuries and fatalities. All breeds of dog have the potential to bite and cause injury (Overall and Love, 2001; Kahn *et al.*, 2003; Collier, 2006), and it has been argued that there is no reliable evidence to suggest that particular breeds are more dangerous than others (Sacks *et al.*, 2000). Duffy *et al.* (2008) suggested that 'it is inappropriate to make predictions about a given dog's propensity for aggressive behaviour based solely on its breed'. Most of the information relating to bite injuries is from emergency department records. Bite-related injuries from large dogs are more likely to be brought into emergency departments, given their ability to inflict more serious injury, and many bites from smaller breeds of dogs may go unrecorded (Duffy *et al.*, 2008). National registrations of dog breeds are often not accurate, and it can be very difficult to verify the breed of dog involved in an attack (Sacks *et al.*, 2000; Duffy *et al.*, 2008). All of these factors make it very difficult to produce accurate statistical analysis of the data relating to dog bite-related injuries and fatalities. Public opinion of so-called 'dangerous' dog breeds is often heavily influenced by media reporting.

It has been found that male dogs bite more frequently than females, particularly intact males, perhaps because of their propensity to roam (Overall and Love, 2001). Most dog bite-related injuries are caused by adult dogs (Overall and Love, 2001), but there is little other data relating to a correlation between a dog's age and tendency to bite. Pain, certain endocrine and neurological conditions, in addition to medications, can make dogs less predictable and more reactive, and therefore more likely to bite (Overall and Love, 2001).

Contrary to popular belief, most dog bites occur within the home and not in a public place (Weiss *et al.*, 1998; Overall and Love, 2001; De Keuster *et al.*, 2006). Having a dog in the household is associated with increased risk of dog bites (Gilchrist *et al.*, 2008). It is reported that 65% of dog bites in children occur within the home (Kahn *et al.*, 2003; De Keuster *et al.*, 2006) and in most cases a familiar dog is involved (reported figures range from 85%–94%) (Brogan *et al.*, 1995; Overall and Love, 2001; Kahn *et al.*, 2003; De Keuster *et al.*, 2006; Cornelissen and Hopster, 2010).

11.3 Comparison between Human Bitemarks, Dog Bitemarks and Bitemarks from Other Species of Forensic Relevance

Bitemarks have certain measurable characteristics, which can be of use when attempting to determine the species of the biter. These include the arch width, the shape of the dental arch, the spacing between the teeth, and the shape and size of the teeth.

Bitemarks can present as a spectrum of injuries, from impact marks to deep lacerations. The human bitemark is typically circular or oval, with a void in the centre, or may represent a more limited portion of the dental arcade (for example, canine to canine). The lower incisors tend to anchor the bitten substrate, while the upper teeth bite down. This may result in scrape marks being present in the portion of the bitemark representing the upper arcade (De Munnynck and Van de Voorde, 2002; Morgan and Palmer, 2007). Human dentition is highly individual, so a human forensic odontologist may be able to reach a strong opinion of association in terms of identification. There are four types of teeth: incisors (I), canines (C), premolars (P) and molars (M). The human dental formula is I2/2, C1/1, P2/2, M3/3, and usually only the rostral dentition is involved in a bitemark.

In contrast to man, both cats and dogs have asymmetrical dental arches (see Fig. 11.1), with the mandibular arcade being both shorter and narrower than the maxillary arcade (with the exception of the brachycephalic breeds, which exhibit mandibular prognathism).

Adult dogs have 42 permanent teeth, whereas adult cats have 30 permanent teeth.

With regard to the rostral dental arch (the portion most often represented in bitemarks) humans have four incisors per dental arcade, whereas dogs have six, but it must be remembered that distortion produced by movement may lead to misinterpretation (Tedeschi-Oliveira *et al.*, 2011).

The size and shape of a dog bitemark can vary considerably depending on the size and breed of the dog. There is less variation within the feline species, although there is considerable size variation between breeds (Clark *et al.*, 1994). Breed variation can cause problems when using standardized measurements to determine the species of biter. For example, a common measurement taken is the inter-canine distance, which in smaller dog breeds can be similar to those of a human, so it is important not to simply rely on a single criterion (Tedeschi-Oliveira *et al.*, 2011). The rostral portion of the dental arch is much narrower in dogs than in humans, and the canine teeth are much larger, with a conical outline. These are used to anchor the prey, while the other teeth tear.

The canine dental formula is I3/3 C1/1, P4/4, M2/3. The incisors are aligned in a shallow arch, terminating in the canines. The dental arcade then angles sharply toward the caudal part of the arcade. The premolars increase in size caudally, whereas the first molar is the largest of the molar teeth. The upper and lower premolars and molars interlock with each other when biting, allowing these teeth to bite and lacerate (Clark *et al.*, 1994).

Dog bites are the most frequently encountered animal bitemark, and dogs have been reported to bite humans eight times more frequently than humans bite each other (Lessig *et al.*, 2006).

The feline dental formula is I3/3 C1/1 P3/2 M1/1. The feline bitemark is much shorter and more rounded than that of the dog. Cats have a tendency to claw their prey, meaning that claw marks are often found in addition to bitemarks (Clark *et al.*,1994).

Rodent bitemarks consist of long grooves caused by the central incisors. These are typically post-mortem findings, but may possibly be seen in a living victim in, for example, cases of severe neglect.

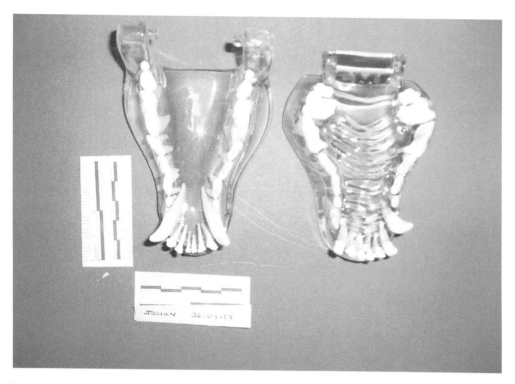

Fig. 11.1. Asymmetric canine dental arcades (copyright David Bailey).

Regardless of the species of biter, there are several factors which can make interpretation more challenging; for example, the level of violence involved in the attack, the size/breed of the biter, the area of the body attacked and positioning at the time. These can all cause distortions and variations to the bitemark (De Munnynck and Van de Voorde, 2002; Morgan and Palmer, 2007). It is often not possible to state that an individual animal is responsible for a particular bite. However, by referring to species characteristics and individual dentition via dental impressions and overlays, it may be possible to rule an individual *out* of the investigation.

11.4 Overview of Forensic Techniques and Methods Used

There are a variety of techniques used to investigate suspected bitemarks. Essential elements include analysis of the mark itself (commonly performed by a forensic doctor, although veterinary surgeons may examine images of the mark) and examination of the suspected biter (performed by a veterinary surgeon). It is assumed that these investigations will be part of a legal investigation, so chain of custody must be maintained and detailed contemporaneous records must be kept. Gloves must always be worn for personal protection and to prevent contamination.

It is important to recognize a patterned injury as a potential bitemark. Dog bites can be variable in appearance and can include many different forms of tissue damage, including crushing (from molar teeth), tissue avulsion, scratches (claw marks), fractures, and penetrating and tearing (often referred to as 'hole and tear') injuries. These wounds are usually three-dimensional in nature.

Ideally a bitemark should be swabbed for saliva before the area is washed, although this may not be possible under some circumstances. Saliva is a good source of canine DNA and although there is not a reference database for dogs, the DNA can be compared to that of the suspected biter to confirm or rule out that dog as being responsible for the bite (Clarke and Vandenberg, 2010). Swabs may also be taken for bacteriology from puncture wounds to detect common oral canine commensals (Bernitz *et al.*, 2012), which may help to confirm that a dog (but not a specific individual) inflicted the bite in question.

A full description of the bitemark location, shape, appearance and the size and type(s) of skin and deeper tissue damage, including any surrounding marks or abrasions, should be documented with both written and photographic evidence. Close-up pictures of the bitemark must include a scale; the American Board of Forensic Odontology (ABFO) No. 2 Bitemark Scale (Fig. 11.2) is a validated measuring tool. It is important that the bite, the scale and the camera are in the same plane to eliminate parallax distortion. The colouration of the tissue surrounding the bitemark should be recorded, as bruising may give a broad indication of the time that has elapsed between the bite occurring and the wounds being analysed.

Alternate light sources such as infrared (IR) and ultraviolet (UV) can make certain areas of the bitemark more distinct, although

photography with these wavelengths does require some specialist equipment (Golden and Wright, 2005). IR can capture superficial extravasation of blood beneath the skin surface (to approximately 3 mm depth). UV can reveal tissue damage deep to healed skin and so can reveal previous trauma. The absorption of the UV wavelength is increased by melanin deposition, which may be enhanced in wounded areas. This technique can be very useful on non-pigmented human skin at least 10 days after an injury but the enhancement may be visible for much longer periods (up to 2 years has been recorded). Using the invert function on commonplace computer photo-manipulation programmes can also highlight subtle changes. Any manipulation of case photographs must be done from a working copy of the images after all the originals have been copied to a non-rewritable CD or other storage form.

The presence of an arch shape makes the recognition of a bitemark easier. The arch shape (often U-shaped in canine bites) and maximum width are important features to record, along with the number of dental impressions visible. Intertooth space, tooth rotations and curvature are important details used to compare a bitemark with the dentition of the suspected biter.

It must be remembered that the suspected biter has a history of aggression and the veterinary examination should be performed on a sedated, anaesthetized, or in some cases euthanized animal.

A full medical history, including, where available, previous behaviour assessments and dental charts, should be obtained. Assessment of the dog's general condition and behaviour should be made, including weight, maximum standing height and body condition score. Any signs of fear or avoidance behaviour by the dog should be recorded, as well as any current or old injuries indicating possible abuse. Radiographs of the whole dog can be very helpful and should be performed. This information may be important when considering possible triggers for a dog bite incident and subsequently for determining the dog's future.

The dog must be examined for any gross evidence of blood, tissue or trace evidence; for example, clothing fibres. The location

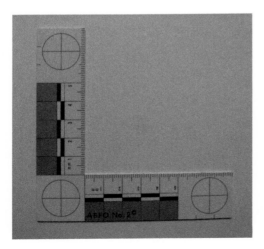

Fig. 11.2. ABFO No. 2 Bitemark Scale (copyright Louise MacLeod).

with the highest possibility of recoverable evidence is likely to be under the nails of digits 2–5 of the front paws, and these areas should be swabbed for DNA.

The dog should be induced to vomit and the vomitus collected and strained to preserve any tissue, fabric or other evidence from within the stomach. Evidence will usually only be recoverable in this manner if the dog is presented to a veterinary surgeon within 6 h of a bite occurring. The dog must be housed as the sole occupant of clean accommodation, with faeces collected for 3 days following a bite incident, as this may also contain evidence for examination.

The dog should have a serum sample taken for rabies serology testing, regardless of the rabies status of the country the bite occurred in. A full external oral exam should be undertaken and marks of trauma or previous surgery recorded. The function of the temporomandibular joint, muscle symmetry and jaw symmetry should be assessed.

A thorough intraoral examination must be performed. Any gross tissue, fabric or other foreign bodies must be collected and retained. Maximum jaw opening is an important measurement to take along with an assessment of the general oral health; for example, stomatitis or fractured teeth may indicate that the dog was experiencing oral pain. Tongue mobility and injuries should be noted and a saliva swab taken for DNA. The dentition should be recorded with photography and a dental chart. In particular any missing, worn, supernumerary, restored or fractured teeth should be noted.

Intercanine width is a frequently used measurement in bitemark comparison (Tedeschi-Oliveira et al., 2011). The authors recommend measurements of both upper and lower sets of canines, recording (for each set) the distance between the coronal tips of the two canine teeth (Fig. 11.3). The interincisal width between the mesial points of the incisal edges of the central incisors is also a useful measurement to have when performing a comparison.

Ultimately what is required is a comparison between the suspected bitemark

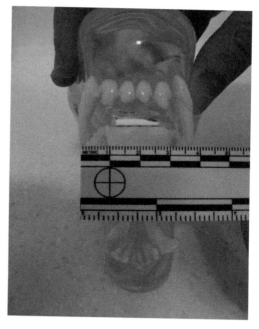

Fig. 11.3. Measurement of intercanine width (copyright Louise MacLeod).

and the dental structures of the suspected biter. This can be achieved by either the generation of a dental cast or acetate overlay. Both of these can be placed over the bitemark or a life-size image of the bitemark, for comparison purposes.

To generate an acetate overlay, plasticine is inserted into the mouth and the jaws closed. The author uses a double layer of plasticine (a thickness of approximately 8 mm) to minimize distortion when the jaws are closed. Canine bitemark investigations will usually centre around the pattern of canine and incisor teeth and it is recommended that one impression is generated of this rostral area of the jaw for both the maxilla and mandible. Four further impressions can then be taken of each of the four quadrants of remaining teeth (premolars and molars). See Figs 11.4–11.6 for examples of an impression set from a canine maxilla. Each impression must be labelled and photographed with a scale in place. Acetate is laid over the impressions and the teeth

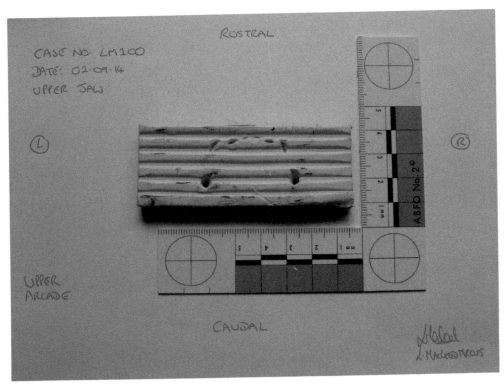

Fig. 11.4. Plasticine impression of the upper jaw – upper arcade (copyright Louise MacLeod).

margins accurately traced, thus generating an overlay.

Dental casts can be taken from a dog's mouth after it has been thoroughly cleaned and all contaminants removed with isopropyl alcohol. Materials such as vinyl polysiloxanes are used (under various trade names), as approved by the American Dental Association, to take impressions. Plaster casts are then made using dental calcined gypsum (Pomara *et al.*, 2011).

Using simple software a three-dimensional (3D)-CAD (computer assisted design) approach to analysing bitemarks may be employed (Thali *et al.*, 2003). The 3D virtual models generated of both the bitemark and suspect dentition can be manipulated on screen to assist in determining a possible association between the two.

Although not commonly performed, other techniques can be very useful in specific cases. Scanning electron microscopy is used to study three-dimensional characteristics of a wound in more detail. Occasionally the bitemark is excised and fixed (with a ring to prevent shrinkage). Any histological analysis must be the final examination performed as it is destructive, but it can be very helpful in assessing inflammatory responses, such as vessel engorgement, haemorrhage and macrophage infiltration, which may help to differentiate ante- and post-mortem changes.

Bitemark analysis encompasses many techniques and must include examination of the suspect biter as a whole not just its dental impression. It may provide class characteristic evidence (which associate the bitemark with some type of dog), but used alone is highly unlikely to detect the 'discernible uniqueness' required to individualize a specific dog. There are currently no large databases of canine dentition for reference. Bitemark analysis has good exclusionary potential for the elimination of suspects.

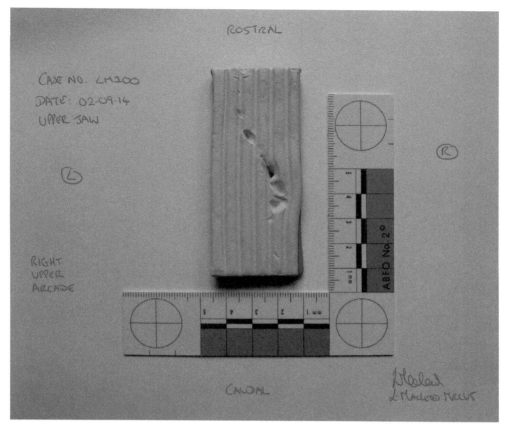

Fig. 11.5. Plasticine impression of the upper jaw – right upper arcade (copyright Louise MacLeod).

11.5 Literature Review

The earliest known bitemark case in the USA saw Reverend George Burroughs sentenced to death in 1692 after being convicted on the strength of bitemark evidence during the Salem Witch Trials (Vale, 2005).

The ABFO was formed in 1976 in order to provide accreditation and evolving standards for experts involved in bitemark analysis (http://www.abfo.org), and its guidelines are used as a basis for the investigation of dog bites in humans (Bailey and Drew, 2013).

As discussed, significant differences exist between human and dog dentition, the forces involved in a bite, and the resultant tissue changes observed in the victim (Dorion, 2005; Lessig *et al.*, 2006; Murmann *et al.*,

2006; Tedeschi-Oliveira *et al.*, 2011; Bernitz *et al.*, 2012). Certain injuries are suggested to be pathognomonic for dog bite wounds (De Munnynck and Van de Voorde, 2002).

Veterinarians have no authority to examine a human. Therefore a multidisciplinary approach is required when a dog is suspected of biting a human (Bernitz *et al.*, 2012; Bailey and Drew, 2013). Human victims of dog bites are frequently treated by medical staff without forensic training (Bailey and Drew, 2013). Lessig *et al.* (2006) and Bailey and Drew (2013) report that the forensic investigation of bite victims may occur sometime after the injury, with the subsequent loss of valuable evidence that could have been recovered at the time. They highlight the difficulties of interpreting poorly documented injuries, such as photographs with

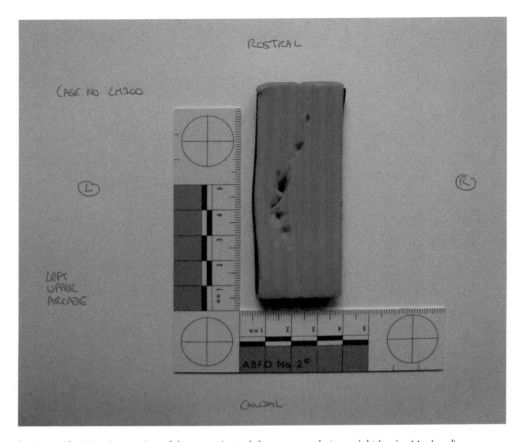

Fig. 11.6. Plasticine impression of the upper jaw – left upper arcade (copyright Louise MacLeod).

no scale in place. Photographic techniques involving reflective UV light may allow a bitemark to be visualized weeks or months after the initial injury (Richards, 2010; Bailey and Drew, 2013).

Human bitemarks frequently feature in the injuries found on sexual assault, child and elder abuse victims (McDowell, 2005). Humans may occasionally inflict bites on themselves (Bernstein, 2005). When presented with an alleged dog-inflicted bitemark in a human, it is necessary to identify the species of the biter, and rule out a human as a cause (Stavrianos *et al.*, 2011).

Intercanine width is a parameter which is commonly compared between suspects and bitemarks to attempt to identify the origin of bite wounds (Murmann *et al.*, 2006; Tedeschi-Oliveira *et al.*, 2011). Tedeschi-Oliveira *et al.* found that humans and dogs

are too similar in this respect to allow this to be used as a sole method for distinguishing between an animal and a human bitemark.

Bowers highlights the rate of false positives in bitemark identification in his critical review of human bitemark analysis techniques, referring to several post-conviction exonerations, after DNA testing of suspects who were imprisoned on the strength of bitemark evidence (Dorion, 2005; Bowers, 2006; Pretty, 2006; Bailey and Drew, 2013).

In cases of dog bites, Bailey and Drew recommend that bitemark analysis be used in combination with other techniques, notably salivary DNA analysis (Bailey and Drew, 2013). It is advisable to collect suitable samples for human and canine short tandem repeat DNA analysis from the victim's wounds, and the suspect dog's mouth (Eichmann *et al.*, 2004; Tsuji *et al.*, 2008; Clarke and Vandenberg,

2010; Bailey and Drew, 2013). Demonstration of reciprocal transfer of DNA between the two parties would be of higher evidential value than bitemark analysis alone (Bailey and Drew, 2013). Rahimi *et al.* (2005) were able to differentiate between bitemarks produced by eight human individuals in an initial study using genotyping of oral bacteria (Rahimi *et al.*, 2005), of which there are over 2000 in an individual's mouth (Pretty, 2006). They are optimistic that this future research could allow this technique to be used in bitemark cases where salivary DNA is unavailable.

Keiser also considered the evidential value of bitemark analysis (Keiser, 2005). He analysed the verifiability of human bitemark evidence using criteria laid down at the Daubert ruling (*Daubert vs Merrell Dow Pharmaceuticals* (92–102), 509 US 579 (1993)), which provides guidance to courts on the admissibility of scientific expert testimony: proven technique, peer review, known error rate and general acceptance. He concludes that uncertainty is a key element of the comparison of the data from the injury and the suspect, and more research is required before the Daubert criteria are fulfilled. He is optimistic about newer molecular methods, such as DNA short tandem repeat analysis and genomic fingerprints from oral bacteria.

Others have also observed the shortage of empirical research and scientific literature available for bitemark analysis compared to other forensic disciplines (Pretty, 2006; Bailey and Drew, 2013). Case studies make up much of the available literature (Pretty, 2006), which is of lower evidential value than empirical research. Pretty reviews the issues that bitemark analysis faces under increased scrutiny since the Daubert ruling (Pretty, 2006).

Case Study 11.1.

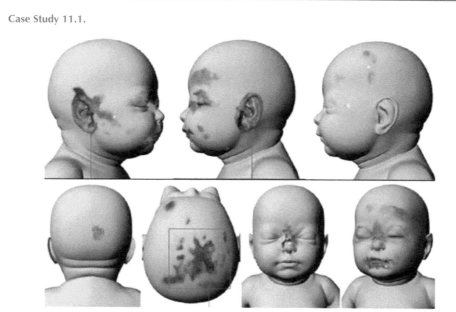

Fig. 11.7. Deceased infant (copyright David Bailey).

The images above represent injuries on a deceased infant who had been subjected to abuse. The expert in the case suspected that some of the injuries were dog bites. There were no neck injuries, suggesting the possibility that they were inflicted by a dog that was being restrained by a lead. The absence of an owner or canine suspect for comparison with the marks prevented any investigation proceeding.

Case Study 11.2.

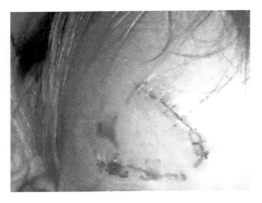

Fig. 11.8. Wound on child's forehead (copyright David Bailey).

The image above is a photograph of a sutured wound on a child's forehead after being allegedly bitten by a dog in a public place. There were no witnesses to a bite incident, and no other evidence was collected. There was no scale used in the photograph supplied, which strongly limited the scope for comparison of the injury with the dentition of any suspect animal.

Pictorial analysis by an expert excluded the possibility of the injury being a bitemark. The injury is not, as it might initially appear, an outline of a dog's dental arcade. If it were, there would be a corresponding injury from the other arcade, and the injury would be likely to be much deeper.

The evidence in this case was insufficient to reach a reliable conclusion.

11.6 Strategies for Prevention and Risk Mitigation

As discussed previously, all dogs can bite and dogs of any breed can be dangerous. Children are most at risk of being bitten by a dog, and are most commonly bitten by a known dog in the home. Strategies for prevention should take these factors into account. In addition to the obvious physical trauma suffered, children who have suffered severe or multiple bites should be considered at risk of developing post-traumatic stress disorder (De Keuster *et al.*, 2006).

Most bites occur because of human misunderstanding of dog behaviour and dog 'language', and therefore education is the key to prevention (Overall and Love, 2001; Kahn *et al.*, 2003; De Keuster *et al.*, 2006). A collaborative approach is needed, with human and veterinary teams working together.

People often misinterpret dog communication signals, and young children score particularly badly (Lakestani *et al.*, 2005). There is also the potential for bilateral misunderstanding, and inappropriate reactions to situations, and again, this is particularly true for children. Dogs can misinterpret human signs; they can be frightened by the unpredictable and uncoordinated movements of children, and loud sounds such as shrill squealing and screaming (Overall and Love, 2001). In a study by Kahn *et al.*, it was estimated that 67% of dog bite-related injuries in children could have been prevented by better education of the child and their parents on safe conduct towards the dog, a factor which is considered by many to be the preventative measure that should have the highest priority (Kahn *et al.*, 2003). In a study in the Netherlands, Cornelissen and Hopster suggested that 'mitigation strategies addressing children should focus on teaching the young how to behave around dogs so that their behaviour does not trigger a dog bite' (Cornelissen and Hopster, 2010). Education of children can take place at home, for example, using books and internet-based education initiatives, such as The Blue Dog©, which are designed to help parents and children learn about the safest way to interact with their dog (De Keuster *et al.*, 2005; Náhlík *et al.*, 2010). Education can also take place at school. Dog bite prevention programme studies have been trialled in the US and Australia, educating children about how to behave around dogs. A study in Australia found that children who had received this teaching, and who had learnt to recognize friendly, angry or frightened dogs, showed more precautionary behaviour around dogs compared to children who had not received this teaching (Lakestani *et al.*, 2005). Adult education programmes are also important, and should address bite prevention, in addition to basic canine behaviour, care and management (Sacks *et al.*, 2000). In cases where people are bitten outside the home, dog owners should be educated and advised to take appropriate measures to prevent dogs causing harm to others, such as keeping dogs on a lead, and muzzled if needed.

It has been shown that children are at a much higher risk of dog bite-related injuries if they are left unsupervised with a dog (Kahn *et al.*, 2003; De Keuster *et al.*, 2006; Náhlík *et al.*, 2010). Parents should be advised that under no circumstances should children be left unattended with a dog (Brogan *et al.*, 1995; Cornelissen and Hopster, 2010), no matter how well-behaved the dog normally is. Sachs *et al.* (1989) said that 'parents and physicians should be aware that infants left alone with a dog may be at risk of death'.

Dogs that have a prior history of aggression or propensity to bite are more likely to bite in the future (Patronek and Slavinski, 2009). Dog owners should seek veterinary advice as soon as they have concerns that their dog may bite or has bitten someone. The medical profession, particularly emergency clinicians, should be giving this advice to any dog bite victims. In addition, provisions should be made to improve behaviour training for veterinarians at universities, and provide continuing professional development courses for practising veterinarians in the area. Aggression in dogs can be fear-based, and adequate socialization of puppies can really help to reduce this problem (Sacks *et al.*, 2000).

There is much controversy in the literature and among experts about the use of breed-specific legislation to reduce the risk of dog bite-related injuries and fatalities. We have already discussed the difficulties in identifying specific breeds that are a problem. After the introduction of the Dangerous Dogs Act (1991) in the UK, a comparative study looking at dog bite-related attendances to emergency facilities before and after the introduction of the Act demonstrated very little change (Klassen *et al.*, 1996). In contrast, a dangerous dog ordinance passed in Multnomah County in Oregon in 1986 preceded a significant reduction in dangerous incidents involving dogs that had previously caused injury to people or other animals through attacks or biting (Oswald, 1991).

A significant problem when analysing dog bite-related incident data is underreporting of incidents and a lack of national reporting systems (Overall and Love, 2001). Enhanced reporting and the creation of a universal database for dog bite incidents, with training for and support from the medical and veterinary professions, would help to identify risk factors more reliably.

11.7 Conclusion

Dog bites can cause a wide range of injuries to a victim. The result can be permanent disfigurement or even death of a victim, although the latter is, fortunately, rare. Dog bite-related wounds can become infected, and there is always the potential for rabies infection. Post-traumatic stress disorder is a frequently encountered sequel to a dog bite attack, particularly in children, and there may be both financial and legal implications. Children are at highest risk of being bitten by a dog, and are more likely to receive more serious injuries as a result of the bite. Most dog bites occur within the home, involving a familiar dog.

The dentition of humans, dogs and other species of forensic interest, for example, cats, can vary widely. There are many factors to consider when examining bite-related injuries, and caution should be used when interpreting such evidence. Bitemark evidence alone is unlikely to be conclusive in an investigation, and should normally only be used to rule an individual out of an investigation, and ideally in combination with other techniques, such as salivary DNA analysis.

A strict protocol should be followed when investigating bitemark cases, using ABFO guidelines. Personnel involved in an investigation should stay within their area of expertise; for example, veterinarians should not perform examinations on human victims. A full history (including dental history) and clinical examination should be performed by a veterinarian of the dog in question. Photographs with a scale in place should be taken.

Emesis should be induced, and faeces collected, and both examined for potential evidence. Saliva swabs should be taken for DNA analysis and bacteriology. Specific measurements, such as intercanine distance, should be recorded. Dental casts or acetate overlay techniques may be used to compare the dental structures of the biter and the bitemark. More advanced techniques are also available for bitemark analysis.

Education, particularly of parents and children, is considered key to reducing the incidence of dog bite-related injuries (Náhlík *et al.*, 2010). This includes teaching both adults and children how to interact with dogs, and read dog 'language', as well as encouraging adequate socialization of puppies, and ongoing training of dogs. A collaborative approach, involving both medical and veterinary professionals, is warranted, and improved recording of dog bite-related injuries is needed. There is much controversy about the effectiveness of breed-specific legislation.

References

Avis, S.P. (1999) Dog pack attack: hunting humans. *The American Journal of Forensic Medicine and Pathology* 20(3), 243–246.

Bailey, D. and Drew, S. (2013) Forensics: bitemark analysis. In: Tiplady, C. (ed.) *Animal Abuse: Helping Animals and People*. CAB International, Oxford, UK, Chapter 23.

Bernitz, H., Bernitz, Z., Steenkamp, G., Blumenthal, R. and Stols, G. (2012) The individualisation of a dog bite mark: a case study highlighting the bite mark analysis, with emphasis on differences between dog and human bite marks. *International Journal of Legal Medicine* 126(3), 441–446.

Bernstein, M.L. (2005) Nature of bitemarks. In: Dorion, R.B.J. (ed.) *Bitemark Evidence*. Marcel Dekker, New York, USA, pp. 59–80.

Bowers, M. (2006) Problem-based analysis of bitemark misidentifications: the role of DNA. *Forensic Science International* 159, 104–109.

Brogan, T.V., Bratton, S.L., Dowd, D. and Hegenbarth, M.A. (1995) Severe dog bites in children. *Pediatrics* 96(5), 947–950.

Calkins, C.M., Bensard, D.D., Partrick, D.A. and Karrer, F.M. (2001) Life-threatening dog attacks: a devastating combination of penetrating and blunt injuries. *Journal of Pediatric Surgery* 36(8), 1115–1117.

Chin, Y., Berkelhamer, J.E. and Herold, T.E. (1982) Dog bites in children less than 4 years old. *Pediatrics* 69, 119–120.

Clark, M.A., Sandusky, G.E., Hawley D.A., Pless, J.E., Fardal, P.M. and Zate, L.R. (1994) Fatal and near-fatal animal bite injuries. *Journal of Forensic Sciences* 36(4), 1256–1261.

Clarke, C. and Vandenberg, N. (2010) Dog attack: the application of canine DNA profiling in forensic casework. *Forensic Science, Medicine and Pathology* 6, 151–157.

Collier, S. (2006) Breed-specific legislation and the pit bull terrier: Are the laws justified? *Journal of Veterinary Behavior* 1(1), 17–22.

Cornelissen, J.M.R. and Hopster, H. (2010) Dog bites in the Netherlands: a study of victims, injuries, circumstances and aggressors to support evaluation of breed specific legislation. *The Veterinary Journal* 186, 292–298.

De Keuster, T., De Cook, I. and Moons, C.P.H. (2005) Dog bite prevention – how a blue dog can help. *European Journal of Companion Animal Practice* 15(2), 136–139.

De Keuster, T., Lamoureux, J. and Kahn, A. (2006) Epidemiology of dog bites: a Belgian experience of canine behaviour and public health concerns. *The Veterinary Journal* 172, 482–487.

De Munnynck, K. and Van de Voorde, W. (2002) Forensic approach of fatal dog attacks: a case report and literature review. *International Journal of Legal Medicine* 116(5), 295–300.

Dorion, R.B.J. (2005) Dog bitemarks. In: Dorion, R.B.J. (ed.) *Bitemark Evidence*. Marcel Dekker, New York, USA, pp. 293–322.

Duffy, D.L., Hsu, Y. and Serpell, J.A. (2008) Breed differences in canine aggression. *Applied Animal Behaviour Science* 114, 441–460.

Eichmann, C., Berger, B., Reinhold, M., Lutz, M. and Parson, W. (2004) Canine-specific STR typing of saliva traces on dog bite wounds. *International Journal of Legal Medicine* 118(6), 337–342.

Gilchrist, J., Sacks, J.J., White, D. and Kresnow M.-J. (2008) Dog bites: still a problem? *Injury Prevention* 14(5), 296–301.

Golden, G.S. and Wright, F.D. (2005) Photography. In: Dorion, R.B.J. (ed.) *Bitemark Evidence*. Marcel Dekker, New York, USA, pp. 87–168.

Kahn, A., Bauche, P. and Lamoureux, J. (2003) Child victims of dog bites treated in emergency departments: a prospective survey. *European Journal of Paediatrics* 162(4), 254–258.

Keiser, J.A. (2005) Weighing bitemark evidence: a postmodern perspective. *Forensic Science, Medicine, and Pathology* 1(2), 75–80.

Klassen, B., Buckley, J.R. and Esmail, A. (1996) Does the dangerous dogs act protect against animal attacks: a prospective study of mammalian bites in the accident and emergency department. *Injury* 27, 89–91.

Kullberg, B.-J., Westendorp, R.G.J., Van't Wout, J.W. and Edo Meinders, A. (1991) *Purpura fulminans* and symmetrical peripheral gangrene caused by *Capnocytophaga canimorsus* (formerly DF-2) septicemia – a complication of dog bite. *Medicine* 70(5), 287–292.

Lakestani, N.N., Waran, N., Verga, M. and Phillips, C. (2005) Dog bites in children. *European Journal of Companion Animal Practice* 15(2), 133–135.

Lessig, R., Weber, M. and Wenzel, V. (2006) Bite mark analysis in forensic routine case work. *EXCLI* 5, 93–102.

McDowell, J.D. (2005) Role of health professionals in diagnosing patterned injuries from birth to death. In: Dorion, R.B.J. (ed.) *Bitemark Evidence*. Marcel Dekker, New York, USA, pp. 31–42.

Meints, K., Racca, A. and Hickey, N. (2010) Child–dog misunderstandings: children misinterpret dogs' facial expressions. In: *Proceedings of the 2nd Canine Science Forum* (Vienna, Austria) 99.

Morgan, M. and Palmer, J. (2007) Dog bites. *British Medical Journal* 334, 413–417.

Murmann, D.C., Brumit, P.C., Schrader, B.A. and Senn, D.R. (2006) Comparison of animal jaws and bite mark patterns. *Journal of Forensic Sciences* 51(4), 846–860.

Náhlík, J., Baranyiová, E. and Tyrlík, M. (2010) Dog bites to children in the Czech Republic: the risk situations. *ACTA VETERINARIA BRNO* 79, 627–636.

Oswald, M. (1991) Report on potentially dangerous dog program: Mutnomah County, Oregon. *Anthrozoos* 15, 44–52.

Overall, K.L. and Love, M. (2001) Dog bites to humans – demography, epidemiology, injury and risk. *Journal of the American Veterinary Medical Association* 218(12), 1923–1934.

Patronek, G.J. and Slavinski, S.A. (2009) Animal bites. *Journal of the American Veterinary Medical Association* 234(3), 336–345.

Peters, V., Sottiaux, M., Appelboom, J. and Kahn, A. (2004) Posttraumatic stress disorder after dog bites in children. *The Journal of Pediatrics* 144(1), 121–122.

Pomara, C., D'Errico, S., Jarussi, V., Turillazzi, E. and Fineschi, V. (2011) Cave Canem, bite mark analysis in a fatal dog pack attack. *American Journal of Forensic Medical Pathology* 32, 50–54.

Pretty, I.A. (2006) The barriers to achieving an evidence base for bitemark analysis. *Forensic Science International* 159, 110–120.

Rahimi, M., Heng, N.C., Kieser, J.A. and Tompkins, G.R. (2005) Genotypic comparison of bacteria recovered from human bite marks and teeth using arbitrarily primed PCR. *Journal of Applied Microbiology* 99, 1265–1270.

Richards, A. (2010) Reflected ultraviolet imaging for forensics applications. Available online at: http://www.company7.com/library/nikon/Reflected_UV_Imaging_for_Forensics_V2.pdf (accessed 25 August 2014).

Sachs, J.L., Sattin, R.W. and Bonzo, S.E. (1989) Dog bite-related fatalities from 1979 through 1988. *Journal of the American Medical Association* 262, 1489–1492.

Sacks, J.J., Kresnow, W. and Houston, B. (1996) Dog bites: how big a problem? *Injury Prevention* 2, 52–54.

Sacks, J.J., Sinclair, L., Gilchrist, J., Golab, G.C. and Lockwood, R. (2000) Breeds of dogs involved in fatal human attack in the United States between 1979 and 1998. *Journal of the American Medical Association* 217(6), 836–840.

Stavrianos, C., Aggelakopoulos, P., Stavrianou, P., Pantelidou, L., Vasiliadis, L. and Grigoropoulos, L. (2011) Comparison of human and dog bitemarks. *Journal of Animal and Veterinary Advances* 10(20), 2649–2654.

Talan, D.A., Citron, D.M., Abrahamian, D.O., Moran, D.J. and Goldstein, E.J.C. (1999) Bacteriologic analysis of infected dog and cat bites. *New England Journal of Medicine* 340(2), 85–92.

Tedeschi-Oliveira, S.V., Trigueiro, M., Oliveira, R.N. and Melani, R.F.H. (2011) Intercanine distance in the analysis of bite marks: a comparison of human and domestic dog dental arches. *Journal of Forensic Odontostomatology* 29(1), 30–36.

Thali, M.J., Braun, M., Markwalder, T.H., Brueschweiler, W., Zollinger, U., Malik, N.J. and Dirnhofer, R. (2003) Bite mark documentation and analysis: the forensic 3D/CAD supported photogrammetry approach. *Forensic Science International* 135, 115–121.

Tsuji, A., Ishiko, A., Kimura, H., Nurimoto, M., Kudo, K. and Ikeda, N. (2008) Unusual death of a baby: a dog attack and confirmation using human and canine STRs. *International Journal of Legal Medicine* 122(1), 59–62.

Vale, G.L. (2005) History of bitemark evidence. In: Dorion, R.B.J. (ed.), *Bitemark evidence*. Marcel Dekker, New York, USA, pp. 1–32.

Weiss, H., Friedman, D. and Coben, J. (1998) Incidence of dog bite injuries treated in emergency departments. *Journal of the American Medical Association* 279, 51–53.

Wise, J.K. and Yang, J.J. (1994) Dog and cat ownership. *Journal of the American Veterinary Medical Association* 204(1), 1166–1167.

12 Report Writing

David Bailey*

*Department of Forensic and Crime Science, Staffordshire
University, Stoke-on-Trent, Staffordshire, UK*

Bias cannot be excluded from the report writer. Bias can be excluded from the report.

12.1 Definition of an Expert

According to the case of *Turner*, in the UK:

> an expert's opinion is admissible to furnish the court with ... information, which is likely to be outside the experience and knowledge of a judge or jury. If on the proven facts a judge or jury can form their own conclusions without help, then the opinion of an expert is unnecessary.[i]

The role of an expert witness is to advise on technical matters of a case as well as respond

---

*Corresponding author: daysbays@yahoo.co.uk

[i] *R vs Turner* [1975] 1 QB 834, 841.

to requests from the opposing party for technical information. They can and are expected to advise on their interpretation of the technical significance of evidence or a report disclosed by the opposing side and then produce a report. After they have produced and submitted a report it is likely that any number of legally trained personnel will look at both reports for the prosecution and defence and then ask the expert(s) to narrow down areas of agreement and disagreement. If the matter cannot be resolved between legal parties at this point, then it is likely the expert will be required to attend court, face cross-examination about his or her own report and be on hand to advise in cross-examination of the opposing expert.

An expert is defined in a legal sense as someone who is able to assist the court where areas of knowledge or expertise outside that of the court would be required. This is an important definition because an expert in court is allowed to provide opinion evidence. This allows them to infer and deduce and make interpretations as to certain facts and matters that are within their area of expertise and considered outside the court's expertise, and with this expectation an expert should have a sound knowledge of their subject matter.

Expert witnesses can provide an opinion on what they see, while a professional witness can provide an explanation of what duties they performed in their professional role without any interpretation of what they did or saw. An eyewitness can provide a verbal description on what they saw with their own eyes without any interpretation.

The following three examples of an expert can all be fulfilled in court by a veterinarian.

1. **Eye witness:** 'I saw a dog hit by a car.'
2. **Professional witness:** 'I treated a dog hit by a car. The dog had cuts and scratches.'
3. **Expert witness:** 'The delay between the dog being hit by a car and presented to the vet with the type of wounds it had would have caused the cuts and scratches to become infected.'

The opinion which the *expert* adduces would assist the court in determining whether the owner of the dog, who (in this hypothetical

example) had delayed consulting the vet after the dog was accidentally hit by a car, was responsible for causing unnecessary pain and suffering to the dog by not having it checked over immediately after the accident. A vet can act as a professional witness and as an expert witness and in the above example it can be assumed that the attending vet (professional witness) did not wish to provide expert opinion against the owner, who may have also been a client of the practice.

12.2 Requirements of an Expert Report

12.2.1 Admissibility versus reliability

All vets are considered and recognized as experts inside a court room in all areas of veterinary science, yet they may not hold or maintain a recognized postgraduate specialism in any field outside a court room. There is no expert admissibility test in any jurisdiction. If you are a qualified veterinarian, then your testimony is admissible as an expert. Beyond this, there are no further tests or requirements that the courts can seek to impose on a veterinary expert opinion or report. There is a reliability test built into the adversarial system, where any claim to any type of expertise in the field of veterinary science will be appropriately tested.

If you are a dog-and-cat vet and you are instructed by a solicitor to write a report on an equine matter, then your evidence will be *admissible* expert evidence to the court – the court cannot stop you or your report at the door if you possess a degree in veterinary science. However, your evidence may not be *reliable* and the adversarial system, in one of its constructed wisdoms, will determine the extent of the *reliability* of any expert evidence, usually under cross-examination. So while *any* vet can be asked to write a report on any subject *that is animal-related* and provide that evidence to a court in the form of a report, the rules of cross-examination allow the reliability of that evidence to be stress-tested to breaking point. A new graduate and a vet with 30 years experience will have the same rules of *admissibility* applied to their report and expertise. But the real test comes when the reliability of that report is subject to polite, thoughtful and probing questioning from opposing counsel.

Many vets acting as expert witnesses do have an existing knowledge and expertise of the subject matter in their chosen field; however, many experts tend to fall below the reliability standards expected of a court. Experts will often pass the admissibility test and then fail to articulate carefully their *analytical reasoning*. This is, in my own view, the key aspect of a report that is required of an expert.

The veterinary expert that may be considered to have a *low reliability* report will write a report that will separate out their observations and conclusions with *their* experience only and not with any attempt at analytical reasoning.

A good report should include an expert's experience and attempt to introduce an independent verification to that view. This can be in the form of journal articles, laboratory report or photographs that demonstrate that the experience of the submitting expert is reliable, as it is also the experience of others and is recognized and verifiable.

Many veterinary experts will write reports that indicate a 'because I say so' approach and this is a failure to make the successful transition from clinical to adversarial veterinary medicine. Unable to remove themselves from a familiar and good-natured clinical disposition where being challenged is unlikely, into the adversarial setting where being challenged with a healthy dose of polite scepticism is the norm and the good-natured element of a convivial consultation rapidly evaporates.

12.3   Rules of Reliability

There is one expert admissibility test: the expert has acquired by study or experience sufficient knowledge of the subject to render his or her opinion of value. There are two elements to the reliability of an expert's report: the report must contain the experience of the expert and it must bridge to other sources of evidence and information that are *accepted and verifiable*.

12.4   Elucidation

An expert witness asked to produce a report is not just a *subject matter expert*. Remember – a court only requires you to be a subject matter expert in order for your evidence to be *admissible*. Once accepted as a recognized expert, then a court report subsequently has a set of more onerous requirements placed on the veterinarian (or other expert) who authored it, above being just a subject matter expert. The criteria that the court will place on the admissibility of an expert's report (subject matter expert) relate to the *reliability* of the report (accepted and verifiable content) and the *elucidation requirements* of the expert (analytical reasoning, ability to communicate, and willingness to alter an opinion in the face of new evidence). This realization of a linear sequence that exists between *acceptance* of a court report produced by an expert, the subsequent *reliability requirements* and the *elucidation requirements* in that report is a large part of understanding the necessary elements for report writing, and to understand a report is not just a regurgitation of your experience and qualifications in a subject. Vets like to describe events or their observations in a report according to their own experiences, yet find it difficult to articulate their interpretation of these descriptions in a legal framework. This is an impediment to the uptake of information by the legal system, which is not schooled in matters veterinary. Even with the necessary acceptability criteria and the requirement for verifiability, a report that is not well reasoned and elucidated will fail to penetrate the court's ears.

As minimum requirements, the four pillars of elucidation are as follows:

1. The necessary ability to reason their argument.
2. The necessary skills to articulate and communicate their findings.
3. The ability to change their mind if they feel that new evidence has been introduced.
4. The ability to describe and interpret the evidence in a critical manner.

These are *the elucidation requirements* of an expert *report* (not necessarily an expert *vet*) and many prosecution and defence experts are exceptionally good vets, but lack the elucidation requirements to be able to assemble and apply knowledge to a report with the reliability and lucidity the courts seek. Nobel prize winners win Nobel prizes, but very few of them are used as expert witnesses, as they fail in their ability to elucidate and articulate in a manner that a court can understand. The ability and skill to elucidate one's argument is beyond the scope of this book; however, there are many useful books on critical thinking that will assist in the pursuit of this skill, a key tenet for forensic and legal scholars.

Many vets feel comfortable regurgitating facts and clinical findings and augmenting their findings with reference to a text or a journal, yet fail in their attempts to link their expertise to sound reasoning and an ability to articulate their points within a legal framework.

Many barristers will often highlight an expert's lack of articulation or reasoning in a submitted report and they will avoid the subject matter that the expert is strong on. It is not just what you say but how you say it and, in a report, how you say it is as vital to the penetration of the report as the expert's veterinary experience.

12.5   Obligations of an Expert

A highly regarded report contains low levels of emotion, and you should not be able to tell which way the expert is leaning. An expert is obliged to deliver what the court wants – independent and unbiased views on matters to assist the court to determine the outcome of a case. An expert does not charge for their opinion, but for the time taken to reach that opinion. Regardless of whether the prosecution or defence instructs them, their opinion should be the same: the court expects this consistency of character and professionalism. A good report appears to be without bias and hides strong personal views in favour of actual content, reasoning

and articulation. The predilection for guilt or innocence of the alleged offender should not be clear to the report reader.

Problems can occur in an adversarial system of justice when defence solicitors or prosecution authorities are required to seek out and instruct an expert. Courts demand good experts, and lawyers for both prosecution and defence insist on good witnesses. Experts sometimes find themselves caught between what the courts require and what the instructing solicitor needs. Whenever you are involved in this type of conflict, it is important to remember that your obligation is to the court: this is the first rule of writing a report. An expert doesn't determine the outcome of the legal dispute – others will. Those others may rely heavily on the expert and the report produced, but the expert should not cross the boundary between writing a report for the benefit of the court and the construction of a report for the benefit of the instructing party.

The rules in report writing are, in order of importance:

*   Write the report for the court and for the benefit of the court.
*   Know your subject matter.
*   Develop the skill of reasoning.
*   Develop the skill of articulating and communication in your reports.
*   Be willing to change your mind if you come across an alternate view.

The following boxes contain examples of fictious reports.

Box 12.1.

My name is Joe Blogs, I qualified from Bristol in 1985. I have been a vet for 30 years.

I saw a cat with fleas on it and this cat was suffering.

J. Blogs

This report is admissible; however, it has low reliability criteria and it has poor elucidation. The presence or absence of unnecessary suffering as a conclusion is up to the court to determine and the vet can assist in this determination, but should avoid the appearance that they are attempting to usurp the role of the court in this finding.

Box 12.2.

My name is Joe Blogs, I qualified from Bristol in 1985. I have been a vet for 30 years.

I saw a cat with fleas on it. See the photo in Appendix A.

I also saw a large amount of flea dirt on the cat and have taken photos of this (Appendix B). Fleas do not normally cause a lot of irritation to a cat; however, in severe infestations they can cause severe discomfort, and if a cat has a flea bite allergy then this can cause a serious clinical condition that needs veterinary attention and intervention (see reference on flea bite allergy in Appendix C).

This report is admissible and it is reliable as it refers to different accepted and verifiable methods to demonstrate the presence of fleas on the cat. However, it lacks the skills of articulation and elucidation that lawyers and courts are used to seeing in their own profession.

Box 12.3.

My name is Joe Blogs, I qualified from Bristol in 1985. I have been a vet for 30 years.

On 3/3/2015 I was asked by the Ulster Society for the Prevention of Cruelty to Animals (USPCA) to examine a cat that had been seized by them from an address known to me. A record of my examination at the time is included in Appendix A. I have since been asked by the USPCA to write a report on the condition of the cat.

I have defined suffering as 'anything significantly greater than minor transient discomfort'. And while suffering is up to the court to determine, this is the definition I used when determining whether suffering was or was not present in the cat that I examined.

There are other definitions of suffering but there is no accepted definition of suffering in the UK that refers to animal welfare and animal cruelty.

I examined the cat and observed a large number of fleas, and a significant amount of flea dirt, on the cat (see photos in Appendix B). The cat appeared to have a flea bite allergy as it had excoriation around its neck, raised papules along its back and symmetrical alopecia. These are three of the cardinal signs of flea bite allergy in a cat (see Appendix C).

Fleas jump onto and bite cats and feed on their blood. The saliva of a flea may cause an allergic reaction in the host animal and, if this is present, then every bite of a flea causes a severe local and systemic inflammatory reaction in the animal. Fleas can be controlled on indoor cats by correct use of environmental sprays. If a cat has a recognized flea bite allergy, an owner should pay attention to the cat's environment and not allow it to become infested with fleas and bitten to the point that this cat was at the time of my examination.

A single flea bite would not cause suffering in a cat according to the definition I have used. However, a large number of flea bites would cause suffering in a cat. A blood test demonstrated that this cat was anaemic (see Appendix D); it is possible that this was due to flea bites, but other causes of anaemia cannot be ruled out.

Multiple flea bites in a cat that has a pre-existing flea bite allergy would be a source of constant, repetitive irritation and inflammation. This would be a cause of suffering in the cat, in my view, according to the definition I have provided. The necessity of this suffering is unclear in my view and cannot be explained by any clinical observation.

This report is admissible, reliable and lucid. The reader of this report may reach the conclusion that the cat was suffering; however, they are unable to determine whether the writer of the report thinks the cat owner is guilty. It is well articulated, definitions are provided and the reasoning is laid out in a logical and sequential manner. The central purpose of a veterinary medico-legal report is to provide the court with an opinion relating to an animal or animal product. The legal consequences, and any recommendations arising from the assessment of the facts relating to the case, are up to the court. The body of the report should set out the actions taken to produce the report and the facts on which the report is based.

12.6   Report Bias

The important rule overriding all other rules of report writing is an understanding of your obligations in your report. Most vets will be at some point asked or instructed by a solicitor to write a report. The first-time vet will be flattered that they have been identified as an 'expert' and will be keen to demonstrate this newly discovered expertise. Unwittingly, and, in some cases, deliberately, some vets may set out to write a biased report on demand because they feel an obligation to their instructing solicitor. This is a bias that occurs in many reports; I call it selection bias. Other dangers are hidden bias (an expert doesn't know of the bias that exists in the report) and coaching bias (an expert is coached in to what to say in a report). It is a skill in a report reader to recognize, search for and identify bias in a submitted report and then to attempt to limit the impact that bias may have on one's own report. It is impossible to eliminate bias altogether, as we all have bias built into us through our accumulation of lifetime experiences. Often these biases accumulate in us from an early childhood stage, e.g. from a school trip to an abattoir. These experiences and biases remain deeply imprinted within us for a lifetime; we may not even be aware that because of that abattoir trip we chose to become a lifelong vegetarian and pursue a lifestyle based on a childhood experience. Bias, it seems, is normal for the proprietor. Scientists try to reduce the inherent bias in any report by talking a bias-free language using statistics. A court report that understands the obligations of the author of the report and introduces a vet's experience (only) is useful but is biased (and unreliable), to the point that the experiences articulated and successfully reasoned in that report are only true according to that vet's experience. What else would anyone expect?

That expert opinion is considered lowest in the evidence hierarchy for retrospective research (Table 12.1) is another anomaly between the standards of the clinical world of evidence-based veterinary medicine and the preference of the courts, which adopt

Table 12.1. The benefits of a strong hypothesis for retrospective research (Harcourt-Brown, 2013). Example of an evidence hierarchy used in medical and veterinary research. The various types of study are listed in order of descending weight of evidence.

Order in Hierarchy	Study Types
1	Systematic reviews and meta-analyses
2	Randomized controlled trials
3	Cohort studies
4	Case-control studies
5	Cross-sectional studies
6	Case reports and case series
7	Expert opinion

expert opinion above all other forms of evidence as the preferred mechanism of dispute resolution. Science, it seems, has six preferred contenders for the delivering of the truth above that of expert opinion, which is too prone to bias yet preferred by the courts. The court prefers the opinion of the expert as it can change; it is dynamic when confronted with variable and shifting information, and no scientific study can do this once the ink has dried. This pliability of expert opinion is what makes it so useful for a court and so disagreeable for scientific studies.

12.6.1   Resilience in a report

Introducing a supporting and relevant article from a journal or a book chapter, a laboratory report or another expert's view allows you to support a proposed view in a report that is *also* reliant on your own experience. This is considered a valuable aspect to a report and helps to reduce bias and articulate a response which is based on your experience as well as backed up by a written article and the experience and finding of others. This golden rule of forensics is learned when collecting evidence and translating it into a report – *have multiple independent sources of evidence in your report.*

To rely solely on your expert opinion leaves the report vulnerable to ambush in the adversarial system. There is only one target – *you,* and in an adversarial system your report, your opinion and you become the focus of more polite but stern questions. Add a journal article (or similar external source of verifiable and accepted information) to demonstrate that your view is shared by others. You may add a report by another expert in the field who you have asked to adduce an opinion. Add a photo to support your description and you now have multiple independent sources of evidence that help to reduce any hidden bias that may be present in your report. As I have said in the epigraph above, bias cannot be excluded from the report writer; bias can be excluded from the report. And now the other side needs to dilute their focus and concentrate on multiple discrete and independent elements of your report and not just one biased opinion from a vet. The matter is a little harder for them to dispute, because your report is reliable and a little more resilient.

12.7 Report Structure and Lucidity

The structure, layout and lucidity of the report is as important as the content. Most vets concentrate on the content only to the point of subject matter expertise, as they are knowledgeable in this area, and ignore the structure. This leaves their report unread or unable to be interpreted, as it is often a clinical report, rather than in a style or structure that a court can digest. Vets are frontloaded through undergraduate training toward the top of the hierarchy of evidence pyramid (see Fig. 4.1) while courts are frontloaded to the bottom of this pyramid. This chapter emphasizes the importance of critical thinking to a report; always remember that articulation and reasoning are as vital as subject knowledge. Bias-proof your report by flanking the content with reference to independent sources. Understand your obligations, but also that lucidity should be the means by which your expertise is delivered into an adversarial legal arena. Most vets suffer from *report over-penetration* – the report makes little impact on the reader because the emphasis is on the regurgitation of years of

clinical experience and rote-learned scientific facts, and there is little focus on the structure, articulation, lucidity and layout of the report.

Vets may not appreciate that non-vets reading the report don't necessarily understand the content and meaning of many veterinary terms or the scientific language and style of veterinary science. Invert the pyramid and you will see what courts prefer.

Criminal law is concerned with justice, fact-finding and the attribution of guilt. The subject matter of veterinary science concerns itself with living animals and animal products and people involved in animal care. Tensions between veterinary science and the law arise because decisions in court are final and binding, but veterinary evidence concerns matters and usually evidence that is dynamic, not least because it is often living and changes over time. Courts find this type of living evidence quite inconvenient and difficult to deal with. The law and courts define animals as property and this, in many ways, is at odds with the way in which many vets deal with animals – i.e. as living beings. The vet writing a court report can then be seen as a translator or interpreter of the information from living and dead pieces of evidence into a form that the court can understand.

12.7.1 Confidentiality and records

As medical professionals, veterinarians are subject to similar obligations to confidentiality when providing a report to court as in ordinary clinical practice. The implications of this principle are, however, somewhat different when the defendant is one's own client. Relevant guidance should be consulted from an individual's governing professional body. Clinical reports and notes do not automatically form part of the defendant's animal's medical records, except by the consent of the defendant or their legal representative. Reports cannot be disclosed to a third party without the consent of the body commissioning the report; however, this is weighed up against the gravity of the offence.

Report writers must ensure safe maintenance of records to include the 3Rs.

1. *Retain* – all documentation until after
any potential appeals.
2. *Record* – keep structured, clear, legible and
comprehensive records in a format suitable
for other instructed experts to consult.
3. *Reveal* – all sources of information must
be disclosed in the report.

All experts should have appropriate indem-
nity insurance; this last requirement is a
demonstration of the emerging frustration of
the courts with experts and report writers in
the UK, where for the first time in 400 years,
experts have recently lost their automatic immunity from prosecution (*Jones vs Kaney*).[ii]

As a vet or animal welfare officer, you
have an obligation to the animal that is central
to the dispute. You also have an obligation to
the animal's owners. As an expert witness,
you have an obligation to the court, but you
are being paid by the instructing solicitor.

Vets also have standards imposed on
them by state or national professional bodies and all people have an innate and naturally biased obligation to themselves.

Expert witnesses are not immune from
prosecution in some jurisdictions, the consequence of which is if you *knowingly* make an
error in your report or testimony, you can expect to be back in court at a later date as a
defendant instructing your own solicitor and
team of independent and objective experts.

Your report is written for the court, not
the client. The obligation to impartiality is
muddied by financial circumstances, professional hubris, and by hidden and known biases. These are discovered when critical
thinking is laid down in the words of the report, the translation of the life of an animal
into a description of a journey of property.
We are now in the judicial world, where animals are regarded as biological machines.
We need to articulate and communicate our
information into a form the court can understand – in law, animals are property and any
emotional sentiment will distract the impact

the report has on a decision involving a living, dead or dying animal.

12.8 Accepting Instructions

Four requirements relating to the admissibility of expert evidence in criminal proceedings have developed at common law,
principally with reference to expert opinion
evidence – this is the Common Law Admissibility Test for expert evidence.

The requirements are that the expert
can provide assistance, relevant expertise,
impartiality and evidentiary reliability.

12.8.1 Assistance

According to the leading case of *Turner*:

> an expert's opinion: is admissible to furnish
> the court with ... information which is
> likely to be outside the experience and
> knowledge of a judge or jury. If on the
> proven facts a judge or jury can form their
> own conclusions without help, then the
> opinion of an expert is unnecessary.[iii]

And this is all an expert is – someone who
knows more than the average person. Being
a vet assumes an expert status in matters
dealing with animals, animal welfare and
animal products and most matters relating
to non-human animals.

12.8.2 Relevant expertise

The individual claiming expertise must be an
expert in the relevant field. This was described in the South Australian case of *Bonython* as a requirement that the individual 'has
acquired by study or experience sufficient
knowledge of the subject to render his [or her]
opinion of value',[iv] a description which has
found favour in England and Wales.[v]

[ii] See http://www.out-law.com/page-11843 for an
outline of the case.

[iii] *R vs Turner* [1975] 1 QB 834, 841.
[iv] *Bonthyon* [1984] 38 SASR 45, 47.
[v] *Stubbs* [2006] EWCA Crim 2312, [2006] All ER (D)
133; *Leo Sawrij vs North Cumbria Magistrates' Court*
[2009] EWHC 2823 (Admin), [2010] 1 Cr App R 22.

For a vet, the relevant expertise is really gained on the same day they receive their degree: a vet with 20 years' experience is considered an expert on a similar level as a new graduate regarding *admissibility* of evidence. How much weight the court attributes to the report of a new graduate and a similar report of a 20-year veteran is up to the court, but the court cannot deny a new graduate or a 20-year veteran the right to *provide* evidence.

12.8.3   Impartiality

The expert must be able to provide impartial, objective evidence on the matters within his or her field of expertise. In the civil case of *Field vs Leeds City Council*,[vi] Lord Woolf, the Master of the Rolls, said that for an expert to be 'qualified to give evidence as an expert', he or she must be able to provide an objective, unbiased opinion on the matters to which his or her evidence relates. More recently, in the case of *Toth vs Jarman*,[vii] the Court of Appeal (Civil Division) recognized that an expert witness 'should provide independent assistance to the court by way of objective unbiased opinion'[viii] and that where an expert witness 'has a material or significant conflict of interest, the court is likely to decline to act on his [or her] evidence, or indeed to give permission for his [or her] evidence to be adduced'.[ix]

An expert's apparent bias does not render their evidence inadmissible in court. It is still allowed into the court. It does, however, affect the weight (or reliability) the court will attribute to that evidence.

A pattern is developing that there are very few restrictions placed on an expert's reports and admissibility of evidence. The court can't stop the expert getting in. There is, however, inbuilt freedom and flexibility to allow varying degrees of emphasis on the different experiences of an expert.

12.8.4   Evidentiary reliability

The expert's opinion evidence must in other respects satisfy a threshold of acceptable reliability.

In *Bonython*[x] this admissibility requirement was described as being 'whether the subject matter of the [expert's] opinion forms part of a body of knowledge or experience which is sufficiently organized or recognized to be accepted as a reliable body of knowledge or experience'.[xi]

The court did not divert from the established position that there is no enhanced reliability test for such evidence. Reliability of expert evidence is nearly always going to be of issue in court. Courts need experts to assist them in their determination of a winner in an adversarial dispute.

12.9   Comparison of Jurisdictions (USA, UK and Australia)

12.9.1   American views of admissibility and reliability

The American courts' views on admissibility standards are based on two main standards: Daubert and Frye.

The Frye Case (1923) involved polygraph evidence (the reliability of which was unclear at the time) and led to a general admissibility standard for scientific evidence.

> Just when a scientific principle or discovery crosses the line between the experimental and demonstrable stages is difficult to define. Somewhere in this twilight zone the evidential force of the principle must be recognized, and while the courts will go a long way in admitting experimental testimony deduced from a well-recognized scientific principle or discovery, *the thing from which the deduction is made must be sufficiently established to have gained general acceptance in the particular field in which it belongs.*
>
> (*Frye vs United States*, 293F. 1013 (DC Cir. 1923); emphasis in original)

---

vi *Field vs Leeds City Council* [2000] 1 EGLR 54.
vii EWCA Civ 1028 [2006] 4 All ER 1276.
viii EWCA Civ 1028 [2006] 4 All ER 1276 at [100], citing *Polivitte Ltd vs Commercial Union Assurance Co. Plc* (1987) 1 Lloyd's Rep 379, 386.
ix EWCA Civ 1028 [2006] 4 All ER 1276 at [102].

---

x *Bonython* [1984] 38 SASR 45.
xi *Bonython* [1984] 38 SASR 45, 47.

The interpretation of Frye has been that the technique or scientific procedure that is being introduced into court must be generally accepted. And while it does help to keep pseudoscience out of the courtroom, it also places great emphasis on the expert's skills, experience and credibility. This discovery by the courts caused them some difficulty, as it placed the experts in a powerful position and took a lot of the decision-making ability from the court and placed it into the hands of the expert. In response, a 1993 ruling balanced the test and in *Daubert vs Merrell Dow Pharmaceuticals*, the US Supreme Court ruled that the 'general acceptance' criterion was insufficient. *An independent* judicial assessment must be carried out to establish a particular technique's acceptability and this then returns the power of the court back to the judge.

The Daubert Test seeks to answer the following.

- Does the evidence rest on a proven and tested technique?
- Has the underlying science been peer-reviewed?
- Is the error rate (reliability) of the technique known?
- Can the technique be explained simply to the court?
- What is the expert's standing in the scientific community and does the technique rely on the expert's special skill?

Although Frye and Daubert do not apply to British jurisdictions, the general principles of Daubert are widely accepted in the adversarial system outside the USA, including in Britain and Australia.

12.9.2 The UK view

There is currently no British statutory scientific reliability test.

There is just one test of admissibility – you must be recognized by a court as an expert, i.e. have a degree in veterinary science or medicine. All vets with a relevant degree are considered by the court as experts and are able to provide admissible evidence to a court. An expert is allowed to provide opinion evidence on the facts before the court.

While any qualified vet can stand up in court and provide evidence as an expert, and once you have passed this admissibility test then you can say whatever you want (as long as you believe it to be true), when the courts apply Frye and Daubert they are really asking your evidence to be accepted (Frye) and verifiable (Daubert). However, outside court, new forensic methods and procedures are generally validated by the following.

- Proof of concept trials and rigorous testing.
- Publication in international peer-reviewed journals.
- Implementation of a quality system (e.g. ISO 17025).
- Accreditation by the UK Accreditation Service (UKAS).

While experts seek guidance from the legal history of Frye and Daubert, there is always an unwritten old-school approach to report writing. Francis Camps (1905–1972), a Home Office pathologist, has suggested that an expert in writing a report must have the following (Camps, 1973).

- Knowledge based on proper training in his/her subject.
- Humility in admitting when there is doubt.
- Courage in desiring to establish the truth.
- Absolute integrity.

The Forensic Science Regulator (for the UK) drafted a code of practice in 2011 for all staff who provide expert evidence and they should:

> have a sufficient level of experience, knowledge, standing in the peer group and, where appropriate, qualifications, relevant to the type of evidence being adduced, to give credibility to reliability of the work undertaken and the conclusions drawn [and] are able to explain their methodology and reasoning, both in writing and orally, concisely and in a way that is comprehensible to a lay person and not misleading.
> (FSR, 2011, Section 25.2.1)

Within UK law, a seminal case illustrates the court's frustration with expert witnesses.

The Ikarian Reefer case (1993) involved a marine insurance claim following the loss of a vessel at sea. The defence claimed the vessel had been deliberately run aground and set on fire with the connivance of the ship's owners. The judge, Mr Justice Cresswell, said of the experts: 'I consider that a misunderstanding on the part of certain expert witnesses in the present case as to their duties and responsibilities contributed to the length of the trial' (Lloyd's Law Reports, 1993, p. 68).

The principles of expert evidence which Mr Justice Cresswell laid down in his judgment in this shipping case have become widely accepted as a classic statement of the duties and responsibilities of expert witnesses. They were endorsed by the Court of Appeal, commended by Lord Woolf in his report on the civil justice system in England and Wales, and have been cited with approval in several subsequent cases. This is not to say, though, that they have won complete acceptance.

Mr Justice Cresswell set out 'seven tenets' on experts' duties and responsibilities:

1. Expert evidence presented to the court should be, and should be seen to be, the independent product of the expert uninfluenced as to form or content by the exigencies of litigation ...
2. An expert witness should provide independent assistance to the court by way of objective unbiased opinion in relation to matters within his expertise ... An expert witness in the High Court should never assume the role of advocate.
3. An expert witness should state the facts or assumptions on which his opinion is based. He should not omit to consider material facts, which could detract from his concluded opinion ...
4. An expert witness should make it clear when a particular question or issue falls outside his expertise.
5. If an expert's opinion is not properly researched because he considers that insufficient data is available, then this must be stated with an indication that the opinion is no more than a provisional one. If the expert cannot assert that the report contains the truth, the whole truth and nothing but the truth without some

qualification, that qualification should be stated in the report.
6. If after exchange of reports, an expert witness changes his view on a material matter having read the other side's expert's report, or for any other reason, such change of view should be communicated (through legal representatives) to the other side without delay and where appropriate to the Court.
7. Where expert evidence refers to photographs, plans, calculations, analyses, measurements, survey reports or other similar documents they must be provided to the opposite party at the same time as the exchange of reports.
(Lloyd's Law Reports, 1993, p. 69)

In the (criminal) case of *R vs Thomas Bowman* (2006), recommendations were made, further to those of Cresswell, about what should go into the expert's report.

1. Details of the expert's academic and professional qualifications, experience and accreditation relevant to the opinions expressed in the report and the range and extent of the expertise and any limitations upon the expertise.
2. A statement setting out the substance of all the instructions received (whether written or oral), questions upon which an opinion is sought, the materials provided and considered, and the documents, statements, evidence, information or assumptions which are material to the opinions expressed or upon which those opinions are based.
3. Information relating to who has carried out measurements, examinations, tests, etc. and the methodology used, and whether or not such measurements, etc. were carried out under the expert's supervision.
4. Where there is a range of opinion in the matters dealt with in the report a summary of the range of opinion and the reasons for the opinion given. In this connection any material facts or matters which detract from the expert's opinions and any points which should fairly be made against any opinions expressed should be set out.
5. Relevant extracts of literature or any other material which might assist the court.
6. A statement to the effect that the expert has complied with his/her duty to the court to provide independent assistance by way of objective unbiased opinion in relation to

matters within his or her expertise and an acknowledgment that the expert will inform all parties and where appropriate the court in the event that his/her opinion changes on any material issues.

7. Where on an exchange of experts' reports matters arise which require a further or supplemental report the above guidelines should, of course, be complied with.[xii]

With a range of court cases and advice given to provide 'clarity' as to the reliability of expert evidence, it may be difficult to keep up to date with what is required. A consolidation of views is usually found in guidance such as CPS guidance for experts and criminal and civil procedure rules, which specify the content of an expert report or statement.

Scientists disagree on many things, but when experts disagree in the court, it can be extremely damaging. In the case of Angela Cannings, who was accused in 2003 of killing her two infant children (who, it later transpired, both died of Sudden Infant Death Syndrome), the court of appeal ruled:

> If the outcome of the trial depends exclusively, or almost exclusively, on a serious disagreement between distinguished and reputable experts, it will often be unwise, and therefore unsafe, to proceed.[xiii]

There is no code of practice or code of conduct to regulate expert witnesses. Once you are a recognized expert in your field, there is nothing stopping you from giving expert evidence. There is, however, guidance provided to courts as to how much weight they should apply to your evidence.

It is the function of the expert witness to provide opinions and to provide a basis on which the opinions rest. Data is derived from the expert's own experience and literature sources and from information obtained from associates. The interpretation and evaluation of this data are mostly subjective – it is rare for an opinion to be based on a statistic or probabilistic study alone.

The attitude required in a report is to abandon the idea of absolute certainty, so

that a fully objective approach to the problem can be made.

Subjective opinions, however firmly based in personal experience, are still at the mercy of factors such as inadequate or atypical experience, some lack of understanding of fundamentals, or even a mental bias of which its possessor may be totally unaware. If it can be accepted that nothing is absolutely certain, then it becomes logical to determine the degree of confidence that may be assigned to a particular belief. It is here that statistics may be useful.

Most, if not all, of our amateurish efforts to justify our own evidence interpretations have been deficient in mathematical exactness and philosophical understanding (Kirk and Kingston, 1964). Statistical analysis provides forensic scientists with a basis for an opinion and an evaluation of the likelihood that their testimony reflects the truth, rather than a personal belief or bias.

The following passage from *Taylor on Evidence* reminds us of the need for impartiality:

> These witnesses are usually required to speak not to facts but to opinions and when this is the case, it is often quite surprising to see with what facility and to what extent their views can be made to correspond with the wishes or the interests of the parties who call them.
>
> (P. H. W., 1932, p. 428)

12.9.3 The Australian view

The high court of Australia has dealt in detail with the skill necessary to qualify a witness as an expert, and with the circumstances in which the testimony of a skilled person is admissible. The putative expert must have undertaken a professional course of study, which has given him or her more opportunity of judging the matters in question than other people, or must have completed the professional study of what has been described by the high court as an organized branch of knowledge relevant to the subject matter of the inquiry. The standard to be applied is somewhat indefinite, and it follows that any medical practitioner may be

---

[xii] *R vs Thomas Bowman* [2006] EWCA 417.
[xiii] *R vs Cannings* [2004] EWCA Crim 01.

admitted to give evidence on any branch of medicine. And one can always be found who will. Courts can't apply stringent limitations on the testimonial capacity of a person who is qualified.

The fundamental characteristic of expert evidence is that it is *opinion* evidence. This means, significantly, that evidence is required to exceed a mere description of events (vets are comfortable with this) and is an interpretation of events (vets are also comfortable with this) within a legal context and framework (vets are unprepared for this). A professional expert may give an opinion of fact, but not an expert opinion. They can't interpret what they have seen.

For example, a professional expert (a police officer) may not say that a vehicle was being driven carelessly. They can only say that a vehicle ended up in a ditch and they can say it happened at 10.15am on Sunday 11 October 2006. An expert opinion may be offered by an accident investigator who is instructed to provide an opinion on the car in the ditch. They can provide an opinion on the speed of the car and the effort the driver made to brake prior to ending up in the ditch.

The court can decide whether, after hearing all this evidence, the car was being driven carelessly. Only the court can make this claim, and only after hearing all the available evidence.

If the relevant legislation has determined that careless driving is against the law, then a fine or sentence can then be imposed on that driver by the court, according to guidelines set out in the legislation.

12.10   Conclusion

Lord Justice Aikens expressed the view that 'the way expert evidence is dealt with in jury trials is one of the system's weaker links'; the Criminal Bar Association opined that the 'current treatment of expert evidence in criminal proceedings has contributed to a significant number of miscarriages of justice, risks continuing to do so, and requires urgent reform'; and the Bar Law Reform Committee felt that the common law approach to expert evidence was 'deeply unsatisfactory'.

(Law Commission, 2011, Section 3.24)

I discovered the importance of self-awareness when studying Forensic Science. Opposing barristers unable to shake your expertise in a dispute will then often attack your character.

It isn't until you are challenged in court or on your report by another expert that you realize how valuable it is to recognize, learn and attempt to master this skill. Being an expert is a recognition of your skills and experience and knowledge, but the guides to expert witness procedures will never mention a sense of self-awareness as a pre-requisite for being an expert. Cross-examining lawyers and solicitors intuitively know this and they exploit it. They will know very little about an expert's subject matter but they tend to avoid this and attack the expert's bias. Questions tend to focus on *why* you said something and *how* you know something, not what you said and whether you know – they do this because they have learned about critical thinking, evaluating arguments and understanding bias. They may not know your subject area, but they don't need to.

References

Camps, F. (1973) *Camps on Crime*. David & Charles, Newton Abbot, Devon, UK.

FSR (Forensic Science Regulator) (2011) *Codes of Practice and Conduct for Forensic Science Providers and Practitioners in the Criminal Justice System*. Forensic Science Regulator, Birmingham, UK. Available online at: https://www.gov.uk/government/uploads/system/uploads/attachment_data/file/118949/codes-practice-conduct.pdf (accessed 21 October 2015).

Harcourt-Brown, T. (2013) The benefits of a strong hypothesis for retrospective research. *Veterinary Record* 173. 447–448.

Kirk, P.L. and Kingston, C.R. (1964) Evidence evaluation and problems in general criminalistics (paper presented at the Sixteenth Annual Meeting of the American Academy of Forensic Sciences, Chicago, USA). *Journal of Forensic Science* 9(4), 434–444.

Law Commission (2011) Expert Evidence in Criminal Proceedings in England and Wales (Law Com No 325). Presented to Parliament pursuant to section 3(2) of the Law Commissions Act 1965. The Stationery Office, London, UK. Available online at: https://www.gov.uk/government/uploads/system/uploads/attachment_data/file/229043/0829.pdf (accessed 22 October 2015).

Lloyd's Law Reports (1993) Vol. 2, Part 1: The 'Ikarian Reefer'. Available online at: http://www.rtpi.org.uk/media/9981/Ikarian-Reefer.pdf (accessed 22 October 2015).

P. H. W. (1932) Review of R. P. Croom-Johnson, and G. F. L. Bridgman, *Taylor on Evidence, 12th edn. The Cambridge Law Journal* 4(3), 428. doi:10.1017/S0008197300132593.

13 The Human–Animal Interaction

Pippa Swan*

Clare Veterinary Group, Ballyclare, Co. Antrim, Northern Ireland, UK

13.1   Introduction

That animals and humans always were, and will continue to be, intricately and inextricably linked is borne out by the arts, from caveman drawings through painting and literature to photography; and by science, from Darwin to current studies of animal biology and behaviour. The relationship includes dependence, respect and affection, as well as power, exploitation and abuse. Our relationships with animals are arguably more complex than our relationships with each other.

13.2   A Historical Context

The beliefs and practices of the past can appear fantastical or incomprehensible. There are numerous accounts of animal killing by the Romans on a vast scale for spectacular entertainment. Animals in Europe were accused of crimes, tried in court and sentenced to torture and death during the 14th and 15th centuries. Wild and domesticated animals would commonly be chained and attacked, or baited, by men and dogs for sport in the 16th century. The desires and thought processes behind these acts may

*Corresponding author: pippaswan@gmail.com

seem anathema to most people today, but their shadows remain. There are still those who kill animals as a pastime and some who find pleasure in the destruction or violent injury of animals. Anthropocentric motives, for bad and good, are still attributed to animals: pests and assistance dogs, for example. Enlightened as most Western cultures consider themselves to be, our relationship with animals can only be understood in the context of our past. The many inconsistencies and contradictions inherent in the ways humans and animals interact have their roots in history.

Foreign visitors to England in the 18th century were often shocked by the type and extent of pursuits involving animals regularly performed by all classes of people. Bull running, where bulls are run through a town until exhausted and then set upon by dogs or thrown off a bridge, and goose pulling, where horsemen attempt to pull off the heads of live greased geese suspended upside down, were regularly performed for sport in Britain. All types of animal fighting were practised, usually to the death. Cats were eaten alive at country fairs, cocks were tied to stakes and had sticks and stones thrown at them until they were dead and school boys would bite the heads off sparrows, tie cats together by the tail and club hamstrung sheep to death (Ryder, 2000). Horses and dogs were used as draught (working) animals and would regularly be subjected to excessively heavy workloads, beatings and mutilations (Radford, 2001). Vast numbers of animals were killed for food, with many of them driven long distances into cities without food or water and then slaughtered by a variety of inhumane methods (Radford, 2001). Calves were hung up alive by their Achilles tendon, hooks stuck through their nostrils and slowly bled to death, pigs were beaten to death in an attempt to improve meat quality, geese with their eyes removed were nailed to boards and force-fed (Ryder, 2000).

While past treatment of animals may seem to modern sensibilities to be foreign and distressing, the fortunes of disempowered humans could be similarly brutal. Criminals, the poor, the mad, slaves, women and children were all treated in ways which would be considered unfair, cruel or capricious now. Animals were another part of society and were accorded status and consideration in line with prevailing cultural attitudes. On an individual level, there were undoubtedly those who demonstrated compassion and kindness to both animals and people.

13.3 Towards Enlightenment and Legislation

By the 18th and 19th centuries, particularly in Great Britain, an increasingly organized and campaigning movement towards more enlightened times began with writers, both secular and theological, starting to challenge the status quo. Improvements in the treatment of animals, women and slaves were sought. Richard Dean in 1767 argued for kinder treatment:

> As Brutes have sensibility, they are capable of pain, feel every bang and cut and stab, as much as he himself (the reader) does, some of them perhaps more, and therefore he must not treat them as stocks or stones or things that cannot feel.
>
> (Dean, 2000, p. 62)

Humphry Primatt, an Anglican priest, wrote in 1776 'Pain is Pain, whether it be inflicted on man or on beast; and the creature that suffers it, whether man or beast, being sensible of the misery of it while it lasts, suffers Evil' (Primatt, 2000, p. 62). The most enduring arguments were made by the well-known philosopher Jeremy Bentham in 1780.

> The day *may* come when the rest of the animal creation may acquire those rights which never could have been withholden from them but by the hand of tyranny. The French have already discovered that the blackness of the skin is no reason why a human being should be abandoned without redress to the caprice of a tormentor. It may come one day to be recognized, that the number of the legs, the villosity of the skin, or the termination of the *os sacrum*, are reasons equally insufficient for abandoning a sensitive being to the same fate. What else should trace the insuperable line? Is it the faculty of reason, or, perhaps, the faculty of

discourse? But a full-grown horse or dog is beyond comparison a more rational, as well as a more conversable animal, than an infant of a day, or a week, or even a month, old. But suppose the case were otherwise, what would it avail? The question is not, Can they *reason*? nor, Can they *talk*? but, Can they *suffer*?

(Bentham, 1907, Ch. 17, fn. 122)

A significant concern for many about practices of animal torment or violence was the effect that participation might have upon those involved. During a parliamentary debate in 1825, the MP Sir Francis Burdett agreed to support a bill against animal fighting and baiting only because he was aware of 'the injurious effect which such scenes had on the morals of society'. And 'he was not legislating on a principle of humanity towards brutes, but for men' (Burdett, 1825, p. 550). He was also, along with many others at the time and since, keen to distinguish the pursuits of the upper classes, such as hunting, from those, such as bull baiting, carried out by those considered less desirable and potentially villainous members of society. That unkindness to animals is undesirable, not just because of the effects on the animals, but because of the desensitizing and dehumanizing effects on the perpetrator, remains in contemporary thinking through the suggested link between animal abuse and domestic violence.

Legislation to reduce the worst excesses of animal cruelty was gradually introduced during the 19th century by Richard Martin, Lord Erskine and John Lawrence, among others. Britain at this time appears to have emerged from being 'the cruellest nation in Europe' to being the leader of a humane reaction (Ryder, 2000). Without a police force to enforce the new laws, Martin established a Society for the Prevention of Cruelty to Animals in 1822, a prosecuting and campaigning body, which was later awarded royal patronage to become the RSPCA. Interest from Queen Victoria and other ladies of society led to concern about animal suffering being regarded as 'feminine' in nature. Over time this has resulted in criticism from those opposed to greater protection of animals being directed at a perceived 'womanly' or overly sentimental approach to animals.

During the second half of the 19th century, science and scientists rose in profile and importance. Vivisection, the dissection of living and usually fully conscious animals, was widely practised across Europe both for scientific discovery and as a form of entertainment by physiologists and physicians. Many found the practice abhorrent and women were instrumental in limiting its prevalence and methods in Britain. Frances Power Cobbe, a writer and social worker, became a prolific and persistent anti-vivisection campaigner. The RSPCA was officially opposed to many of the methods employed by vivisectionists, but was regarded as being weak and ineffectual in tackling it. Influential scientists made a powerful case for vivisection furthering knowledge and emphasised its potential to alleviate human suffering. Cobbe organized petitions signed by prominent members of the aristocracy, the church and the ruling classes and set up her own society, latterly the British Union for the Abolition of Vivisection, to lobby and submit Bills for the regulation of vivisection to Parliament. Queen Victoria made her opposition to the dissection of conscious animals known to government ministers and made a donation to the RSPCA specifically for their campaign. A Royal Commission into the subject was eventually set up in 1876. Its members were at times so horrified by the descriptions provided by scientists that they were convinced that some form of control was needed. Dr Emanuel Klein, a lecturer at St Bartholomew's Hospital, explained that:

> when dogs are operated upon they are fastened down by broad bands, their limbs being extended and secured – when he finds inconvenience from the cries of the animal he uses chloroform – as rabbits do not howl or scratch he never anaesthetises them.
>
> (RSPCA and Royal Commission, 1876, pp. 178–179)

The Commission eventually concluded that the use of animals in legitimate research was not, in itself, immoral, but limits must be placed and certain practices should be banned. Scientists then, and sometimes now, were keen to dissociate science from moral considerations, suggesting that it was a discipline apart, without value judgements and so should not be constrained. As recently as 1990, an American neurosurgeon, Robert J. White, stated that 'animal usage is not a moral or ethical issue and elevating the problem of animal rights to such a plane is a disservice to medical research and the farm and dairy industry' (White, 1990, p. 43). While some were arguing that animals could and should be used in science because they were unlike people, and therefore outside moral consideration, another influential scientist, Charles Darwin, was arguing how much like animals humans are. The full implications of his conclusions on the close relationship between ourselves and other animals were not fully appreciated then and perhaps still have yet to be.

After some progress in the treatment of animals and their legal standing in the late 19th and early 20th centuries, the immense and profound effects of the First and Second World Wars effectively halted any further significant progress. It was not until the 1960s and 1970s that philosophers began to take a serious interest in animals and their status in society. Influential work was published by Ruth Harrison, Peter Singer, Richard Ryder, Tom Regan and Bernard Rollin, among many others. Increasing awareness of animal consciousness and, crucially, legislation to enforce consideration and protection became the norm for many countries round the world by the early 21st century.

13.4   The Status of Animals

Throughout all the changes outlined during the last few hundred years, the status of animals as property has not changed in most countries. Although generally the infliction of suffering is prohibited, an owner still commands total control over the destiny and purpose of that animal's life. They may use it, or kill it, within certain limits, in any way they choose. There are advantages and disadvantages to this status and it has a profound effect on any ethical debate about the possibility of animals possessing any inherent rights within society. The main advantage is that an animal owner can be identified

and obliged by law to care and provide for their animals during the time they are deemed responsible, and they can also be held responsible for any abuse or suffering the animals may experience. Otherwise who would be responsible for providing for their needs or protecting their welfare? Disadvantages emerge when owners use their animals in ways which others find morally repugnant, such as performing tricks for entertainment or for the mass production of food or fur.

13.5   Moral Considerations

Most people these days find it self-evident that animals fall within the moral circle. That animals are capable of feelings and emotions to which we can relate makes it necessary to treat them well. Philosophers have spent some considerable time examining and describing the nature of our relationship with animals from many perspectives, and have outlined the ways in which it is wanting and should be changed. Debates in ethical theory about the type and extent of any desirable or acceptable restrictions on human behaviour have offered different, and sometimes contradictory, answers. The pragmatic result is that on a personal, cultural and legislative level the treatment of animals is determined by a mixture of moral concern, practicality and self-interest.

The approach of those in the developed world to most ethical problems is based on Utilitarian theory. This requires that we act in a way which brings about the best consequences for all those affected by the outcome. This, of course, still requires some agreement on what might be considered the 'best' consequences, and whether the extreme suffering of a few can be outweighed by huge benefits to the majority. It also relies on our ability to accurately predict what the consequences of any action will be since the outcome determines its moral acceptability. Such cost–benefit analyses are usually the basis for new legislation and form an integral part of much decision making in the public and commercial sector. In many situations the costs are easily mitigated or obviously justified by the proposed benefits.

Hence the use of animals by their human owners is acceptable, since their interests are often mutual. The ownership of pets potentially has an overall positive benefit for both, with the provision of affectionate care adequately compensating for a reduction in freedom and self-determination. Similarly, the use of animals in sport, assistance or law enforcement is considered an acceptable trade-off between useful outcomes, a fulfilling life and meeting their needs.

A problem for some about an exclusively Utilitarian view is the fate of a minority or the weak. The infliction of significant or enduring suffering on one individual so that many others may experience pleasure may satisfy the equation but still leave us feeling uncomfortable. Another view is that individuals have inherent value and the correct action depends not on its consequences but on appropriate, respectful treatment of them. The idea that individuals, who exist as ends in themselves, must not be treated as means to another's end was suggested by Kant (1724–1804; Kart *et al.*, 2002) and is echoed today by those who promote the idea of animal 'rights'. The idea that certain negative consequences cannot be outweighed by a proposed benefit is also found in the law and popular culture. A ban on the use of the great apes in research has been passed in the EU because they are considered the closest species to human beings, having the most advanced social and behavioural skills (Directive 2010/63/EU, para. 18). In New Zealand and Spain, great ape species have been granted basic rights (The Week, 2013). Many people are opposed to the killing of animals for fur or the use of circus animals on moral as well as purely welfare grounds.

Christianity and Judaism promote a view of humans as fundamentally different, being made in the image of God, from the rest of animal kind and uniquely possessing a soul. Man is given 'dominion' over the animals of the earth, air and sea in the Bible and the nature of this dominion is debated by those within the church to this day. Islam largely views animals in relation to man, although they can be regarded as sacred or 'Muslim'. A conservative interpretation of religious texts forms the basis for a view of animals as existing for the purposes of man and so justifies their use for the betterment of mankind. These views still percolate into current thinking and the attitudes of individuals and governments.

Much of the 'worth' of animals in society is related to their relative importance to humans. Concern about the treatment of animals is therefore related to the effect on the humans most affected by it. The harm inflicted by abusing an animal therefore is not, or not only, to the animal itself, but also to the owner or person who is personally attached to it. They may experience not just material loss but psychological distress. By this reasoning, we have few direct duties towards animals, only indirect ones governed by our moral duties to each other. The law generally provides more protection for those animals which are important to humans, whether financially or emotionally, than for those which are not. Animals regarded as pests, for example, may be killed in ways which would not be considered acceptable for other species. Similarly, the harm caused by deliberate animal abuse is not just considered undesirable because of the animal's suffering, but because of the effect of such behaviour on the person committing it and the implications for their relationship with vulnerable people such as women and children. Animals are now considered as potential 'sentinels' in the detection of domestic violence (National Link Coalition, n.d.).

13.6   Human Attitudes

The psychological, sociological and cultural aspects of the wide spectrum of human–animal interactions have been considered by a large number of researchers and writers. An expansive analysis of the existing literature is beyond the scope of this chapter. One attempt to categorize the various attitudes which humans hold towards or about animals was made by Kellert (1980), using questionnaires to assess the attitudes, knowledge and behaviour of more than 3000 randomly selected Americans. A scale of nine basic attitudes is described in Table 13.1.

Table 13.1. The nine basic human attitudes towards animals as described by Kellert (1980).

Attitude	Description	% of US Population Strongly Oriented
Naturalistic	Primary interest in and affection for wildlife and the outdoors.	10%
Ecologistic	Primary concern for the environment and the interrelationships between wildlife species and natural habitats.	7%
Humanistic	Principle interest and strong affection for individual animals, principally pets and large mammals.	35%
Moralistic	Primary concern for the right and wrong treatment of animals, with strong opposition to exploitation or cruelty towards animals.	20%
Scientistic	Primary interest in physical attributes and biological functioning of animals.	1%
Aesthetic	Primary interest in the artistic and symbolic characteristics of animals.	15%
Utilitarian	Primary concern for the practical and material value of animals or the animal's habitat.	20%
Dominionistic	Primary interest in the mastery and control of animals, typically in sporting situations.	3%
Negativistic/ Neutralistic	Active or passive avoidance of animals due to indifference, dislike or fear.	37%

Some of these attitudes were positively correlated, as one might expect, since certain beliefs are linked and based on underlying themes, and others were negatively correlated. These underlying themes could be simplified into:

> two broad and conflicting dimensional perceptions of animals. The moralistic and utilitarian attitudes clash around the theme of human exploitation of animals ... the negativistic and humanistic attitudes tend to clash, although in a more latent fashion, around the theme of affection for animals.
> (Kellert, 1980, pp. 89–90)

These themes have been distilled by Serpell (2004) into two primary motivations: affection towards animals, or 'Affect', and economic or pragmatic considerations, or 'Utility'. Affect and Utility, he suggests, can be represented in two dimensions by a continuum between positive and negative as shown in Fig. 13.1.

Some animals appear to fit easily into the upper-right quadrant, such as assistance dogs. They are both highly useful and generally held in great regard by their owners and society. Animals regarded as pests might be expected to occupy the lower-left quadrant

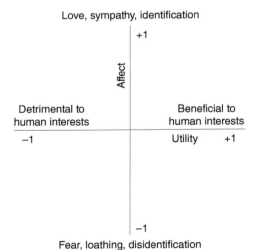

Fig. 13.1. Diagrammatic representation of the postulated relationship between the primary affect and utility attitude dimensions.

since they are considered to cause problems for humans and often provoke feelings of revulsion and antipathy. Problems, or potentially conflict, can arise when animals are especially useful, but do not always engender affectionate feelings – farmed chickens, for example, are held in high regard for their usefulness, but are not particularly loved. On the other hand, endangered species such as the tiger or orang-utan pose problems of significant imposition on human resources, but evoke great affection. For many people there is an inherent difficulty in reconciling their affectionate feelings towards animals with their relative utility, since animal use invariably raises issues of welfare and killing.

People's basic attitudes to and perceptions about animals are influenced or modified by many factors. Serpell suggests three categories of 'attitude modifiers': animal attributes, individual human attributes and cultural factors. Certain types of physical appearance or behaviour makes some animals likely to produce a positive emotional response in people. An aesthetically pleasing physical form, looking 'cute', and behaviours to which we can, or believe we can, relate will raise their status and hence consideration. Those who deliberately harm such animals will be judged harshly. Even legally sanctioned harms, such as the killing of non-native species (e.g. grey squirrels) or culling populations for disease control (e.g. badgers), may cause considerable outrage and conflict.

The attitudes of individuals towards animals can be expected to vary with gender, age, level of education, urban or rural existence, childhood experience, religiosity and personality. Broadly speaking, women, younger adults, the higher educated, urban dwellers, those who kept childhood pets and the less religious have higher levels of positive Affect. Conversely men, older adults, the poorly educated, rural dwellers and the more religious tend to have higher levels of positive Utility. The nature of past, or ongoing, relationships with animals will also modify people's attitudes: some may have experience of abusive childhood–animal interactions or be heavily reliant on animals to make a living (Serpell, 2004).

As previously outlined, the cultural attitudes of the past still affect our beliefs about animals today and a great deal of baggage still encumbers the relationship. Religion colours attitudes, with the utility of animals for man emphasized in most cases, and some animals given additional significance, such as cows in Hinduism or pigs in Islam and Judaism. Some cultures revere certain types of interaction: hunting, for food or trophies, or bull fighting may be considered a noble and enriching pursuit by those involved. Popular culture and the media also significantly influence attitudes, and the relative coverage given to certain types of animals or types of animal use may sway people's opinions about how and what animals are. Certain types of dog are labelled as 'dangerous'; anthropomorphized animals, such as meerkats, squirrels and penguins, are used in advertising campaigns; and children's literature is full of animal characters. The production of fur for clothing generates significant levels of disapprobation, whereas the keeping of battery chickens or production of leather is broadly accepted, despite comparable welfare and moral concerns. Science also continues to modify attitudes. Television programmes describing the latest discoveries about animal capabilities and the intricate balance of animal species in the environment affects the attitudes of much of society. Intensive animal farming and slaughter or the use of laboratory animals cause conflicts of affect and utility and are much less commonly portrayed. Scientific study of animals still highlights the very many similarities between ourselves and animals, but also raises significant concerns by using animals in research or applying scientific and medical principles to further refine the already highly technological use of animals for food.

13.7 The Range of Relationships

While there is much to say about humans' collective relationship with animals, it is at the individual level that forensic practitioners generally become involved. The need for forensic science by the judicial system in the resolution of a legal dispute usually relates to an individual person and their interaction, whether brief or prolonged, with an animal or small group of animals. Commonly this involves the infliction, or omission, of particular acts by the individual *on* an animal, but could also include the infliction of injury *by* an animal; dog bites, for example. Personal relationships with animals can range from those characterized by deep affection and close bonding, through benign and practical utility, to feelings of fear, antipathy and the deliberate infliction of harm.

13.8 Positive Human–Animal Relationships

There are numerous stories of dog owners rescuing dogs from drowning in situations which endanger their own lives, sometimes resulting in their own death (WGRZ, 2014). In the serious bush fires in Australia in 2009, the time taken to persuade people to leave animals increased the risks for evacuees and rescuers and several people died while trying to save dogs, horses and cattle from the flames (Thompson, 2013). There is increasing recognition of the range and richness of benefits that companion animals can bring to humans. Studies have confirmed that the presence and companionship of animals, particularly dogs and cats, can reduce or ameliorate the effects of loneliness, isolation and negative life events. They have a beneficial effect on self-esteem, child development, social interaction and have a suggested additional therapeutic effect on those with autism or learning difficulties (Mills and Hall, 2014). Companion animals, for many, would be regarded as family members. Animals in the context of a close and 'loving' relationship will be generally treated with affection and consideration and could be regarded as being at the most positive end of the affection and utility spectrum. Working animals used by law enforcement agencies and the armed forces and assistance dogs are often uniquely useful because of their innate skills or level of training.

For a significant number of people, their relationship with animals may be of an impersonal, loosely benign or utilitarian nature without the need to seek out or maintain contact. Animals are used for leisure and sporting activities, such as showing, the racing of horses, dogs and pigeons, show jumping and hunting. These animals are less likely to be regarded as significant individuals in themselves, since the purpose for which they are kept often assumes a greater emphasis.

13.9 Animal Cruelty

It is perhaps not surprising, given the prevalence of socially permitted, animal-targeted violence in the past, that animals are still the occasional recipients of deliberately inflicted abuse. A relatively limited number of studies have examined the reasons why some people abuse animals, often with the focus of determining whether such people also pose a risk to others. Kellert and Felthous (1985) questioned groups of aggressive criminals, non-aggressive criminals and non-criminals about their past experiences with animals and proposed nine animal cruelty motivations:

- To exert control.
- Retaliation against an animal.
- To satisfy prejudice against an animal.
- To express aggression.
- To enhance one's own aggressiveness.
- To shock people.
- Retaliation against another person.
- To displace hostility.
- Non-specific sadism.

The relative frequency of these motivations was further explored by Hensley and Tallichet (2005) by sending questionnaires to prison inmates in the Southern USA (Table 13.2).

There are inherent problems with studies investigating 'animal cruelty', since the definition of precisely what, and to whom, is considered cruel treatment (physical, psychological, what species? involving death?) is somewhat subjective, and self-reporting by perpetrators is vulnerable to both under- and over-representation. None the less, anger and fun seem to be the main motivators for animal cruelty, with dislike, fear and the imposition of control being important, and possibly contributory, factors, since inmates

Table 13.2. Frequencies and percentages of inmates who committed childhood and/or adolescent animal cruelty and their motivations for engaging in these acts (n = 112).

Motivation	Number	Percentage
For fun	43	38.4
Out of anger	54	48.2
Dislike for the animal	25	22.3
Shock people	5	4.5
Fear of animal	24	21.4
Impress someone	11	9.8
Revenge against someone	16	14.3
Control the animal	25	22.3
Sex	16	14.3
Imitation	17	15.2

could select more than one motivation. Other findings were that inmates from an urban background were more than four times more likely to have abused out of fun, and that those who abused alone were seven times more likely to have abused out of anger. The abuse of animals has been considered for the past 20 years as one of several potential diagnostic factors when diagnosing Conduct Disorder in children by the American Psychiatric Association (2013). Conduct Disorder is one of the most frequently diagnosed conditions in outpatient and inpatient mental health facilities for children and a substantial proportion continue to show behaviours which in adulthood then meet criteria for Antisocial Personality Disorder. Children with Conduct Disorder typically have little empathy or concern for the feelings and well-being of others, often destroy property and are often aggressive to people and animals. Researchers have also tried to link certain types of childhood behaviour with adult violence, some studies point to a connection between a 'triad' of behaviours in boys – bedwetting, firesetting and cruelty to animals – and the committing of violent aggressive crimes in adulthood (Miller, 2001). The presence of a 'violence graduation hypothesis', whereby abusers start their careers, often as children, with animals and then progress on to increasing levels of aggression and violence, is a matter of some debate, with some authors challenging the simplistic 'chicken

and egg' theory and instead linking animal abuse with other complex and more generalized deviant behaviour (Arluke et al., 1999).

13.10 Family Violence and The Link

The proposed relationship of animal abuse and other sorts of interpersonal abuse, violence and neglect, especially towards children, forms the basis for 'The Link' (National Link Coalition, n.d.). Acknowledgement of 'The Link' between child maltreatment, elder abuse, domestic violence and animal abuse forms the basis for a suggestion that social and health services, veterinary practitioners and animal welfare organizations should work together. They need to identify, and intervene in, those situations where a 'red flag' – neglect or non-accidental injury of an animal, for example – indicates that other family members may be at risk. Using this approach, anyone aware of, or investigating, an incident of animal abuse, where that animal lives as part of a family, should alert social services or health professionals to the possibility of other family victims. In an echo of the sentiments of Thomas Aquinas (1225–1274), who wished to forbid cruelty towards animals, 'to remove a man's mind from exercising cruelty towards other men, lest anyone, from exercising cruelty upon brutes, should go on hence to human beings' (Aquinas, 2000, 29), the modern focus is to regard the mistreatment of animals as part of a wider social problem, the significance of which is greater than just concern for the animals involved.

Arluke has argued that childhood animal abuse may be for many children a form of 'dirty play', which, along with other sorts of potentially undesirable childhood activities, enables children to act out certain adult behaviours as part of their development and may reflect the conflicting values of society when it comes to animals. After a series of detailed interviews with university students reflecting on childhood animal cruelty, he states:

When respondents reflected on and grappled with what their animal abuse said about them, the stories they told themselves about themselves were no more or less contradictory than those writ big across our society's ambiguous and shifting canvas of human–animal relationships.

(Arluke, 2002)

Many animal abusers, in common with some child abusers, may express high levels of affection for the animals they abuse. In chaotic and violent households with poorly functioning parental models, animals may find themselves scapegoated as an outlet for anger, used as a instrument of control through the threat of harm or destruction, or categorized as a 'bad' animal when compared to others in the house. Some poor treatment of animals may originate from a lack of familiarity with their needs, conflicts over the provision of their care, unrealistic expectations about their abilities, and unfamiliarity with effective ways of achieving desired behaviour (Deviney *et al.*, 1998).

13.11   Hoarding and Bestiality

A problem of, sometimes extreme, animal welfare concern, related to professed strong animal affection is that of animal hoarding. This phenomenon has been increasingly recognized since the 1980s, mainly in the USA, with a relatively limited number of researchers specifically addressing the topic. An animal hoarder has been defined as:

> someone who accumulates a large number of animals; fails to provide minimal standards of nutrition, sanitation, and veterinary care; and fails to act on the deteriorating condition of the animals (including disease, starvation, and even death) or the environment (severe overcrowding, extremely unsanitary conditions) or the negative effect of the collection on their own health and well-being and on that of other household members.
>
> (Patronek, 1999)

There are suggestions by mental health professionals that animal hoarding is an extension of the pathological hoarding of inanimate objects where control and identity are sought in the excessive accumulation and acquisition of objects, often those things considered 'rubbish' by others. The demographics of the different types of hoarding show some variations, however; animal hoarders tend to be female, middle-aged or older, not in work, and do not begin their hoarding behaviour early in life. Both object and animal hoarders tend to live in single-person households, are socially isolated and have a history of traumatic life events, with dysfunctional and chaotic childhood homes (Frost *et al.*, 2011). While animal hoarding is now recognized by many as a psychopathological problem in its own right, it may also be accompanied by other psychiatric disorders, and its diagnosis and treatment is exceptionally complex. Animal hoarders typically identify strongly with animals and may describe their relationship with them as being equivalent to, or better than, their relationships with people. The reasons for having so many animals may be due to passive acquisition, usually due to uncontrolled breeding; or active, where animals such as strays or those in need of 'rescue' are sought. Perhaps the most striking feature of animal hoarders is:

> that in the face of professed love and desire to care for animals, there can be tremendous animal neglect and suffering. Invariably, an animal hoarder will ignore, minimize, or deny adverse events as obvious as starvation, severe illness, and death along with environmental effects of the hoarding, such as household destruction.
>
> (Patronek and Nathanson, 2009)

Hoarders' profound lack of insight into the reality of the situation for themselves and their animals, and their need for control, makes resolution particularly difficult. Animal hoarders strongly resist attempts to remove animals from them, have an extremely high recidivism rate and will invariably begin acquiring replacement animals at the earliest opportunity even after prosecution (Williams, 2014).

Since incidents of animal hoarding often require the involvement of a wide range of agencies: environmental health, housing, social services, police, fire, mental health and animal welfare, the challenges of dealing with the problem can be significant, since there could well be a poor understanding of the responsibilities, and legal authority, of each different agency. This can be further complicated by unpredictable responses of the public and media to those hoarders who may be portrayed as selfless animal lovers who have been unfairly punished for attempting to save animals (Williams, 2014).

One final area where the intentions of humans may be judged as deluded, perverse or even malicious is bestiality. In most cultures it is, and always has been, a great taboo, generating feelings of moral revulsion. In many jurisdictions, the performance of any sexual acts involving animals is outlawed regardless of the details of the specific act. The subject is generally not discussed, and there have been limited studies into its prevalence and practice. In situations involving violence and injury, it may be that there is merely an added sexual dimension to animal abuse carried out for reasons of anger, fun, retaliation or sadism, as discussed previously. Some acts may be the result of experimentation by children or young adults, either as a result of their own childhood sexual abuse or along the lines of 'dirty play'. There have, however, been some more recent studies into a proposed 'zoophilia', which, while it may involve sexual acts between humans and animals, or 'bestiality', implies an emotional and affectionate dimension to the relationship. The area is by its nature difficult to research,

since self-reporting about acts generally abhorred by society is likely to be fraught with inaccuracy. There does seem to be a group of people who view human–animal sexual relations as part of a spectrum of available sexual experiences and as an expression of warm feelings towards animals. Caucasian men more commonly practice bestiality than women, with dogs of both sexes being the most common species involved, along with horses and farm animals of either sex (Beetz, 2008). For many, there are both moral and welfare concerns about whether animals can ever 'consent' to such acts, even if there is no apparent infliction of pain or use of force or coercion, and they appear to be willing or unconcerned.

13.12   Conclusion

Because animals are part of, and sometimes central to, the lives of so many people, veterinary forensic practitioners will find themselves required in a wide variety of situations. Human–animal relationships are far from fading in importance or reducing in number, despite progressive urbanization and industrialization. With increasing protection for animals being sought by legislation around the world and the recognition of important connections in our interactions with animals and with each other, the need for veterinary forensics will become increasingly necessary.

References

American Psychiatric Association (2013) *Diagnostic and Statistical Manual of Mental Disorders,* 5th edition. American Psychiatric Publishing, Washington, DC, p. 472.

Aquinas, T. (2000) Summa Contra Gentiles iii. p113. In: Ryder, R.D. *The Christian Legacy: Medieval Attitudes. Animal Revolution.* Berg, Oxford, UK.

Arluke, A. (2002) Animal abuse as dirty play. *Symbolic Interaction* 25(4), 405–430.

Arluke, A., Luke, C. and Ascione, F. (1999) The relationship of animal abuse to violence and other forms of antisocial behavior. *Journal of Interpersonal Violence* 14(9), 963–975.

Beetz, A.M. (2008) Bestiality and zoophilia: a discussion of sexual contact with animals. In: Ascione F.R. (ed.) *The International Handbook of Animal Abuse and Cruelty; Theory, Research and Application.* Purdue University Press. West Lafayette, Indiana, pp. 201–220.

Bentham, J. (1907 (1789)) Of the limits of the penal branch of jurisprudence. In: Bentham, J. *Introduction to the Principles of Morals and Legislation.* Clarendon Press, Oxford, UK. Available online at Library of Economics and Liberty: http://www.econlib.org/library/Bentham/bnthPMLNotes3.html (accessed 12 January 2015).

Burdett, F. (1825) *Parliamentary History and Review*. Longman, London, UK.

Dean, R. (2000 (1767)) An essay on the future life of brutes. In: Ryder, R.D. (ed.) *Animal Revolution*. Berg, Oxford, UK.

Deviney, E., Dickert, J. and Lockwood, R. (1998) The care of pets within child abusing families. In: Lockwood, R. and Ascione, F.R. (eds) *Cruelty to Animals and Interpersonal Violence*. Purdue University Press, West Lafayette, Indiana, pp. 305–313.

Directive 2010/63/EU, para. 18. Available online at: http://eur-lex.europa.eu/legal-content/EN/TXT/?uri=CELEX:32010L0063 (accessed 27 October 2015).

Frost, R., Patronek, G. and Rosenfield, E. (2011) Comparison of animal and object hoarding. *Depression and Anxiety* 28, 885–891.

Hensley, C. and Tallichet, S.E. (2005) Animal cruelty motivations: assessing demographic and situational influences. *Journal of Interpersonal Violence* 20, 1429–1443.

Kant, I., Wood, A.W. and Schneewind, J.B. (2002) *Groundwork for the Metaphysics of Morals*. Yale University Press.

Kellert, S.R. (1980) American attitudes toward and knowledge of animals: an update. *International Journal for the Study of Animal Problems* 1, 87–119.

Kellert, S.R. and Felthous, A.R. (1985) Childhood cruelty toward animals among criminals and noncriminals. *Human Relations* 38, 1113–1129.

Miller, C. (2001) Childhood animal cruelty and interpersonal violence. *Clinical Psychology Review* 21(5), 735–749.

Mills, D. and Hall, S. (2014) Animal-assisted interventions: making use of the human-animal bond. *Veterinary Record*. 174(11), 269–273.

National Link Coalition (n.d.) What is the link? Available online at: http://nationallinkcoalition.org/what-is-the-link (accessed 6 May 2014).

Patronek, G.J. (1999) Hoarding of animals: an under-recognized public health problem in a difficult-to-study population. *Public Health Reports* 114, 81–87. Available online at: http://www.ncbi.nlm.nih.gov/pmc/articles/PMC1308348/pdf/pubhealthrep00029-0083.pdf (accessed 12 January 2015).

Patronek, G.J. and Nathanson, J.N. (2009) A theoretical perspective to inform assessment and treatment strategies for animal hoarders. *Clinical Psychology Review* 29, 274–281.

Primatt, H. (2000 (1776)) The duty of mercy and the sin of cruelty to brute animals. In: Ryder, R.D. *Animal Revolution*. Berg, Oxford, UK, pp. 14–15, p. 62.

Radford, M. (2001) The first legislation. In: Radford, M. *Animal Welfare Law in Britain: Regulation and Responsibility*. Oxford University Press, Oxford, UK.

RSPCA and Royal Commission (1876) *Vivisection*, 2nd edn. Smith, Elder & Co., London, UK. Available online at: https://ia600302.us.archive.org/18/items/vivisection00unkngoog/vivisection00unkngoog.pdf (accessed 26 January 2016).

Ryder, R.D. (2000) The age of enlightenment: the eighteenth century. In: Ryder, R.D. *Animal Revolution: Changing Attitudes Towards Speciesism*. Berg, Oxford, UK, pp. 59–74.

Serpell, J.A. (2004) Factors influencing human attitudes to animals and their welfare. *Animal Welfare* 13, S145–S151.

Thompson, K. (2013) Save me, save my dog. *Australian Journal of Communication* 40(1), 123–124.

Week, The (2013) Should apes have legal rights? 3 August. Available online at: http://theweek.com/articles/461480/should-apes-have-legal-rights (accessed 9 January 2015).

WGRZ (2014) WNY man dies saving his drowning dog in Florida. Available online at: http://www.wgrz.com/story/news/2014/05/25/wny-man-dies-saving-his-drowning-dog-in-florida/9583867 (accessed 25 May 2014).

White, R.J. (1990) *Hastings Center Report* 20(6). Wiley-Blackwell (on behalf of Hastings Center), Garrison, New York.

Williams, B. (2014) Animal hoarding: devastating, complex, and everyone's concern. *Mental Health Practice* 17(6), 35–39. Available online at: http://journals.rcni.com/doi/pdfplus/10.7748/mhp2014.03.17.6.35.e868 (accessed 12 January 2015; requires log-in).

Index

Note: Page numbers in **bold** type refer to **figures**; page numbers in *italic* type refer to *tables*; and page numbers followed by 'n' refer to notes.